Blastomycosis

CURRENT TOPICS IN INFECTIOUS DISEASE

Series Editors:

William B. Greenough III
Division of Geographic Medicine
The Johns Hopkins University School
of Medicine
Baltimore, Maryland

Thomas C. Merigan
Head, Division of Infectious Disease
Stanford University Medical Center
Stanford, California

A Continuation Order Plan is available for this series. A continuation order will bring delivery of each new volume immediately upon publication. Volumes are billed only upon actual shipment. For further information please contact the publisher.

Blastomycosis

Edited by

Yousef Al-Doory, Ph.D.

George Washington University
* School of Medicine and Health Sciences*
Washington, D.C.

and

Arthur F. DiSalvo, M.D.

Nevada State Health Laboratory
Reno, Nevada

PLENUM MEDICAL BOOK COMPANY
New York and London

Library of Congress Cataloging-in-Publication Data

Blastomycosis / edited by Yousef Al-Doory and Arthur F. DiSalvo.
     p. cm. -- (Current topics in infectious disease)
  Include bibliographical references and index.
  ISBN 0-306-43958-1
  1. Blastomycosis. ·2. Blastomyces dermatitidis. I. Al-Doory,
Yousef, 1924- II. DiSalvo, Arthur F., 1932- . III. Series.
  [DNLM: 1. Blastomyces. 2. Blastomycosis. WC 450 B644]
QR201.B55B53 1992
616.9'69--dc20
DNLM/DLC
for Library of Congress   91-39241
                                      CIP

ISBN 0-306-43958-1

Printed in the United States of America

To

J. Fred Denton, M.D.

and

Norman F. Conant, Ph.D.

Contributors

Yousef Al-Doory, Ph.D., 12150 Long Ridge Lane, Bowie, Maryland

Robert W. Bradsher, M.D., Division of Infectious Diseases, Department of Medicine, University of Arkansas for Medical Sciences, Little Rock, Arkansas

Elmer Brummer, Ph.D., Department of Medicine, Santa Clara Valley Medical Center, San Jose, California

Guy D. Campbell, M.D., Clinical Professor of Medicine, University of Mississippi, School of Medicine, Jackson, Mississippi

William A. Causey, M.D., Clinical Associate Professor of Medicine, University of Mississippi, School of Medicine, Jackson, Mississippi

Francis W. Chandler, D.V.M., Ph.D., Department of Pathology, Medical College of Georgia, Augusta, Georgia

George C. Cozad, Ph.D., Department of Botany and Microbiology, University of Oklahoma, Norman, Oklahoma

Arthur F. DiSalvo, M.D., Nevada State Health Laboratory, Reno, Nevada

Norman L. Goodman, Ph.D., Department of Pathology, Albert B. Chandler Medical Center, University of Kentucky, Lexington, Kentucky

Leo Kaufman, Ph.D., Division of Mycotic Diseases, Centers for Disease Control, Atlanta, Georgia

Bruce S. Klein, M.D., Departments of Pediatrics and Internal Medicine, University of Wisconsin at Madison, Madison, Wisconsin

Alfred M. Legendre, D.V.M., University of Tennessee, Department of Urban Practice, College of Veterinary Medicine, Knoxville, Tennessee

Alan M. Sugar, M.D., Department of Medicine, Boston University Medical Center, Boston, Massachusetts

John C. Watts, M.D., Division of Surgical Pathology, Department of Anatomic Pathology, William Beaumont Hospital, Royal Oak, Michigan

Foreword

Blastomycosis remains the most enigmatic of human mycotic infections. The enigmas encompass the natural habitat of the etiologic agent, extent of exposure and subclinical infections in endemic areas, distribution of endemic foci throughout the world, inconsistency of serologic evaluation of infected patients, and varying response of such patients to standard treatment regimens.

In spite of diligent investigations by many competent investigators, we still do not know the ecological niche inhabited by the etiologic agent. We have many tantalizing clues but no definite answers. Nor do we know the extent of the endemic areas in the world for this disease. Skin testing, so useful in defining the distribution of histoplasmosis and coccidioidomycosis, has been of no value in mapping endemic areas for blastomycosis. Even the serologic evaluation of known cases of the disease has been too erratic in results to be useful as a diagnostic or prognostic procedure.

The enigmas of blastomycosis go straight to the disease itself. There is an extensive literature on the debate concerning the presence and extent of subclinical infections. Case report series demonstrate that such transient infections do occur but, unlike other mycoses, the extent to which this phenomenon is common in the general population still cannot be assessed. Even the diagnosis of established disease is a major clinical problem. Serologic procedures are unreliable: the organism may take from 2 days to 12 weeks to grow out in culture (and then be difficult to identify positively), so that observing the fungus in tissue is the only "rapid" procedure, although the latter is fraught with difficulties as well.

It becomes apparent from looking at the list of unknowns regarding blastomycosis that a compendium of known information and evaluations of evidence relevant to these enigmas is greatly needed. This present volume will fill the gap in our appreciation of this disease.

A study of the Contents demonstrates that all major aspects of blasto-mycosis are covered: history, taxonomy and biology, clinical aspects of natural infections in humans and animals as well as experimental infections, the very complex immunological responses elicited by infection, the variation in virulence of different isolates, the great enigmas of distribution and endemicity in human and animal infections, and, finally, the frustratingly contradictory pathology and clinical types of disease are analyzed and clarified. Each of the authors is an experienced and recognized expert in the field. The editors of this volume are experienced not only in medical mycology but also in the writing and communication of that science so the resulting consistency of style contributes greatly to the quality of the volume. This book is therefore a most valuable summation of present knowledge of the subject and will be a reference of great worth for years to come.

John W. Rippon

Preface

Blastomycosis is one of the major systemic mycotic diseases, with a worldwide distribution and a significant rate of mortality. At the same time, it is the most difficult mycotic disease to identify. The causative fungus, *Blastomyces dermatitidis,* is the most difficult agent to isolate from sources in nature where it is expected to be found.

The expansion of scientific research, the accumulation of data, and the increased number of medical, veterinary, and microbiological journals in various languages make it cumbersome for an interested professional to gain comprehensive knowledge of specific mycotic diseases by referring to the few general texts available in medical mycology. For this reason, we believe that a monograph on each major mycotic disease is needed. This need has been recognized, and separate monographs have been published on coccidioidomycosis, histoplasmosis, paracoccidioidomycosis, cryptococcosis, aspergillosis, candidiasis, chromomycosis, and mycetoma. Furthermore, with the rate of accumulation of information regarding certain diseases, we believe that such monographs should be updated periodically. No monograph, however, has been available for blastomycosis.

Our aim is to bring together in this volume all accessible data on *B. dermatitidis* and blastomycosis. We believe this can best be accomplished by having each chapter written by an authority in the field.

Our thanks are extended to the chapter authors as well as to those who permitted the reproduction of photographs and/or quoted material as indicated in source lines accompanying the material.

Endorsement of products or manufacturers named in the text is disclaimed by the editors and the authors. These names are used for identification purposes only.

Yousef Al-Doory, Ph.D.
Arthur F. DiSalvo, M.D.

Publisher's note: The spelling "mold" has been used throughout this volume, as it is our policy to employ American spelling in all our titles. We do acknowledge that many authorities in the fields of microbiology and medicine, including the editors of this volume, prefer the spelling "mould."

Contents

Chapter 3

VIRULENCE OF *BLASTOMYCES DERMATITIDIS* 31

Elmer Brummer

Chapter 4

THE ECOLOGY OF *BLASTOMYCES DERMATITIDIS* 43

Arthur F. DiSalvo

Chapter 5

THE EPIDEMIOLOGY OF BLASTOMYCOSIS 75

Arthur F. DiSalvo

Chapter 6

Chapter 7

Chapter 10

PATHOLOGIC FEATURES OF BLASTOMYCOSIS 189

Francis W. Chandler and John C. Watts

Chapter 11

EXPERIMENTAL BLASTOMYCOSIS 221

George C. Cozad

Chapter 12

Chapter 13

1

Introduction

Yousef Al-Doory

Blastomycosis is a chronic granulomatous and suppurative mycotic disease contracted by the inhalation of the airborne conidia of the dimorphic fungus *Blastomyces dermatitidis.* The primary infection is usually pulmonary and is often inapparent. The disease disseminates from the lungs to other organs of the body, frequently to the skin and bones.

1. HISTORY

The history of blastomycosis began in May 1894 at the meeting of the American Dermatologic Association. T. C. Gilchrist presented the pathology he observed in a biopsy specimen. The tissue, received from Dr. Duhring, was from a patient with a scrofuloderma of the hand. Gilchrist reported that he found "certain bodies" distributed throughout the histopathological section that were characterized by having buds similar to the yeasts. However, no culture was obtained from this case. In 1896, Gilchrist published his findings of the same case[1] and named the disease "blastomycetic dermatitis." He concluded that the case was identical to one reported by Busse[2]

Blastomycosis, edited by Yousef Al-Doory and Arthur F. DiSalvo, Plenum Medical Book Company, New York, 1992.

several months earlier. Busse's patient, as it was reported, had an infection caused by *Saccharomyces hominis,* and the yeast was isolated from the lesion. However, later studies proved that Busse's case was actually a cryptococcosis.

Gilchrist and Stokes reported in July 1896[3] another case of a patient referred to Gilchrist by Dr. Halsted. The case was a 33-year-old man with a tentative diagnosis of lupus vulgaris in which they suspected that the infection was caused by *Oidium.* The lesions started behind the ear and spread to most of the face. During the next several years, lesions appeared on the hand, scrotum, thigh, and back of the neck, in that order. The active lesions were characterized by elevated borders with minute epidermal abscesses, which left scars upon healing. KOH wet mounts from the pustules showed the budding yeasts clearly. Cultures from the same lesions produced a mold with fluffy mycelium.

In their second publication on the same case in 1898,[4] they renamed the fungus *Blastomyces dermatitidis* and concluded that it was certainly different from that of Busse's case where the isolated agent was a yeast rather than a mold. Gilchrist was able to produce the disease in the lungs and other organs of experimental animals by inoculating them with a suspension of the isolated mold.

In the next few years, the awareness of the disease by the medical community produced reports of its presence in various regions of the United States with most cases from the Chicago area. Accordingly, the disease then was called "Chicago disease." In 1901, H. T. Ricketts described 15 cases in the Chicago area and named the causative agent *Oidium dermatitidis.*[5] Another 13 cases were described by Hektoen in 1907.[6] In 1908, Montgomery and Ormsby[7] reported seven new cases of blastomycosis and reviewed the other cases that had been reported from Chicago, Iowa, Indiana, Wisconsin, Ohio, Maryland, New York, Germany, and France. In their report they described the systemic nature of the disease beyond its limitation of cutaneous boundaries. Fontaine *et al.*[8] further reported in 1909 the first case from Tennessee in an Austrian woman living in Memphis. In their report they detailed the histopathological appearance of the fungus in tissues in various organs of the dead patient.

In 1914, Stober[9] published a thorough study on the pathological, bacteriological, and clinical features of systemic blastomycosis, its progress in patients as well as its therapy and prognosis. He also described the mycology and the natural habitat of *B. dermatitidis* and its relation to patients. Wade and Bel[10] further detailed the progress of the disease in patients and presented a report of five new cases and a review of the previous 43 reported cases.

2. THE DISEASE

Blastomycosis originally was called "Chicago disease," then "Gilchrist's disease," and, more recently, "North American blastomycosis." The latter name was established erroneously with the belief that the disease was limited to North America. Since its worldwide distribution has been established, the disease is presently known as "blastomycosis."

Blastomycosis has been reported from several countries in Asia, Europe, Africa, and the Americas. The majority of cases in the world occur in the eastern half of North America. Africa is considered to be second, with cases reported in 16 African countries. Furthermore, cases have been reported from Europe and Asia (India and the Middle East).

The route of infection in blastomycosis and the type of disease produced was misunderstood. Until 1950, it was assumed that there were two types of disease, cutaneous and systemic, with different routes of infection: the first through contact directly to the skin and the second through the inhalation of the fungal conidia. However, Schwarz and Baum in 1951 published a detailed study of histopathological specimens from both types of infection.[11] They suggested that all forms of the disease originated from a primary pulmonary infection that is established by the inhalation of the fungal conidia. This was further confirmed by Busey[12] and Schwarz and Salfelder.[13]

At present, most of the evidence indicates that once the pulmonary infection is established, the disease progresses in one of the following patterns: (1) severe pulmonary symptoms; (2) inapparent pulmonary infection that in rare cases resolves spontaneously[14,15]; (3) disseminating to produce systemic disease involving multiple organs; (4) disseminating to a single organ where it remains occult for several years; (5) producing chronic cutaneous disease that may involve the bones.

Blastomycosis occurs in both human beings and animals. Regardless of race, the disease occurs in men more than women, similar to most other mycotic diseases. Age of onset varies, with the youngest patients reported being 5 and 7 months old[16] and the oldest over 80 years.

Dogs are the most susceptible domestic animals. The infection rate in dogs is estimated at about ten times the human rate. However, the disease is unknown among other domestic animals except that it has been reported occasionally in cats. The first case recognized in a goat was diagnosed by this author from autopsy tissues received from Dr. Howard W. Larsh. Histopathological sections of the lung showed an extensive dissemination of the fungal yeasts throughout the tissue (Fig. 1). On the other hand, the incidence of the disease is difficult to ascertain in wild animals. However, it has been reported in captive dolphins, a sea lion, ferrets, a polar bear, and African lions.

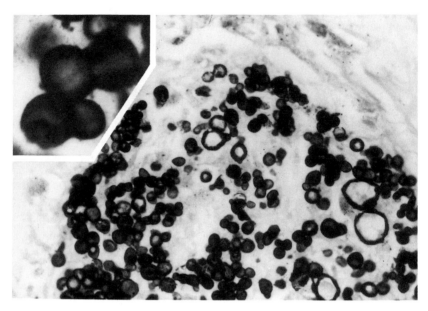

FIGURE 1. Histopathological section from a goat lung with pulmonary blastomycosis. Inset shows an enlarged view of a typical yeast cell of *Blastomyces dermatitidis*. (Giemsa stain, ×250.)

Blastomycosis in its acute, chronic, or disseminated form does not present a distinct diagnostic feature. It is frequently confused with crypto-coccosis, coccidioidomycosis, and paracoccidioidomycosis. Furthermore, it occurs in endemic areas of other systemic mycoses where the general clinical symptoms are similar; this of course will extend the differential di-agnosis. However, separate studies by Almeida, Benham, and Conant have helped eliminate most of its confusion with histoplasmosis and paracoccidioidomycosis.[17,18]

Without a dependable skin test, it is impossible to determine if there is a benign subclinical form of blastomycosis similar to that found in histoplas-mosis and coccidioidomycosis. The lack of such a skin test and the difficulty of isolating *B. dermatitidis* from natural substrates lead to uncertainty of the exact geographic distribution of blastomycosis. Furthermore, the low speci-ficity and sensitivity of the standard immunologic tests add to the difficulty of having a reliable serological test for blastomycosis. However, the develop-ment of antigen A in 1973[19] and its incorporation in the complement fixa-tion, immunodiffusion, enzyme immunosorbent assay, Western blot, and fluorescent antibody assays led to the development of a more reliable test for the early diagnosis of blastomycosis.[20,21] Further antigen purification is still needed to exclude the undesired cross-reactive components of the antigen.

The latest development of DNA and RNA probes for the various pathogenic fungi, including *B. dermatitidis,* is expected to produce more accurate and faster testing for blastomycosis than the presently available techniques.

The mortality rate of untreated blastomycosis depends on the disease manifestations. Iodide, stilbamidine, and X rays were used in past therapies with very limited success. The case fatality of chronic pulmonary and disseminated blastomycosis was 100% prior to the availability of specific therapy. Amphotericin B, since its development by Harrell and Curtis in 1957,[22] is considered to be the main therapeutic agent for blastomycosis. The oral imidazole antifungal agents, such as ketoconazole and itraconazole, have been used in the last several years with encouraging therapeutic results. However, due to the relapse of the disease in many patients treated with these drugs and in cases of chronic and disseminated manifestation, amphotericin B may still be the drug of choice. A dependable, reliable antifungal drug without undesirable side effects is still needed for the treatment of blastomycosis and other systemic mycoses.

3. THE FUNGUS

Blastomyces dermatitidis, the causative agent of blastomycosis (with over 20 synonyms), is assumed to be a soil saprophyte in nature, even though its epidemiologic and ecologic distribution is the least known compared to causative agents of other systemic mycoses. Accumulated data indicate that the fungus is nourished on soil with high organic content, abundant moisture, acid pH, and possibly enrichment with animal excreta.[23] Studies by McDonough *et al.*[24] showed that the fungal yeasts and mycelia rapidly disappear when placed in soil, while conidia survive for several weeks. They also found[25] that conidia are released from mycelia only when wetted. Other studies have shown that the organism grows on decaying organic material and the conidia are distributed when such material is disturbed.[23,26]

The fungus has two forms: a sexual form (teleomorphic or perfect state) and an asexual form (anamorphic or imperfect state). The sexual form was described in 1967 by McDonough and Lewis[27] and named *Ajellomyces dermatitidis,* while the asexual form is known as *Blastomyces dermatitidis.* The latter grows in mammalian tissues as thick-walled budding yeasts with a single bud. At room temperature the fungal colonies appear as a dry white mold with spherical or ovoid conidia. In 1907, Hamburger[28] published a detailed study of the mycology of blastomyces in which he emphasized that temperature is the main factor in the transformation of the fungus from one form to another.

Much knowledge has been accumulated during the past several decades through extensive research on the taxonomy, physiology, and biochemistry of the yeasts and other fungi but little effort has been directed specifically toward the study of *B. dermatitidis.* Actually, the basic mechanism controlling form transition of this fungus from yeast to mold and vice versa is still unknown. An increasing interest in this disease and the continued advancement in clinical medicine and laboratory techniques is expected to enhance the future advances in the understanding of this fungus.

REFERENCES

1. Gilchrist TC: A case of blastomycetic dermatitis in man. *Johns Hopkins Hosp Rep* 1:269, 1896
2. Busse O: Ueber parasitare zelleinschlusse und ihre zuchtung. *Zentralbl Bakteriol* 16:175–180, 1894
3. Gilchrist TC, Stokes WR: The presence of an *Oidium* in the tissues of a case of pseudo-lupus vulgaris. Preliminary report. *Johns Hopkins Hosp Bull* 7:129–133, 1896
4. Gilchrist TC, Stokes WR: A case of pseudo-lupus vulgaris caused by *Blastomyces. J Exp Med* 3:53–83, 1898
5. Ricketts HT: Oidiomycosis of the skin and its fungi. *J Med Res* 6:373–547, 1901
6. Hektoen L: Systemic blastomycosis and coccidioidal granuloma. *JAMA* 49:1071–1077, 1907
7. Montgomery FH, Ormsby OS: Systemic blastomycosis. *Arch Intern Med* 2:1–41, 1908
8. Fontaine BW, Haase M, Mitchell RH: Systemic blastomycosis. Report of a case. *Arch Intern Med* 4:101–117, 1909
9. Stober AM: Systemic blastomycosis. A report of its pathological, bacteriological and clinical features. *Arch Intern Med* 13:509–556, 1914
10. Wade HW, Bel GS: A critical consideration of systemic blastomycosis. *Arch Intern Med* 11:103–130, 1917
11. Schwarz J, Baum GL: Blastomycosis. *Am J Clin Pathol* 21:999–1029, 1951
12. Busey JF: Comparative study of the Veterans Administration. Blastomycosis. I. A review of 195 collected cases in Veterans Administration hospitals. *Am Rev Respir Dis* 89:659–672, 1964
13. Schwarz J, Salfelder K: Blastomycosis: A review of 52 cases. *Curr Top Pathol* 65:165–200, 1977
14. Recht LD, Philips JR, et al: Self-limited blastomycosis: A report of thirteen cases. *Am Rev Respir Dis* 120:1109–1112, 1979
15. Sarosi GA, King RA: Follow-up of an epidemic of blastomycosis. *Am Rev Respir Dis* 116:785–788, 1976
16. Jones JW: Report of a case of cutaneous blastomycosis in a child. *Emory Med* 3:22–23, 1925
17. Benham RW: Fungi of blastomycosis and coccidiodal granuloma. *Arch Dermatol* 30:385–400, 1934
18. Conant NF: Laboratory study of *Blastomyces dermatitidis* Gilchrist and Stokes 1898. *6th Pacific Sci Congr* 5:853–862, 1939
19. Kaufman L, McLaughlin D, Clark M, et al: Specific immunodiffusion test for blastomycosis. *Appl Microbiol* 26:244–247, 1973

20. Green JH, Harrell WK, Johnson J, et al: Preparation of reference antisera for laboratory diagnosis of blastomycosis. *J Clin Microbiol* 10:1–7, 1979
21. Green JH, Harrell WK, Johnson J, et al: Isolation of an antigen from *Blastomyces dermatitidis* that is specific for the diagnosis of blastomycosis. *Curr Microbiol* 4:293–296, 1980
22. Harrell ER, Curtis AC: The treatment of North American blastomycosis with amphotericin B. *Arch Dermatol* 76:561–569, 1957
23. Klein BS, Vergeront JM, et al: Isolation of *Blastomyces dermatitidis* in soil associated with a large outbreak of blastomycosis in Wisconsin. *N Engl J Med* 31:529–534, 1986
24. McDonough ES, Van Prooien R, et al: Lysis of *Blastomyces dermatitidis* yeast phase cells in natural soil. *Am J Epidemiol* 81:86–94, 1965
25. McDonough ES, Wisniewski TR, et al: Preliminary studies on conidial liberation of *Blastomyces dermatitidis* and *Histoplasma capsulatum*. *Sabouraudia* 14:199–204, 1976
26. Kitchen MS, Reiber CD: An urban epidemic of North American blastomycosis. *Am Rev Respir Dis* 115:1063–1066, 1977
27. McDonough ES, Lewis AL: *Blastomyces dermatitidis:* Production of the sexual stage. *Science* 156:528–529, 1967
28. Hamburger WW: A comparative study of four strains of organisms isolated from four cases of generalized blastomycosis. *J Infect Dis* 4:201–209, 1907

2

Taxonomy and Biology of *Blastomyces dermatitidis*

Alan M. Sugar

1. INTRODUCTION

Blastomyces dermatitidis is a dimorphic fungus, growing in the environment in a mycelial form and in mammalian tissue in a yeast form. In common with other dimorphic fungi, the life cycle of *B. dermatitidis* is not dependent upon entering a living host and establishing infection and disease. On the contrary, infection of living beings is an accidental occurrence. One corollary of this concept is that fungal dimorphism did not evolve as a response to survival at the higher temperatures of the infected animal. While ambient environmental temperatures (specifically in the soil) may fluctuate to reach those present in potential mammalian hosts, mean mammalian body temperatures most probably exceed those in the environment, although exact data on this point are not readily available. Therefore, there must be some other explanations for the evolution of fungal dimorphism, which presently remain unknown.

In addition to growth in mycelial and yeast forms (dimorphism), *B. dermatitidis* displays a sexual state that, according to convention, is identi-

Blastomycosis, edited by Yousef Al-Doory and Arthur F. DiSalvo, Plenum Medical Book Company, New York, 1992.

fied by a different genus name. The anamorphic (= asexual, imperfect) state was initially discovered in 1896 by Gilchrist and Stokes,[1] but it took another 70 years for the teleomorphic (= sexual, perfect) state, *Ajellomyces dermatitidis,* to be identified.[2] While some information is available on the physiology of this fungus and some interesting work on taxonomy has appeared, the strengths of the molecular biologic approach to fundamental issues involving *B. dermatitidis* have not yet been focused on this organism. In contrast, a thorough review of the growing body of literature on the basic biology of *Histoplasma capsulatum* has been published.[3] This information will provide for interesting comparisons once similar data derived from *B. dermatitidis* have been generated.

The purpose of this chapter is to review the taxonomy and basic biology of *B. dermatitidis,* stressing information of most interest to the medical mycologist. While a vast literature concerning the physiology and biochemistry of yeast and other fungi has been growing each year, a relatively small number of such studies have been performed specifically with *B. dermatitidis.* Only information directly obtained from *B. dermatitidis* will be included in this chapter. The reader interested in more detailed discussions of fungal physiology/biochemistry is referred to other sources.[4–13] A recent review of the biology of dimorphism of *B. dermatitidis* has also appeared.[14]

2. TAXONOMY

Many microorganisms are reclassified from one genus or species to another, as new information becomes available. Similarly, *B. dermatitidis* has been known by other names throughout the years. A summary of these synonyms is provided in Table 1. As detailed below, *B. dermatitidis* is likely to remain the permanent name of this medically important organism.

Using the strict criteria of the taxonomist, *Blastomyces* is not a legal name, since that genus name had been previously used for another organism, *Blastomyces luteus.* The latter fungus, however, has been reclassified into a different genus, *Aleurisma flavissima,*[15] leaving *Blastomyces* available. Controversy exists concerning whether *Blastomyces* should be placed into *Zymonema* or *Chrysosporium.* Both of these alternative genera are heterogeneous in their composition and experts disagree whether the fungus we know as *B. dermatitidis* should properly be classified as either of these. A proposal to unify the genera *Histoplasma* and *Blastomyces* has been made because both produce echinulate conidia as visualized by electron microscopy.[16] Further, these authors suggest that a subgenus, *Echinulatum,* should be created and integrated into *Chrysosporium.* The details of the arguments for and against reclassifying *B. dermatitidis* as a species of *Zymonema* or

TABLE 1
Obsolete Synonyms for *Blastomyces dermatitidis*[a]

Oidium dermatitidis (Ricketts, 1901)
Cryptococcus gilchristi (Vuillemin, 1902)
Zymonema gilchristi (de Buermann et Gougerot, 1909)
Cryptococcus dermatitidis (Brumpt, 1910)
Mycoderma gilchristi (Janin, 1913)
Mycoderma dermatitidis (Brumpt, 1913)
Glenospora gammeli (Pollaci et Nannizzi, 1927)
Acladium gammeli (Ota, 1928)
Blastomycoides dermatitidis (Castellani, 1928)
Blastomycoides tulanensis (Castellani, 1928)
Endomyces capsulatus (Dodge et Ayers, 1929)
Geotrichum dermatitidis (Basgal, 1931)
Monosporium tulanense (Agostini, 1932)
Aleurisma tulanense (Ota et Kawatsure, 1933)
Glenospora brevis (Castellani, 1933)
Endomyces capsulatus var isabellinus (Moore, 1933)
Torulopsis dermatitidis (Alemeida, 1933)
Endomyces dermatitidis (Moore, 1933)
Gilchristi dermatitidis (Redaelli et Ciferri, 1934)
Aleurisma breve (Dodge, 1935)
Trichosporium gammeli (Dodge, 1935)
Zymonema capsulatum (Dodge, 1935)
Scopulariopsis americana (Broc et Haddad, 1952)
Chrysosporium dermatitidis (Carmichael, 1962)

[a] From Rippon.[56]

Chrysosporium are beyond the scope of this chapter. Moreover, such controversies tend to confuse the importance of the organism as an etiologic agent of a significant mycosis. Since the genus *Blastomyces* is otherwise vacant and because the illness recognized by clinicians called blastomycosis is associated with the organism called *B. dermatitidis,* practicality dictates that the organism continue to be referred to as *B. dermatitidis.* Should "legalization" of this genus by the International Code of Botanic Nomenclature be desired, a formal proposal for conservation of the name *Blastomyces* will be required.

Having briefly reviewed the complexities of placement of *B. dermatitidis* in the genus *Blastomyces,* a discussion of the species therein is much less convoluted. A single species, *B. dermatitidis,* is recognized. A report of a variant of *B. dermatitidis* referred to as *B. dermatitidis* var. *nanum* has appeared.[17] This variety produces small (2–5 μm) yeast cells in tissue, but otherwise appears to be similar to the classic species. Whether these small yeast forms arise as a result of genetically programmed events or whether they arise from environmental factors, including the host immune response, is not clear and is important when considering if the creation of a new variety of the species *dermatitidis* is required. Thus, *B. dermatitidis* is the prototype and the only species currently recognized as a member of this genus.

The teleomorph of *B. dermatitidis* was described in 1967[2] and named *A. dermatitidis* in 1968.[18] The taxonomic status of this species is based largely on the morphology of its reproductive apparatus and surrounding structures: the specialized fruiting bodies called cleistothecia (= ascomata), asci, ascospores, and peridial hyphae. *A. dermatitidis* is now considered to be a member of the order Onygenales, family Onygenaceae, whose species possess the ability to degrade keratin, have projections on the walls of the ascospores, and produce conidia by rhexolysis (separation of conidia from the cells from which they were formed by fracturing of the wall between two septa[19]).

Recent analysis of the relationship of *A. dermatitidis* and the teleomorph of *H. capsulatum, Emmonsiella capsulatus,* has given rise to two opposing views. In the first, propounded by Kwon-Chung, *Ajellomyces* and *Emmonsiella* each represent a distinct genus.[20,21] However, McGinnis and Katz[22] have suggested that the anatomic differences between the two are not sufficient to support the creation of an additional genus. Thus, these investigators consider the genus *Ajellomyces* to contain two species—*A. dermatitidis* and *A. capsulatus*—and the genus *Emmonsiella* is discarded. Until more isolates are studied and more direct markers of relationships are available, e.g., DNA probes and restriction endonuclease enzyme patterns, the question of the taxonomic relationships of the teleomorphs of *B. dermatitidis* and *H. capsulatum* must remain tentative. That the anatomy of the sexual stages of *Histoplasma* and *Blastomyces* are so similar is in striking contrast to the differences of the yeast forms found in infected tissue and to the differences in organ localization in disseminated disease (see Chapter 10).

3. MORPHOLOGY

3.1. Teleomorph (Perfect or Sexual State)

Ajellomyces dermatitidis grows as a mold and is identified on the basis of its characteristic reproductive apparatus. When + and − strains come into contact, swollen cells, or knobs, develop; these represent the nascent ascocarp. Specialized hyphae then emanate from the knobs to form the spiral hyphae that identify the organism as *Ajellomyces*. As shown in Fig. 1A, these spirals are arranged in a radial array surrounding the ascocarp. These spirals are seen at higher magnification in Fig. 1B. The peridial hyphae, which by definition grow between the spiral hyphae, have a different shape than that

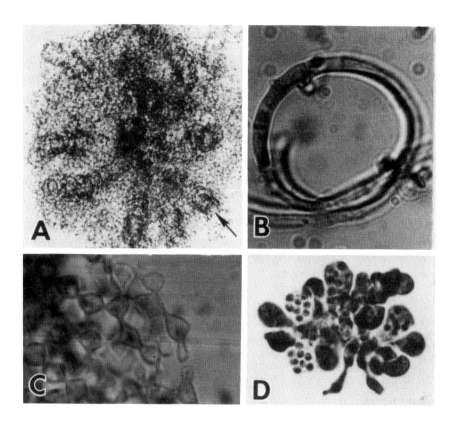

FIGURE 1. Morphology of *Ajellomyces dermatitidis*. (A) Ascocarp with radially arising spirals (arrow) and peridial hyphae interconnecting the spirals (×100; reprinted by permission, *Science* **156**:528–529, 1967). (B) A coil of the spiral hyphae (×1200). (C) A network of obtuse diamond-shaped cells of the peridial hyphae (×1200). (D) A cluster of asci containing ascospores (×1400; reprinted by permission, *Mycologia* **60**:76083, 1968). (Figures courtesy of Dr. K. J. Kwon-Chung.)

found in nonreproductive areas of the fungus. These diamond-shaped cells are shown in Fig. 1C. Typically, each ascus contains eight ascospores (Fig. 1D). More detailed information concerning the cellular and molecular anatomy of the reproductive structures of this teleomorph is not available.

3.2. Anamorph (Imperfect or Asexual State)

In the asexual state, *B. dermatitidis* grows in either mold or yeast form. Temperature is said to be the most important factor controlling the dimorphic transition of *B. dermatitidis.*[23] In contrast, biochemical manipulations can force dimorphic switching of *H. capsulatum* at uncharacteristic temperatures.[24] However, several investigators have noted that the ability of *B. dermatitidis* yeasts grown at 37°C to always form yeasts has not been uniform and some strains may develop hyphae at 37°C in certain situations. For example, Salvin noted that yeast-phase *B. dermatitidis* grown in a peptone semiliquid medium for 2 weeks at 37°C would produce abortive hyphae.[25] Years later, Domer reported that *B. dermatitidis* yeast form would begin to germinate, producing hyphae, after two transfers in glucose yeast extract broth, even when the temperature was maintained at 37°C.[26] Formation of yeast or mycelia at different ambient temperatures was found to be both strain and culture medium dependent.[27] Furthermore, we have observed that the yeast-form cells of certain strains of *B. dermatitidis* (e.g., ATCC 26199) form more elongated and hyphal appearing cells than do others (e.g., ATCC 26197), which appear more spherical in shape. The implications of the differences in morphology are not clear and the biologic relevance of yeast cell shape to virulence still needs to be investigated.

The mycelia are typically thin, septate hyphae that produce conidiophores that branch at right angles to the main hyphal segment (Fig. 2). The solitary aleurioconidia are small (2–10 μm in diameter) and may be oval or pyriform in shape. Occasional conidia produce a "dumbbell" configuration. Under the light microscope the conidia appear smooth, although under the electron microscope they have been described as having a rough surface (echinulate).[16] Both African and North American isolates produce similar appearing conidia, so they cannot be differentiated on the basis of this criterion. *B. dermatitidis* conidia are similar in structure to the microconidia of *H. capsulatum,* but *B. dermatitidis* does not form tuberculate macroconidia as does *Histoplasma.* The appearance of *B. dermatitidis* mycelia is not pathognomonic for the organism and definitive identification depends on examination of the yeast form in cultures incubated at 37°C or exoantigen testing.[28]

The microscopic appearance of the yeast form of *B. dermatitidis* is characteristic and it is unlikely to be confused with other pathogenic fungal species. The yeasts are large (8–15 μm in diameter) and, under light microscopy, one can definitively identify the organism as *B. dermatitidis* based on the doubly refractile cell wall and the broad-based attachment of the daughter bud (Fig. 3).

3.3. Summary

It is unlikely that additional studies that focus only on morphology will have a significant impact on our understanding of the basic biology of this fungus. Correlative studies, in which the function of specific intracellular

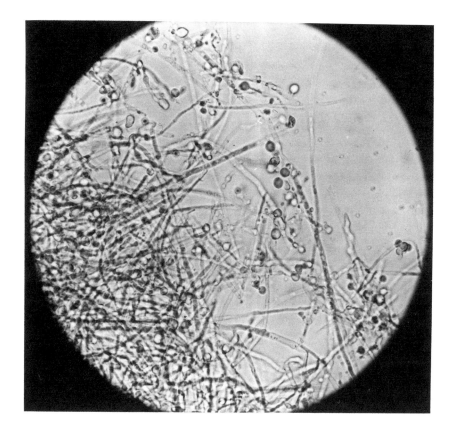

FIGURE 2. Low-power photomicrograph of *B. dermatitidis* mycelia and the round to oval-shaped conidia. The conidia are carried at the terminus of conidiophores. (Courtesy of Dr. J. W. Rippon.)

structures is examined, should help to elucidate the critical events controlling dimorphism and virulence.

4. ULTRASTRUCTURE

Not surprisingly, the composition and arrangement of cellular components of *B. dermatitidis* differ depending on the medium in which the fungus is grown. For example, Zaharee *et al.* have demonstrated marked effects of different media on the electron microscopic appearance of cell wall and cytoplasm, glycogen and lipid content, and development of intracytoplasmic membranes.[29] These effects occurred in yeast, intermediate transitional

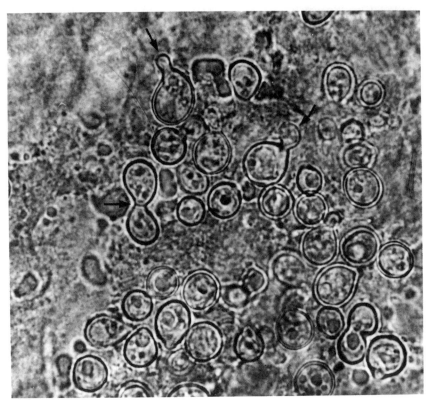

FIGURE 3. Characteristic *B. dermatitidis* yeast cells demonstrating the single bud attached to the parent cell with a broad-based attachment (arrows) and doubly refractile cell walls. (Courtesy of Dr. J. W. Rippon.)

forms, and mycelia. Thus, if meaningful comparisons of different studies on the morphology and biochemistry of *B. dermatitidis* are to be made, the incubation conditions and media used must be carefully defined. Of note was the identification of hyphae growing within dead yeast cells in brain heart infusion (BHI) preparations. Intrayeast hyphae are rarely found in dimorphic pathogenic fungi and are of unclear significance.[29]

Most studies of *B. dermatitidis* have been directed to comparisons of morphological and biochemical characteristics of the two prominent phases of the organism, yeast and mycelia, in an attempt to discern differences between the two and perhaps clues to the mechanisms responsible for dimorphism. However, the nature of these mechanisms remains elusive. Moreover, there are few studies of the intermediate cells that bridge the transition between true mycelia and yeast, so that their importance in the life cycle and pathogenicity of *B. dermatitidis* is unknown.

4.1. Cytoplasm

There are no known unique features of the organization of the cytoplasm of *B. dermatitidis* yeast and hyphae compared to other fungal cells. Distributed throughout the cytoplasm, one can find the usual organelles: endoplasmic reticulum, Golgi bodies, mitochondria, vacuoles, lipid bodies, and Woronin bodies.[29,30] Glyoxysomes and peroxisomes have not been described in *B. dermatitidis* or other medically important dimorphic fungi.[3] Since peroxisomes are thought to be a major cellular repository site for catalase, lack of peroxisomes should be further confirmed because we have found that both yeast and conidia produce significant amounts of catalase (unpublished observations). Some details of the organization of the cytoplasm and internal organelles are seen in Fig. 4. One of the most interesting aspects of this photomicrograph is the demonstration of what appear to be microbodies, which have not been definitively documented to be present on *B. dermatitidis.* The function of these microbodies is not known.

4.2. Ribosomes

Electron microscopic study of *B. dermatitidis* ribosomes obtained from two different non-ATCC strains showed them to be similar in size to those isolated from *H. capsulatum.*[31] Moreover, ribosomes recovered from mycelia were smaller than those isolated from yeasts in both species. These differences were present in preparations positively or negatively stained (with 1% uranyl acetate or shadowed with carbon/platinum, respectively) and thus were thought not to represent artifact.

4.3. Nuclear Cytology

Blastomyces dermatitidis is multinucleate in the yeast phase[32,33] with the number of nuclei varying from two to five per cell. There seems to be a rough correlation between size of the cell and number of nuclei and nuclear division was noted to be independent of budding of the yeast cell.[32] Resting nuclei have been seen to migrate into newly formed buds and nuclear division seems to proceed independently from that of the cell.[32] Nucleoli have also been described.[29] The exact number of chromosomes within each nu-

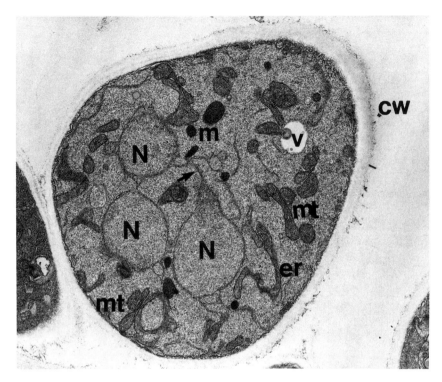

FIGURE 4. Thin section of *B. dermatitidis* yeast showing multiple nuclei (N) with communications of the nuclear membranes with the endoplasmic reticulum (er; arrow), numerous mitochondria (mt), poorly stained cell wall (cw) and, probably, microbodies (m). (×14,600.) (Courtesy of Dr. R. G. Garrison.)

cleus is not known, but estimates suggest the presence of four to six chromosomes per nucleus.[32]

Mycelia are also typically multinucleate, with different numbers of nuclei occupying each hyphal cell.[32] DeLamater suggested that there were more nuclei present in the actively growing apical ends of hyphae than older, more proximal hyphal fragments.[32]

More detailed study of the cellular anatomy of *B. dermatitidis* yeast cells demonstrated the existence of connections between the outer limiting membranes of the nuclei in each cell.[33] Furthermore, the nuclear membranes are also contiguous with the plasma membrane and the membranes of other intracellular organelles (e.g., mitochondria, endoplasmic reticulum). Presumably, these interconnections between the different intracellular compartments facilitate communication within the cell. However, the role of this extensive membrane system in the basic biology of the fungus is not known.

4.4. Yeast-to-Mycelia Conversion

In a study of a single strain of *B. dermatitidis,* Garrison *et al.* described the ultrastructural changes occurring during the conversion of the yeast form to mycelia.[30] Within 6 h of switching the temperature of suspension cultures of yeast from 37°C to 24–26°C, multiple infolding and layering of the plasma membranes could be identified by electron microscopic observation. This intracytoplasmic membrane system appeared to be derived *de novo* from the preexisting plasma membrane and has been generally associated with cell division and formation of septa.[30] Intermediate forms were seen 12–18 h after the temperature shift. These cells had an intercellular septum with Woronin bodies on both sides. The cell wall of the intermediate forms was thinner than that of the yeast cells from which they arose. After 18–24 h, hyphal cells were clearly recognized. These cells contained increased amounts of glycogen, the granules of which tended to associate with the intracytoplasmic membrane systems formed earlier.

4.5. Summary

The intracellular anatomy of *B. dermatitidis* yeast and mycelia appears to be similar to that of other eukaryotes, in general, and other dimorphic fungi, in particular (as reviewed by Maresca and Kobayashi[3]). However, due to the differences in shape of yeast cells and mycelia, the arrangement of intracellular organelles may differ. Functional correlates of the similarities and differences between species and morphologic forms have not yet been made.

5. GENETICS AND REPRODUCTION

As described above, *B. dermatitidis* grows in both perfect and imperfect states. Thus, reproduction of the teleomorph occurs through mating of different sexual types. The anamorph reproduces either by propagation of the mycelium and production of conidia in the mycelial form or by budding in the yeast form.

5.1. Teleomorph

An analysis of the incompatibility system of *A. dermatitidis* was reported by Kwon-Chung.[34] She made several pertinent observations. First, the ability to mate and produce fertile cleistothecia was dependent upon the production of a buff to yellowish brown pigment and the production of the pigment and fertility were rapidly lost as the culture aged in the laboratory. Second, *A. dermatitidis* showed a 1:1 ratio of + versus − mating types, i.e., this organism demonstrates a bipolar incompatibility system. While this system would seem to be ideal for classical genetics experiments, no such reports have appeared in the literature and the use of the *A. dermatitidis* for furthering understanding of the basic elements of heredity and reproduction of this organism remains untapped.

5.2. Anamorph

Mycelia grow by extension of the apical ends of hyphae. Reproduction is by means of conidia that are produced at the terminus of conidiophores or can be found attached to the lateral aspects of hyphae. The conidiophores arise at right angles from hyphae and each bears a single conidium. Conidia incubated at room temperature will germinate and produce hyphae, whereas when incubated at temperatures above 35°C, they undergo phase transition and yeast are formed.

While not well studied, yeast appear to reproduce by binary fission.[29,32] As is true for other pathogenic fungi, the factors controlling cell cycle and cell division are unknown and may be different from those responsible for initiation and maintenance of dimorphic transition.

5.3. Summary

Even though the discovery of *A. dermatitidis* paved the way for investigation into the genetics of the organism, very little has been done to define genetic differences and similarities among different strains. It is likely that the initial attempts to study the mechanisms controlling cell cycle and the different growth phases will utilize molecular biologic techniques, rather than more classic approaches directed to isolating ascospores from individual asci. Such studies may ultimately identify factors responsible for the ability of the fungus to cause disease as well as basic mechanisms of cell growth and reproduction.

6. PHYSIOLOGY

Most of the available information specifically derived from *B. dermatitidis* has been obtained using classical biochemical techniques without the benefits of modern biochemical and biomolecular technology. Nevertheless, the results provide some insight into some of the basic nutritional requirements and biochemical pathways of the organism.

6.1. Growth Requirements

6.1.1. Vitamins

Studies in this area have yielded conflicting results. Biotin was found in one study to be absolutely required for growth of both mycelia and yeast of six isolates.[35] Since fresh isolates could survive at least one passage through biotin-deficient medium, it was postulated that biotin was stored within the cells. Even in complex medium, biotin was required for growth. However, other studies have indicated no requirement for biotin or other vitamins.[6,25,36] Methodologic details might account for these disparate results. However, considering the report that both yeast and mycelia can grow and undergo phase transition in tap water,[37] nutritional requirements for maintenance of viability of this fungus must be minimal. Whether specific substances can enhance growth and thereby affect fungal virulence has not been addressed and remains unanswered.

6.1.2. Amino Acids

While absolute requirements for individual amino acids have not been demonstrated, as might be expected, growth could be stimulated by organic nitrogen sources.[23,25]

6.2. Chemical Composition

Most of our understanding of the biochemistry of *B. dermatitidis* comes from studies of the composition of the cell wall of the organism and not from dynamic study of cellular metabolism and biosynthetic pathways. Comparison of data obtained from both mycelial and yeast forms indicates that significant differences exist.

6.2.1. Cell Wall

The cell walls of *B. dermatitidis* yeast and mycelia have been extensively analyzed with regard to their protein, lipid, and carbohydrate composition.[26,30,38–46] Concordant with data obtained on the effects of growth medium on cellular ultrastructure (see above), marked effects of medium on content of individual chemical moieties have been reported.[47] Specifically, the amount of detectable fatty acids and extractable lipids obtained from both yeast and mycelia changed with different media. An increase in the amounts of fatty acids and lipids was seen in cells grown in Halliday/McCoy medium (HMM) as compared to modified Levine/Ordal medium (LOM). HMM is identical to LOM except that it contains biotin. This one difference, however, cannot explain the differences in lipid content since both brain heart infusion and Sabouraud dextrose also contain biotin and no similar increase in lipids and fatty acids was seen in either mycelia or yeast grown in these media.[47] In contrast, the percentage of carbohydrate and protein recovered from whole yeast or mycelial cells was not affected by the growth media.[47] The differences in lipid content are particularly interesting in light of the finding that yeast cells of a virulent strain of *B. dermatitidis* (in a mouse pneumonia model) contained higher amounts of lipid than did yeast of an avirulent strain, even though both were grown in identical media under the same conditions.[48]

Several investigators have compared the composition of cell walls of yeast and mycelia.[26,38,39,43] Mycelial cell walls were found to have a higher content of hexose sugars compared to yeast, predominantly glucose, but with measurable amounts of galactose and mannose, in a molar ratio of 1.0:0.1:0.2, respectively. In contrast, only glucose was detected on paper chromatograms of cell wall hydrolysates.[38] Mycelia contained 50% more hexoses than did yeast. However, in these studies, the growth media and conditions of incubation of the fungus were not specified.

In contrast, Domer prepared cell walls of *B. dermatitidis* mycelia and yeast that were grown in soy dialysate medium.[26] Using thin-layer chromatography, only glucose and mannose could be detected. Amounts of total hexose measured in yeast cells were comparable to that found by Kanetsuna and Carbonell,[38] but only 20–38% total anthrone hexose was found in mycelia in Domer's study, compared to 51% measured by Kanetsuna and Carbonell. The reason for these differences may be strain related or due to methodological differences.

The cell wall of both morphological forms of *B. dermatitidis* contains glucan and chitin, as do the cell walls of most other fungi. The predominant neutral sugar found in the cell wall is glucose (predominantly as glucan) and the only amino sugar is *N*-acetylglucosamine (as chitin).

In the yeast form of *B. dermatitidis,* 95% of the glucan is α, whereas mycelia contain 60% α and 40% β.[38] This is similar to *Paracoccidioides brasiliensis:* mycelial cell walls contain more β glucan than yeast.[38] The explanation for this switch in predominant glucan type during the mycelia-to-yeast transition is thought to be based on preferential synthesis of α glucan with the increase in temperature, as has been shown in *P. brasiliensis,*[49] presumably because of activation of α glucan synthetase activity at the higher temperatures.

Gow and Gooday have studied the morphology and chromatographic behavior of chitin in several different species of fungi, including *B. dermatitidis.*[50] Chitin fibrils isolated from *B. dermatitidis* mycelia were similar to those obtained from *H. capsulatum* and *P. brasiliensis,* but longer than those isolated from *Candida albicans.* Due to aggregation of the fibrils, quantitative analysis of fibril length could not be done with the material recovered from the endemic fungal pathogens. The infrared spectra of chitin isolated from each species were identical, suggesting that the chitin obtained from these four fungi were chemically similar.

In an attempt to retrieve serologically useful antigenic material from *B. dermatitidis* yeasts, several groups of investigators have extracted alkali-soluble, water-soluble material (ASWS) from yeast cell walls. The resulting preparation has been found to elicit and detect cell-mediated immune responses to the fungus.[41] This preparation has been found to contain at least four components that absorb at 280 nm. One of these fractions was superior to crude ASWS in skin tests in detecting infection with *B. dermatitidis.*[40] However, even though the performance of this preparation has been studied as an immunological reagent, details of its chemical composition (other than it contains protein and carbohydrate) remain a mystery.

The composition of the cell walls of both phases of *B. dermatitidis* following alkali extraction was studied by Roy and Landau.[39] Using similar weights of starting material, the content of total amino acids and cysteic acid (representing cysteine and cystine) was found to exceed that present in yeast cells. However, hexosamines predominated in the yeast cells. Both phases contained similar amounts of neutral sugars. Individual amino acids were present in higher amounts in mycelia than in yeasts, with the exception of histidine, which was present in comparable amounts in both growth phases.

A protein comprising 5% of the protein in the yeast cell wall, with a molecular mass of 120,000 daltons, has been described by Klein and Jones.[51] The most notable aspect to this newly defined molecule is that it seems to be restricted to *B. dermatitidis* yeast cell walls. Use of this 120-kDa protein as the antigen in a radioimmunoassay gave promising preliminary results in the initial report, discriminating between infection with *Coccidioides immitis* and *H. capsulatum* from *B. dermatitidis.* Further work with this molecule should shed light on its identity and its usefulness as a clinical diagnostic reagent.

Lipid obtained by extracting whole cells or from cell walls has been characterized in several studies.[44–46] Peck and Hauser found that extractable lipids made up approximately 9% of the weight of dried yeast cells.[44] From 24 to 34% of the extractable lipids were phosphatides, with the predominant fatty acids being palmitic, stearic, oleic, and linoleic acids. This was confirmed by Domer and Hamilton,[46] who found that oleic and linoleic acids accounted for 75–80% of the total extractable fatty acids recovered from yeast and mycelia. However, oleic acid predominated in the yeast phase, whereas a higher percentage of linoleic acid was recovered from mycelial cells. In comparing the fatty acid composition of cell walls and the remainder of the homogenized cell, cell walls contained more oleic acid than did the corresponding non-cell-wall cellular fractions. Extractable lipids from *B. dermatitidis* and *H. capsulatum* were similar in composition.

Domer and Hamilton reported that lipid comprised approximately 2% of the yeast phase cell wall, whereas mycelial cell walls contained negligible lipid.[46] In contrast, after the cell wall was removed from homogenized preparations, the remaining "cell sap" of yeast was found to contain 12–18% extractable lipid and in similar mycelial preparations, less than 5% was determined to be extractable lipid.[46]

DiSalvo and Denton determined the lipid content of four different strains of *B. dermatitidis* mycelia and yeasts.[45] The amount of lipid recovered from each strain correlated with the virulence of the isolate in mice, with the most virulent strain possessing the most extractable lipid (12 versus 7% in an avirulent isolate). Mycelia contained approximately twice as much lipid as did the corresponding yeast phase. Since whole cells were used in those studies, one cannot localize the lipids to any particular location in the fungal cell and the explanation for correlation of virulence with lipid content is unclear.

6.2.2. Cell Membrane

Specific studies of the chemical composition of cell membranes of *B. dermatitidis* yeast and mycelial phases have not been done. However, there is no reason to suspect that the basic details of the composition of the cell membrane of this fungus differ from those found in other fungi.

6.2.3. Cytoplasm

Composition of the cytoplasmic compartment of *B. dermatitidis* has been determined primarily in the course of studies to identify antigens suitable for use in immunodiagnostic assays.[52] Most commonly, cells have been disrupted by physical means and the cellular debris removed by centrifugation. The resulting supernatants have been characterized by their ability to elicit delayed-type hypersensitivity reactions, but the chemical composition of these preparations has not been reported (reviewed by Young and Larsh[52]). If useful antigens are detected, detailed analyses of their composition should follow.

6.2.4. Nucleus

Taylor studied cultures grown on a synthetic agar medium containing salts, biotin, iron, and glucose.[53] He determined DNA and RNA content of yeast and mycelia after up to 35 days of incubation at 37°C for yeast and 27°C for mycelia. While DNA content of both phases was stable at approximately 5 μg DNA/mg dry wt for the duration of the experiment, RNA content of yeastlike cells exceeds that in mycelia 4- to 12-fold. Maximum RNA content of yeastlike cells approached 120 μg/mg dry wt from 6 to 10 days of incubation and then decreased to a stable concentration of 40–60 μg/mg dry wt after 10 to 15 days of incubation. Functional correlates of these changes are still not known.

In a later study, Bawdon *et al.* measured the DNA base composition of both morphological forms of *B. dermatitidis* and *H. capsulatum.*[54] Based on results from two and five strains, respectively, they determined the guanine plus cytosine content of nuclear DNA obtained from yeast-form *B. dermatitidis* to be 48.2% and of mycelial-form, 48.3%. This was similar to the values obtained for *H. capsulatum,* 47.4 and 47.0%, respectively. These data provided additional support for the notion that these two fungi were phylogenetically closely related and members of the Gymnoascaceae.

6.3. Summary

Studies of the growth requirements and cell composition of both growth forms of *B. dermatitidis* have uncovered remarkable similarities to other dimorphic fungi, especially *H. capsulatum* and *P. brasiliensis.* This is not surprising since these organisms are closely related phylogenetically. While data obtained during the course of experiments with any one of the dimorphic fungi may be applicable to the others, from the medical point of view, there are enough differences in the clinical illnesses and histopathology of their respective illnesses that each organism should be specifically studied, if unique features responsible for virulence are to be found.

7. DIMORPHIC PHASE TRANSITION

In studies extending observations made with *H. capsulatum,* Medoff *et al.*[55] documented the physiological changes that occur during mycelial-to-yeast-phase transition induced by shifting the incubation temperature from 25°C to 37°C, primarily focusing on mitochondrial respiration. The results were remarkably similar to those obtained with *H. capsulatum* and *P. brasiliensis.* These investigators divide the temperature-induced changes into three stages: (1) uncoupling of oxidative phosphorylation with decreases in intracellular ATP concentration, respiration rate, and electron transport components; (2) resting, dormant, with no measurable respiration; and (3) recovery phase with increase in respiration and concentrations of ATP and electron transport components, during which the yeast morphology appears. During the second stage, the dormant cells require cysteine, as do the other two dimorphic fungi, for the operation of electron shunt pathways that bypass the blocked cytochrome system. Removal of cysteine or other sulfhydryl-containing compounds effectively blocks progression of the fungus into stage 3 and, therefore, inhibits completion of phase transition. Other than these observations, further details of the biochemical events affected by dimorphic phase transition have been defined in *H. capsulatum,* and the interested reader is referred to a thorough discussion of this topic in a recent review by Maresca and Kobayashi.[3] Obviously, much work remains to be done with *B. dermatitidis* to determine the relationship between the heat shock response and phase transition, and the role of potential pathways (e.g., polyamine synthesis, guanine nucleotide activity, activation of phase-specific genes) in initiating or regulating phase transition.

8. SUMMARY

While much has been learned over the past 100 years concerning the taxonomy, biochemistry, and physiology of *B. dermatitidis,* the basic mechanisms controlling phase transition are unknown. Moreover, there are significant gaps in our knowledge of fundamental physiologic processes that regulate the growth and reproduction of both phases of this fungus. Advances in these areas may have repercussions on our understanding of why and how this organism can cause disease and may aid in the identification of *B. dermatitidis*-specific "virulence factors." The utility of *A. dermatitidis* in studying the genetics of this fungus remains unexplored. However, advances in the understanding of the closely related pathogen *H. capsulatum*[3] and an increasing interest in blastomycosis in clinical medicine and in the laboratory, may be reflected in future advances in our understanding of this most interesting fungal pathogen.

ACKNOWLEDGMENTS. The author thanks Dr. Michael Rinaldi for his invaluable assistance in reviewing the details of taxonomy and Drs. K. J. Kwon-Chung, R. G. Garrison, and J. W. Rippon for generously providing the photomicrographs used in this chapter.

REFERENCES

1. Gilchrist TC, Stokes WR: The presence of an oidium in the tissues of a case of pseudo-lupus vulgaris. *Johns Hopkins Hosp Bull* 7:129–133, 1896
2. McDonough ES, Lewis AL: *Blastomyces dermatitidis:* Production of the sexual stage. *Science* 156:528–529, 1967
3. Maresca B, Kobayashi GS: Dimorphism in *Histoplasma capsulatum:* A model for the study of cell differentiation in pathogenic fungi. *Microbiol Rev* 53:186–209, 1989
4. Szaniszlo PJ, Jacobs CW, Geis PA: Dimorphism: Morphological and biochemical aspects, in Howard DH, Howard LF (eds): *Fungi Pathogenic for Humans and Animals.* New York, Marcel Dekker, 1983, p 323
5. SanBlas G, SanBlas F: Molecular aspects of fungal dimorphism. *CRC Crit Rev Microbiol* 11:101–127, 1984
6. Gilardi GL, Laffer NC: Nutritional studies on the yeast phase of *Blastomyces dermatitidis* and *B. brasiliensis. J Bacteriol* 83:219–227, 1962
7. Griffin DH: *Fungal Physiology.* New York, John Wiley & Sons, 1981
8. Matsumoto K, Uno I, Ishikawa T: Genetic analysis of the role of cAMP in yeast. *Yeast* 1:15–24, 1985
9. Cole GT: Models of cell differentiation in conidial fungi. *Microbiol Rev* 50:95–132, 1986
10. Kukuruzinska MA, Bergh MLE, Jackson BJ: Protein glycosylation in yeast. *Annu Rev Biochem* 56:915–944, 1987
11. Nasmyth K, Shore D: Transcriptional regulation in the yeast life cycle. *Science* 237:1162–1170, 1987
12. Jennings DH: Translocation of solutes in fungi. *Biol Rev* 62:215–243, 1987
13. Guarente L: Regulatory proteins in yeast. *Annu Rev Genet* 21:425–452, 1987
14. Domer JE: *Blastomyces dermatitidis,* in Szaniszlo PJ (ed): *Current Topics in Infectious Disease: Fungal Dimorphism.* New York, Plenum Press, 1985, p 51
15. Rippon JW: Blastomycosis, in *Medical Mycology. The Pathogenic Fungi and the Pathogenic Actinomycetes,* ed 3. Philadelphia, WB Saunders, 1988, p 474
16. Vermeil C, Bouillard C, Miegeville M, et al: The echinulate conidia of *Blastomyces dermatitidis* Gilchrist and Stokes and the taxonomic status of this species. *Mykosen* 25:251–253, 1982
17. Rippon JW, Ajello LA, Maraganore M, et al: Small form blastomycosis mimicking histoplasmosis. *Abstracts of the Annual Meeting of the American Society for Microbiology* 1986:F-44
18. McDonough ES, Lewis AL: The ascigerous stage of *Blastomyces dermatitidis. Mycologia* 60:76–83, 1968
19. Currah RS: Taxonomy of the Onygenales: Arthrodermataceae, Gymnoascaceae, Myxotrichaceae, and Onygenaceae. *Mycotaxon* 24:1–216, 1985
20. Kwon-Chung KJ: Studies on *Emmonsiella capsulata* 1. Heterothallism and development of the ascocarp. *Mycologia* 65:109–121, 1973
21. Glick AD, Kwon-Chung KJ: Ultrastructural comparison of coils and ascospores of *Emmonsiella capsulata* and *Ajellomyces dermatitidis. Mycologia* 65:216–221, 1973

22. McGinnis MR, Katz B: *Ajellomyces* and its synonym *Emmonsiella*. *Mycotaxon* 8:157–164, 1979

23. Levine S, Ordal ZJ: Factors influencing the morphology of *Blastomyces dermatitidis*. *J Bacteriol* 52:687–694, 1946

24. Gilardi GL: Nutrition of systematic and subcutaneous pathogenic fungi. *Bacteriol Rev* 29:406–424, 1965

25. Salvin SB: Phase-determining factors in *Blastomyces dermatitidis*. *Mycologia* 41:311–319, 1949

26. Domer JE: Monosaccharide and chitin content of cell walls of *Histoplasma capsulatum* and *Blastomyces dermatitidis*. *J Bacteriol* 107:870–877, 1971

27. Clemons KV, Hurley S, Treat-Clemons LG, et al: Variable colonial phenotypic expression of *Blastomyces dermatitidis* (Bd). *Abstracts of the Annual Meeting of the American Society for Microbiology* 1989:F-43

28. Kaufman L, Standard PG, Weeks RJ, et al: Detection of two *Blastomyces dermatitidis* serotypes by exoantigen analysis. *J Clin Microbiol* 18:110–114, 1983

29. Zaharee MH, Wilson TE, Scheer ER: The effect of growth media upon the ultrastructure of *Blastomyces dermatitidis*. *Can J Microbiol* 28:211–218, 1982

30. Garrison RG, Lane JW, Field MF: Ultrastructural changes during the yeastlike to mycelial-phase conversion of *Blastomyces dermatitidis* and *Histoplasma capsulatum*. *J Bacteriol* 101:628–635, 1970

31. Bawdon RE, Fiskin AM, Garrison RG: Ultrastructural aspects of cytoplasmic ribosomes from *Histoplasma capsulatum* and *Blastomyces dermatitidis* as revealed by heavy metal staining. *Mycopathologia* 86:155–163, 1984

32. DeLamater ED: The nuclear cytology of *Blastomyces dermatitidis*. *Mycologia* 40:430–445, 1948

33. Edwards GA, Edwards MR: The intracellular membranes of *Blastomyces dermatitidis*. *Am J Bot* 47:622–632, 1960

34. Kwon-Chung KJ: Genetic analysis on the incompatibility system of *Ajellomyces dermatitidis*. *Sabouraudia* 9:231–238, 1971

35. Halliday WJ, McCoy E: Biotin as a growth requirement for *Blastomyces dermatitidis*. *J Bacteriol* 70:464–468, 1955

36. Levine S, Ordal ZJ: Factors influencing the morphology of *Blastomyces dermatitidis*. *J Bacteriol* 52:687–694, 1946

37. Sheiban ZB: Morphological conversion of *Blastomyces dermatitidis* in tapwater. *Bull. WHO* 51:423, 1974

38. Kanetsuna F, Carbonell LM: Cell wall composition of the yeastlike and mycelial forms of *Blastomyces dermatitidis*. *J Bacteriol* 106:946–948, 1971

39. Roy I, Landau JW: Composition of the alkali resistant cell wall material of dimorphic *Blastomyces dermatitidis*. *Sabouraudia* 10:107–112, 1972

40. Lancaster MV, Sprouse RF: Isolation of a purified skin test antigen from *Blastomyces dermatitidis* yeast-phase cell wall. *Infect Immun* 14:623–625, 1976

41. Deighton F, Cox RA, Hall NK, et al: In vivo and in vitro cell-mediated immune responses to a cell wall antigen of *Blastomyces dermatitidis*. *Infect Immun* 15:429–435, 1977

42. Hall NK, Deighton F, Larsh HW: Use of an alkali-soluble water-soluble extract of *Blastomyces dermatitidis* yeast-phase cell walls and isoelectrically focused components in peripheral lymphocyte transformations. *Infect Immun* 19:411–415, 1978

43. Roy I, Landau JW: Protein constituents of cell walls of the dimorphic phases of *Blastomyces dermatitidis*. *Can J Microbiol* 18:473–478, 1972

44. Peck RL, Hauser CR: Chemical studies of certain pathogenic fungi. I. The lipids of *Blastomyces dermatitidis*. *J Am Chem Soc* 60:2599–2603, 1938

45. DiSalvo AF, Denton JF: Lipid content of four strains of *Blastomyces dermatitidis* of different mouse virulence. *J Bacteriol* 85:927–931, 1963

46. Domer JE, Hamilton JG: The readily extracted lipids of *Histoplasma capsulatum* and *Blastomyces dermatitidis*. *Biochim Biophys Acta* 231:465–478, 1971

47. Massoudnia A, Scheer ER: The influence of medium on the chemical composition of *Blastomyces dermatitidis*. *Curr Microbiol* 7:25–28, 1982

48. Brass C, Volkmann CM, Philpott DE, et al: Spontaneous mutant of *Blastomyces dermatitidis* attenuated in virulence for mice. *Sabouraudia* 20:145–158, 1982

49. Kanetsuna F, Carbonell LM, Azuma I, et al: Biochemical studies on the thermal dimorphism of *Paracoccidioides brasiliensis*. *J Bacteriol* 110:208–218, 1972

50. Gow NAR, Gooday GW: Ultrastructure of chitin in hyphae of *Candida albicans* and other dimorphic and mycelial fungi. *Protoplasma* 115:52–58, 1983

51. Klein BS, Jones JM: Isolation, purification, and radiolabelling of a novel 120-kD surface protein on *Blastomyces dermatitidis* yeasts to detect antibody in infected patients. *J Clin Invest* 85:152–161, 1990

52. Young KD, Larsh HW: Antigens and chemical composition of *Blastomyces dermatitidis*. *Mycopathologia* 78:47–63, 1982

53. Taylor JJ: Nucleic acids and dimorphism in *Blastomyces*. *Exp Cell Res* 24:155–158, 1961

54. Bawdon RE, Garrison RG, Fina LR: Deoxyribonucleic acid base composition of the yeast-like and mycelial phases of *Histoplasma capsulatum* and *Blastomyces dermatitidis*. *J Bacteriol* 111:593–596, 1972

55. Medoff G, Painter A, Kobayashi GS: Mycelial- to yeast-phase transitions of the dimorphic fungi *Blastomyces dermatitidis* and *Paracoccidioides brasiliensis*. *J Bacteriol* 169:4055–4060, 1987

56. Rippon JW: Blastomycosis, in *Medical Mycology: The Pathogenic Fungi and the Pathogenic Actinomycetes,* ed 3. Philadelphia, WB Saunders, 1988, pp 499–500

3

Virulence of *Blastomyces dermatitidis*

Elmer Brummer

Virulence of disease-producing organisms is generally defined as the ability to produce a rapid course of infection or disease. Therefore, virulence of an organism can be considered to be its degree of disease-producing capacity.

1. *IN VIVO*

1.1. Measurement of Virulence

Different methods can be utilized to measure or compare the virulence of pathogenic strains or isolates of an organism. Determination of the minimal lethal dose (MLD) is one of these methods. This is accomplished by infecting groups of a standard susceptible host, e.g., a mouse strain of certain age and sex, with graded doses of the pathogen via a certain route. The most virulent isolate will have the lowest MLD. These data can also be used to determine the LD_{50} (50% lethal dose) of an isolate or strain. When cumulative deaths are plotted against $\log_{10}$ of the doses, the LD_{50} is the point on the

Blastomycosis, edited by Yousef Al-Doory and Arthur F. DiSalvo, Plenum Medical Book Company, New York, 1992.

dose scale at which the line intersects the 50% mortality point. This dose would be expected to produce death in half of the animals inoculated.

Another method that can be used to express relative strain virulence of a pathogen is determination of the mean survival time (MST) in groups of animals infected with a constant lethal dose of the strain or isolate. Alternatively, the time (days) to 50% mortality can also be used as an index of virulence. Both of these methods have been used to measure virulence of *Blastomyces dermatitidis*.

1.2. Basis of Pathogenicity

Pathogenicity and even virulence of many microbial pathogens, especially bacteria, has been causally associated with toxins (exotoxins and endotoxins), enzymes, capsules, and other virulence factors.[1] On the other hand, the thermally dimorphic fungal pathogens have a unique adaptation that enables them to parasitize and cause death in mammalian hosts. The saprophytic forms of these fungi grow in nature at ambient temperatures and under certain conditions form conidia or arthroconidia, which if inhaled can transform into a parasitic yeast form at body temperature in a few hours. Pathogenicity is clearly associated with the new yeast form because they resist killing by human polymorphonuclear neutrophils (PMNs), which readily kill the mycelial form *in vitro*.[2]

Virulence, and even loss of pathogenicity, in thermally dimorphic fungal pathogens has been reported.[3-7] Although identification of virulence factors in these pathogens has been attempted in different laboratories,[4,8,9] they have been elusive and much remains to be determined.

Investigating pathogenicity of the thermally dimorphic fungus *B. dermatitidis* is complicated by the fact that it has only been isolated from nature by host infection. However, we do not know whether pathogenic and nonpathogenic strains exist in nature. Information regarding this awaits development of a method to isolate *B. dermatitidis* directly from nature and which does not depend upon selection of pathogenic strains by the mouse inoculation method of Denton *et al.*[10] or natural animal[11] or human[12,13] infection.

1.3. Virulence of Isolates

1.3.1. Soil

All isolates of *B. dermatitidis* at their time of isolation were pathogenic by nature of the isolation process; however, their degree of pathogenicity or virulence is an available object of study. When *B. dermatitidis* (KL-1) was originally isolated from soil by Denton *et al.*,[10] they compared its virulence in mice to a human and a sea lion (SL-1) isolate.[14] A yeast-form suspension of KL-1 was adjusted spectrophotometrically and compared to similar suspensions of other isolates by intravenous (i.v.) injection of 0.5 ml suspension per mouse. It was found that the group of mice inoculated with KL-1 had the shortest mean time of survival and KL-1 was considered to be the most virulent compared to the other isolates.[4]

As more *B. dermatitidis* isolates (ten) were obtained from soil samples by the mouse isolation method,[15] Denton and DiSalvo compared virulence of soil isolates in mice to five isolates of *B. dermatitidis* cultured from patients with blastomycosis. All ten soil isolates were found to be highly virulent in mice causing 50% mortality in 7 to 14 days. By comparison, four of five human isolates produced 50% mortality in mice after 13 to 53 days and one human isolate failed to produce deaths before 135 days.[4]

1.3.2. Human

Virulence of human *B. dermatitidis* isolates has been confirmed in mice by a number of investigators using the pulmonary route instead of the i.v. route of infection. Harvey *et al.*[16] in 1978 infected groups of young (15–20 g) male BALB/c mice intranasally (i.n.) with the yeast form of five different isolates of *B. dermatitidis* and reported that two were virulent (90 to 100% mortality in 30 days, MST = 23 days), two were attenuated (20 to 29% mortality in 30 days), and one (GA-1) was avirulent.

The conidia of *B. dermatitidis* were also shown to cause blastomycosis in mice (Denton and DiSalvo[17]). This was confirmed when Williams and Moser[18] infected mice intratracheally (i.t.) with conidia. Using this system, they tested 13 different clinical isolates of *B. dermatitidis* by the i.t. inoculation of 6- to 8-week-old BALB/c male mice with 10^4 conidia. They found that the virulence of these isolates varied widely with MST of 24 to 134 days.[19] Virulence of these isolates fell into three categories: (1) five isolates with MST of 24 to 31 days (virulent), (2) five isolates with MST of 65 to 107 days (attenuated), and (3) two isolates with MST of 130 to 134 days (very attenuated). One isolate reported previously[18] was again avirulent[19] and did not cause gross pathology or deaths in 285 days. Taken together, these studies on virulence of *B. dermatitidis* isolates established that virulence in *B. dermatitidis* can be variable. These data opened a new area of investigation; namely, a search for virulence factor(s), which will be addressed later.

1.4. Stability of Virulence

1.4.1. Loss

One explanation for variations of virulence in *B. dermatitidis* isolates is that these variations reflect stable inherent genetic differences of isolates within the species. However, with studies of virulence in other microorgan-

TABLE 1
Loss of Virulence by an Isolate of *B. dermatitidis*

Isolate (source)	Year tested	Mortality[a] at 90 days	Survivors culture +
KL-1 (Med. College Georgia)	1962	18/20[b]	2/2
KL-1 (S.C. Dept. Health)	1986	3/20[c]	17/17
KL-1 (Inst. Med. Res.)	1986	0/20[c]	0/20
KL-1 (ATCC 26198)	1986	0/20[c]	0/20

[a] Swiss white mice infected i.v. with 0.5 ml of yeast-form *B. dermatitidis.*
[b] Number of mice dead/number of mice infected.
[c] Two-tailed Fisher exact test; $p < 0.001$ compared to KL-1 tested in 1962.

isms it has been observed that some pathogens apparently lose their virulence subsequent to cycles of growth on laboratory medium. Two cases in particular illustrate this point. To maintain the virulence of *Legionella pneumophila,* it was necessary to pass the organism in guinea pigs.[20] Recently, it was shown that *in vitro* passages on supplemented Mueller–Hinton agar selected out stable avirulent variants of *L. pneumophila* isolate, whereas *in vivo* passage maintained the virulent form.[21] A similar situation has been reported for *Coccidioides immitis,* a thermally dimorphic fungal pathogen. Virulence was markedly attenuated after 84 serial passages *in vitro,* e.g., LD_{20} increased from 20 arthroconidia to 3.7×10^5 arthroconidia. Virulence in this isolate was "regained" after passage in mice.[5]

This phenomenon of virulence loss was observed with two isolates of *B. dermatitidis,* KL-1 and MCG-1.[22] KL-1 and MCG-1 were virulent when isolated from soil by the mouse inoculation method.[10,15] Subsequent to cycles of *in vitro* growth and storage over a 10-year period followed by deposit at ATCC as ATCC 26198 (KL-1), it is now avirulent as tested in the mouse i.v. infection model (Table 1) and in the i.n. pulmonary infection model.[22] MCG-1 was also avirulent in the mouse i.n. pulmonary infection model. Virulence in these two isolates was not restored after five serial passages in mice.[22] When five recent patient isolates and a recent soil isolate were tested within 1 year of isolation, they were all virulent in mice.[22]

1.4.2. Attenuation

Changes in virulence in ATCC 26199 when the yeast form was stored at $-70°C$ for greater than 12 months were observed. At two different times, i.e., 1982 and 1984, when samples were retrieved and tested *in vivo,* virulence was found to be attenuated (unpublished data). The 1982 attenuated variant of ATCC 26199 was deposited as ATCC 60915. It is not known at this time whether an attenuated variant of an isolate represents a mixture of virulent organisms or a single distinct variant with reduced capacity to cause disease. If the former is the case, then like *L. pneumophila*,[21] it may be possible to retrieve the virulent form by animal passage.

It is of interest to note that clinical isolates used in experiments by Moser *et al.*[19] were stored at −70°C prior to testing. The possible influence of such unspecified storage time on virulence should be considered in interpretation of results from such experiments.

1.4.3. Preservation

A patient isolate deposited at ATCC within 1 year of isolation in 1970 (ATCC 26199) has retained virulence for 15 years as stored by the freeze-liquid nitrogen method used by ATCC. Purchase and testing of this isolate from ATCC in 1982, 1984, and 1986 has documented stability of virulence in ATCC 26199 when stored by this method.[22]

1.5. Correlates of Virulence

1.5.1. Replication in Lungs

Differences between ATCC 26199 (virulent) and ATCC 26199A (attenuated) in their ability to replicate in the lungs of infected mice were examined in young (15 g) BALB/c mice by Brass *et al.*[3] Low doses of the attenuated variant (20 CFU) could not be recovered from the lungs of infected mice 48 h later, whereas the parent isolate (90 CFU) replicated more than 10-fold in 48 h. When higher doses of the attenuated variant (10,000 CFU) were used to infect young mice, the CFU per lung decreased 100-fold in 4 days while CFU per lung increased to the extent of 10,000 CFU per lung at day 18. These findings suggest, but do not prove, that the attenuated variant may consist of a mixture of the avirulent variant plus the virulent parent isolate and infection with high doses may result in selection of virulent-type cells that go on to produce disease.

1.5.2. Subcutaneous Replication Model

A subcutaneous model of *B. dermatitidis* infection was developed during immunological studies in mice.[23] ATCC 26199 replicated fivefold subcutaneously in nonimmunized mice during the first week of infection and then gradually was eliminated over the next 3 weeks. This process resulted in protection against lethal pulmonary challenge with ATCC 26199 and tenfold reduction of CFU of subcutaneously injected ATCC 26199 in 1 week and clearance in 2 weeks.[23]

Similar studies with different isolates of *B. dermatitidis* showed that the virulent ATCC 26199 replicated fivefold during 1 week of subcutaneous infection, whereas avirulent GA-1 did not replicate and was cleared in 1 week.[24] The CFU of the attenuated variant of ATCC 26199 decreased three-fold in 4 days but was not cleared in 7 or 14 days.[24] The subcutaneous model of infection reflected early events described by Brass *et al.*[3] in the lungs of mice infected with these isolates.

2. IN VITRO

2.1. Macrophages

2.1.1. Virulence and Replication

In studies on the interaction of murine macrophages and *B. dermatitidis* yeast cells *in vitro,* it was found that resident peritoneal macrophages surrounded and inhibited the replication of *B. dermatitidis.*[25] Compared to replication of *B. dermatitidis* in medium alone and as measured by the number of CFU, macrophages in 24-h cocultures inhibited replication by 24%. If peritoneal macrophages were elicited by prior intraperitoneal (i.p.) injection of fetal bovine serum or concanavalin A, they exhibited enhanced ability to inhibit replication of *B. dermatitidis,* i.e., 49 and 64%, respectively.[25]

When virulent, attenuated, and avirulent strains of *B. dermatitidis* were studied in this system, replication of strains was inhibited to about the same extent in 24-h cocultures.[24] However, when coculture time was extended to 72 h the virulent isolate escaped from inhibition of replication, e.g., coculture of CFU were not significantly different from control CFU.[24] In contrast, replication of attenuated and avirulent strains continued to be inhibited in 72-h cocultures. These findings suggested that virulence of *B. dermatitidis* in mice might be associated with capacity to circumvent certain defensive actions of macrophages. However, generalizations about virulence from the results with this set of isolates should be made with caution until more sets of isolates are tested.

Murine macrophages, activated by prior treatment with lymphokines or γ-interferon, were able to kill (reduce inoculum CFU) isolates of *B. dermatitidis* in short-term 4-h assays.[26–28] Killing by activated macrophages was shown to be mediated by mechanisms that did not depend on products of the oxidative burst.[29] Since avirulent, attenuated, and virulent isolates were killed to the same extent (32 to 35%) by activated pulmonary macrophages,[27] virulence of ATCC 26199 in mice did not appear to be associated with resistance to killing by activated macrophages.

2.1.2. Human Monocytes and Macrophages

Human monocytes, like resident murine peritoneal macrophages, inhibited replication of both virulent and avirulent strains of *B. dermatitidis* in 24-h cocultures.[30] In 72-h cocultures, human monocytes continued to inhibit the replication of both virulent and the avirulent isolates 45 and 63%, respectively. The virulent isolate did not escape from monocyte inhibition of replication as it had done when cocultured with murine macrophages.[24]

Human monocyte-derived macrophages, monocytes cultured *in vitro* for 9 days, were more efficient than monocytes in inhibiting replication of *B. dermatitidis* isolates.[30] Replication of the virulent and avirulent strains was inhibited 85 and 88%, respectively, in 72-h monocyte-derived macrophage cocultures. These contrasting results of murine and human macrophages with respect to escape from inhibition of replication by a virulent isolate of *B. dermatitidis* illustrate the possible dangers of extrapolating results from a murine system to a human system.

Killing (reduction of inoculum CFU) of *B. dermatitidis* isolates by human monocytes or monocyte-derived macrophages was not observed in the system described above, although inhibition of replication was easily demonstrated. Using a different method to assess viability (exclusion of methylene blue), monocyte-derived macrophages were reported to kill the yeast form of *B. dermatitidis in vitro*.[31] Additional studies are warranted to verify these results and also to determine whether activated human monocytes or monocyte-derived macrophages are equally fungicidal for all isolates of *B. dermatitidis*. To date there are no published reports about the capacity of lymphokine- or γ-interferon-activated monocytes or monocyte-derived macrophages to kill *B. dermatitidis*.

2.2. PMNs

2.2.1. Virulence and Replication

Studies on the interaction of *B. dermatitidis* isolates and human PMNs showed that human PMNs were not able to kill yeast-form *B. dermatitidis in vitro*.[2,30] Instead, an opposite effect was observed in 24- and 72-h cocultures, namely, enhancement of *B. dermatitidis* replication in the presence of human PMNs. Replication of a virulent isolate of ATCC 26199 was significantly enhanced compared to an avirulent isolate in cocultures with human PMNs.[30]

Similar results were obtained when *B. dermatitidis* isolates were cocultured with murine PMNs elicited i.p. with thioglycollate. In 24-h PMN cocultures, replication of a virulent isolate was enhanced by 60%, whereas replication of an avirulent isolate was enhanced by 34%.[32] Even lysates of murine PMNs or of human PMNs had an enhancing effect on replication of *B. dermatitidis* isolates compared to tissue culture medium.[30,32] Coculturing of *B. dermatitidis* isolates with lymph node cells or their lysates did not have this effect.[30]

Taken together, these findings suggest that accumulation and death of PMNs in *B. dermatitidis* lesions favor replication of a virulent isolate and may partially account for its virulence. Additional studies with a greater number of virulent and avirulent isolates in this system are needed in order to determine whether PMN enhancement of replication is generally associated with virulent isolates.

2.2.2. Virulence and Susceptibility to Killing

Murine PMNs elicited with specific antigen i.p. in *B. dermatitidis* immunized mice were found to be highly fungicidal for yeast-form *B. dermatitidis*.[33] PMNs (5×10^5) were able to kill 80 to 90% of a small inoculum (400–700 CFU) of a virulent isolate in 4 h. Killing of *B. dermatitidis* by immunologically elicited PMNs was dependent upon products of the oxidative burst of PMNs because catalase, a scavenger of hydrogen peroxide, abrogated killing.[34]

Murine PMNs elicited i.p. with thioglycollate were found to have impaired fungicidal activity ($3 \pm 5\%$) compared to PMNs elicited with caseinate ($82 \pm 3\%$) or proteose peptone ($50 \pm 10\%$).[35] On the other hand, murine peripheral blood PMNs were able to kill *B. dermatitidis* ($38 \pm 11\%$), but to a lesser extent than elicited PMNs.[35] This finding correlated with those in a cell-free hydrogen peroxide–myeloperoxidase–halide system where a virulent, an attenuated, and an avirulent isolate had comparable susceptibility to killing.[36]

In summary, virulence of *B. dermatitidis* does not appear to be associated with resistance to killing by murine peripheral blood PMNs, or PMNs elicited immunologically. Moreover, resistance of virulent isolates is not dependent on insensitivity to products of the oxidative burst of PMNs.

3. VIRULENCE FACTORS

3.1. Lipids and Phospholipids

A popular concept of microbial pathogenicity in the 1950s was that microbial lipids mediated pathological reactions during infection. With an avirulent and a virulent isolate as a starting point, DiSalvo and Denton[4] investigated lipids in *B. dermatitidis* as a virulence factor(s). They found that the virulent isolate (SL-1) had more extractable lipid (12.3%) than the avirulent isolate (GA-1), which had 6.8%.[4] Although these findings showed an association between lipid content of *B. dermatitidis* isolate and virulence, it does not necessarily follow that there is a causative relationship.

More recently, similar but more extensive studies were done by Brass *et al.*[37] using a virulent (ATCC 26199) and an attenuated mutant isolate of ATCC 26199. Analysis showed that the virulent isolate had three times less total lipid than the attenuated mutant, but the virulent isolate had double the phospholipid and linoleic fatty acid content. The significance of these findings relative to virulence factors is difficult to ascertain at this time. In these studies,[37] the isolates were indistinguishable relative to growth on various media, utilization of sugars as a sole carbon source, or sugar fermentation. However, the virulent isolate differed from the avirulent mutant by escape from growth inhibition with low concentrations of bile and failure to hydrolyze esculin.[37] Again it is difficult to assess the significance of these differences in terms of virulence of these isolates in mice.

3.2. Cell Wall Composition

Another approach to identify the virulence factor(s) in *B. dermatitidis* is the analysis of the chemical composition of cell walls from different isolates.[38,39] Differences in cell wall composition between a virulent and an avirulent strain were found, namely, cell walls of the virulent strain contained more chitin, protein, and alkali-insoluble material (β 1,3-glucan) but less alkali-soluble material (α 1,3-glucan) than cell walls from an avirulent isolate.[38]

It is of interest to note that the α 1,3-glucan content of *B. dermatitidis* cell walls did not correlate with virulence in the above study. This contrasts with two other thermally dimorphic fungal pathogens, i.e., *Paracoccidioides brasiliensis* and *Histoplasma capsulatum*, where high α 1,3-glucan cell wall content correlated with yeast morphology and virulence of *P. brasiliensis*[7,40] and *H. capsulatum.*[6] In the case of the avirulent mutant of *P. brasiliensis* which had a hyphal rather than a yeast morphology, the cell wall glucan was primarily β 1,3-glucan.[7,40] Similarly, the cell walls of an avirulent spontaneous mutant of *H. capsulatum* consisted almost exclusively of β 1,3-glucan and lacked α 1,3-glucan.[8] Whether the correlation of virulence with α 1,3-glucan cell wall content is a general phenomenon in these fungi is not known and will require additional studies of more paired virulent and avirulent strains. Moreover, it is not known how α 1,3-glucan could affect macrophage defenses and metabolism.

REFERENCES

1. Symposium: Biochemical aspects of microbial pathogenicity. *Ann NY Acad Sci* 88:1021–1318, 1960
2. Schaffner A, Davis CE, Schaffner T, et al: In vitro susceptibility of fungi to killing by neutrophil granulocytes discriminate between primary pathogenicity and opportunism. *J Clin Invest* 78:511–524, 1986
3. Brass C, Volkmann CM, Philpott DE, et al: Spontaneous mutant of *Blastomyces dermatitidis* attenuated in virulence. *Sabouraudia* 20:145–158, 1982
4. DiSalvo AF, Denton JF: Lipid content of four strains of *Blastomyces dermatitidis* of different mouse virulence. *J Bacteriol* 85:927–931, 1963
5. Levine RB, Pappagianis D, Cobb JM: Development of vaccines for coccidioidomycosis. *Mycopathologia* 41:171–185, 1970
6. Klimpel KR, Goldman WE: Isolation and characterization of spontaneous avirulent variants of *Histoplasma capsulatum*. *Infect Immun* 55:528–533, 1987
7. San Blas G, San Blas F, Serrano LE: Host–parasite relationship in the yeast-like form of *Paracoccidioides brasiliensis* strain IVIC Pb 9. *Infect Immun* 15:343–346, 1977
8. Kimpel KR, Goldman WE: Cell walls from avirulent variants of *Histoplasma capsulatum* lack alpha 1,3-glucan. *Infect Immun* 56:2997–3000, 1988
9. San Blas G, San Blas F: Variability of cell wall composition in *Paracoccidioides brasiliensis:* A study of two strains. *Sabouraudia* 20:31–40, 1982
10. Denton JF, McDonough ES, Ajello L, et al: Isolation of *Blastomyces dermatitidis* from soil. *Science* 133:1126–1127, 1961
11. Sarosi GA, Eckman MR, Davies SF, et al: Canine blastomycosis as a harbinger of human disease. *Ann Intern Med* 91:733–735, 1979
12. Baker RD: Tissue reactions in human blastomycosis: An analysis of tissue from twenty three cases. *Am J Pathol* 18:479–495, 1942
13. Gilchrist TCA: A case of blastomycosis in man. *Johns Hopkins Hosp Rep* 1:269–298, 1896
14. Williamson WM, Lombard LS, Getty RE: North American blastomycosis in a northern sea lion. *J Am Vet Med Assoc* 135:513–515, 1959
15. Denton JF, DiSalvo AF: Isolation of *Blastomyces dermatitidis* from natural sites at Augusta, Georgia. *Am J Trop Med Hyg* 13:716–722, 1964
16. Harvey RP, Schmid ES, Carrington CC, et al: Mouse model of pulmonary blastomycosis: Utility, simplicity, and quantitative parameters. *Am Rev Respir Dis* 117:695–703, 1978
17. Denton JF, DiSalvo AF: Respiratory infection of laboratory animals with conidia of *Blastomyces dermatitidis*. *Mycopathol Mycol Appl* 36:129–136, 1968

18. Williams JE, Moser SA: Chronic murine pulmonary blastomycosis induced by intratracheally inoculated *Blastomyces dermatitidis* conidia. *Am Rev Respir Dis* 135:17–25, 1987

19. Moser SA, Koker PJ, Williams JE: Fungal strain dependent alterations in the time course and mortality of chronic murine pulmonary blastomycosis. *Infect Immun* 56:34–39, 1988

20. McDade JE, Shephard CC: Virulent to avirulent conversion of Legionnaires' disease bacterium (*Legionella pneumophila*): its effect on isolation techniques. *J Infect Dis* 139:707–711, 1979

21. Catrenich CE, Johnson W: Virulence conversion of *Legionella pneumophila*: A one-way phenomenon. *Infect Immun* 56:3121–3125, 1988

22. Brummer E, DiSalvo AF, Stevens DA: Virulence in *Blastomyces dermatitidis:* Influence of in vitro passage and storage methods, *The XI Congress of ISHAM, Montreal, Program and Abstracts*, p 169, 1991.

23. Morozumi PA, Brummer E, Stevens DA: Protection against pulmonary blastomycosis: Correlation with cellular and humoral immunity in mice after subcutaneous nonlethal infection. *Infect Immun* 37:670–678, 1982

24. Brummer E, Morozumi PA, Philpott DE, et al: Virulence of fungi: Correlation of virulence of *Blastomyces dermatitidis* in vivo with escape from macrophage inhibition of replication in vitro. *Infect Immun* 32:864–871, 1981

25. Brummer E, Morozumi PA, Stevens DA: Macrophages and fungi: In vitro effects of method of macrophage induction, activation by different stimuli, and soluble factors on *Blastomyces*. *J Reticuloendothel Soc* 28:507–518, 1980

26. Brummer E, Morrison CJ, Stevens DA: Recombinant and natural gamma-interferon activation of macrophages in vitro: Different dose requirements for induction of killing activity against phagocytizable and nonphagocytizable fungi. *Infect Immun* 49:724–730, 1985

27. Brummer E, Stevens DA: Activation of pulmonary macrophages for fungicidal activity by gamma-interferon or lymphokines. *Clin Exp Immunol* 70:520–528, 1987

28. Brummer E, Sugar AM, Stevens DA: Activation of peritoneal macrophages by concanavalin A or *Mycobacterium bovis* (BCG) for fungicidal activity against *Blastomyces dermatitidis* and effect of specific antibody and complement. *Infect Immun* 39:817–822, 1983

29. Brummer E, Stevens DA: Fungicidal mechanisms of activated macrophages: Evidence for nonoxidative mechanisms for killing *Blastomyces dermatitidis. Infect Immun* 55:3221–3224, 1987

30. Brummer E, Stevens DA: Opposite effects of human monocytes, macrophages, and polymorphonuclear neutrophils on replication of *Blastomyces dermatitidis* in vitro. *Infect Immun* 36:297–303, 1982

31. Drutz DJ, Frey CL: Intracellular and extracellular defences of human phagocytes against *Blastomyces dermatitidis* conidia and yeast. *J Lab Clin Med* 105:737–750, 1985

32. Brummer E, Stevens DA: Enhancing effect of murine polymorphonuclear neutrophils (PMN) on the multiplication of *Blastomyces dermatitidis* in vitro and in vivo. *Clin Exp Immunol* 54:587–594, 1983

33. Brummer E, Sugar AM, Stevens DA: Immunological activation of polymorphonuclear neutrophils for fungal killing: Studies with murine cells and *Blastomyces dermatitidis* in vitro. *J Leukocyte Biol* 36:505–520, 1984

34. Brummer E, Sugar AM, Stevens DA: Enhanced oxidative burst in immunologically activated but not elicited polymorphonuclear leukocytes correlates with fungicidal activity. *Infect Immun* 49:396–401, 1985

35. Brummer E, McEwen JG, Stevens DA: Fungicidal activity of murine inflammatory polymorphonuclear neutrophils: Comparison with murine peripheral blood PMN. *Clin Exp Immunol* 66:681–690, 1986

36. Sugar AM, Chahal RS, Brummer E, et al: Susceptibility of *Blastomyces dermatitidis* strains to products of oxidative metabolism. *Infect Immun* 41:908–912, 1983
37. Brass C, Volkman CM, Klein HP, et al: Pathogen factors and host factors in murine blastomycosis. *Mycopathologia* 78:129–140, 1982
38. Cox RA, Best GK: Cell wall composition of two strains of *Blastomyces dermatitidis* exhibiting differences in virulence in mice. *Infect Immun* 5:449–453, 1972
39. Kanetsuna F, Carbonell LM: Cell wall composition of the yeast-like and mycelial forms of *Blastomyces dermatitidis*. *J Bacteriol* 106:946–948, 1971
40. San Blas G, San Blas F: *Paracoccidioides brasiliensis:* Cell wall structure and virulence—A review. *Mycopathologia* 62:77–86, 1977

4

The Ecology of *Blastomyces dermatitidis*

Arthur F. DiSalvo

1. INTRODUCTION

Understanding the epidemiology of blastomycosis depends on comprehension of the ecology of *Blastomyces dermatitidis.* This interrelationship, without a doubt, is real. There is a paucity of data on both the ecology and the epidemiology of this disease. The present assumptions of these concerns either are based on analogy with other systemic pathogenic fungal infections or are postulated from the meager data available.

Although some facets of the epidemiology of blastomycosis have been derived from studies of sporadic cases and a few clusters of patients, there are gaps in knowledge that will be clarified when the ecology of the agent is defined. It is probable that there is a benign subclinical form of blastomycosis similar to that found in histoplasmosis and coccidioidomycosis. The geographic distribution of the latter diseases has been outlined by skin testing and by soil isolations of the etiologic agents. Such tools led to the recognition that not all cases of these mycoses were fatal disseminated infections, but

Blastomycosis, edited by Yousef Al-Doory and Arthur F. DiSalvo, Plenum Medical Book Company, New York, 1992.

rather the majority were minor respiratory disorders. These means are not available for blastomycosis.

This chapter will consider the ecology of the terricolous fungus *B. dermatitidis*. The geographic distribution, probable sources in nature, infectious particles, and limited information on the ecological niche will be discussed. Factors that may influence the survival and dissemination of the fungus and the present method of its isolation from the environment will be reviewed.

2. SOURCE IN NATURE

There are few infectious agents for which the ecological niche remains unresolved. *B. dermatitidis* is one of these. The ecology of *B. dermatitidis* is based on 20% investigation (or facts) and 80% speculation (analogy and extension of the limited data). A complete description of the environmental factors that affect *B. dermatitidis* remains to be achieved. The natural habitat of this organism has long baffled mycologists. The reservoir appears to be material with a high organic content, with or without soil. Despite intensive efforts for the past 30 years to define this arcane source, there have been few substantial results. The only clues to the source of this organism lie in the limited description of the substrates from which the organism has been infrequently isolated.

The natural reservoirs of some pathogenic fungi such as *Histoplasma capsulatum, Cryptococcus neoformans,* and *Coccidioides immitis* are more precisely defined. *H. capsulatum* is associated with organic matter such as bat droppings, chicken droppings, or the soil of blackbird roosts contaminated with these droppings. The association between *Cryptococcus neoformans* and pigeon droppings has been well established and *Coccidioides immitis* is found in desert soils, particularly around animal burrows. By analogy, one would assume that *B. dermatitidis* also has its reservoir in a similar habitat. However, such a relationship is only apparent.

It is assumed that *B. dermatitidis* is a soil saprophyte that presumably exists as a mold in nature. The organism probably thrives in a nidus that is high in organic material and, under specific conditions of temperature and humidity, the mycelium will grow resulting in the production and liberation of conidia. Desiccation of the substrate with subsequent disturbance of the site by anthropurgic activity or by the wind presumably results in an infectious aerosol of conidia and mycelial fragments. Schwarz and Baum have ably demonstrated that blastomycosis is most likely acquired by inhalation.[1]

Speculation on the source of *B. dermatitidis* began shortly after the first report of the disease. In 1901, Ricketts wrote a treatise on blastomycosis reviewing the literature and presenting the occupation, activities, and possible sources of infection of 12 new patients he reported.[2] *B. dermatitidis* is still being sought in similar ecological niches.

As early as 1914, Stober observed that *B. dermatitidis,* in the laboratory, grew on paper, cardboard, cotton, sawdust, fruit, and vegetables.[3] He also investigated the residence of many patients with blastomycosis in the Chicago area, eight of whom lived in rooms with wooden floors that were directly on the earth, in basements with wet floors and walls or that contained some decayed wood. From two of these domiciles he obtained "cultures of a mold which differ in only a few respects from the blastomycetes. . . ." He also stated, "It would also be hazardous to do more than suggest an identity between the molds grown from decaying boards and walls in these dwellings and the blastomycetes, although in many respects points of similarity were demonstrated, such as morphology, cultural reaction, pathogenicity and vaccine reaction." Seventy years later we still cannot state much more than that.

Several investigators have suggested that there is a strong association between water and the exogenous saprophytic source of *B. dermatitidis.* In 1962, Greer reported on 810 cases of blastomycosis occurring in the continental United States during the previous 25 years.[4] He compared various geographic and climatic factors between the five states without any reported cases of blastomycosis and the five states with the greatest incidence of the disease. The former states had a water-to-land-surface-area ratio of 0.7% and an average rainfall of 24 inches while the respective values for the states with the highest incidence of blastomycosis were 3.4% and 45 inches.

The first isolates from naturally infected environmental samples were reported by Denton and DiSalvo in 1964.[5] Ten of three hundred fifty-six samples yielded *B. dermatitidis.* All samples were collected from along 1 mile of road in an area composed of the flood plain of the Savannah River south of Augusta, Georgia. Two small creeks passed through this area to flow into the Savannah River.

In 1969, Borelli *et al.* described the pattern of freshwater systems in the United States and the geographical distribution of salamanders belonging to the genus *Necturus* (mud puppies).[6] They suggested that the salamander may play a role in the ecology of *B. dermatitidis.*

In 1970, Furcolow *et al.* published an extensive review of the prevalence and incidence of blastomycosis in dogs and human beings.[7] Their study reviewed the literature from 1885 to 1968. They found a high incidence of human and canine cases south of the Ohio River and east of the Mississippi River and raised the question of the ecologic relationship between blastomycosis and the proximity to water.

McDonough and Kuzma have suggested that foggy weather may be a prelude to infection.[8] They support this hypothesis with the association of canine and human cases of blastomycosis in Wisconsin related to possible exposure to the ecologic niche during periods of fog. They cite an earlier demonstration that moisture appears to facilitate the release of conidia from the mycelium of *B. dermatitidis* as support for this theory.[9]

Archer also investigated canine blastomycosis in Wisconsin in 1985. He found that 137 of 200 dogs studied (68.5%) lived within 500 yards of water.[10] Twenty five of these dogs resided along four waterways: the Plover River, Pigeon River, Eagle River, and Namekegon River. The latter two rivers were the sites of two outbreaks of human blastomycosis.[11,12] The maps in that report illustrate the location of each affected dog along the waterway. Similarly, Harasen and Randall described and illustrated the location of eight dogs with blastomycosis in Regina, Saskatchewan.[13] All eight dogs resided within two blocks of the Wascana Creek, which meanders through the town. They also noted that this area served as a rest stop for migrating Canada geese, thus the area was heavily contaminated with avian droppings.

Bakerspigel *et al.* reported the isolation of *B. dermatitidis* from an oil field worker in Canada and his work site in 1986.[36] The patient worked in a shed that contained large bags of diatomaceous earth. The air was constantly laden with this dust and therefore was sprinkled daily with water.

Finally, five of the twelve outbreaks of human blastomycosis occurred along the Namekegon, Crystal, Tomorrow, Bigfork, and Eagle rivers. Each of these outbreaks will be discussed in detail in Chapter 5.

3. EXPERIMENTAL ECOLOGY

In attempts to identify the ecological niche of *B. dermatitidis,* investigators have tried to grow the fungus on a variety of substrates. The work of Stober has been mentioned above.[3] Bark, sapwood, and heartwood from four varieties of trees common to the endemic area for blastomycosis were examined.[14] All species and most types of wood, when sterilized, supported the growth of *B. dermatitidis.* McDonough and Hierl studied the growth on oak leaves.[15] Growth only occurred after the application of human airway secretions or saliva on the leaves. They reasoned that these substances provided nutrients and inhibited competing bacteria. The authors suggested that this growth-enhancing factor may aid in the survival of *B. dermatitidis* in nature as animal saliva on forest litter may be the key to survival of this fungus amidst other competitive organisms.

Denton and DiSalvo, in unpublished data, were able to grow and recover *B. dermatitidis* on potato. The potato was placed in Kolle flasks and autoclaved. After cooling, the potato was inoculated with *B. dermatitidis* strain FC-1. Ninety days later a portion of the potato was suspended in 15 ml of saline. White Swiss albino mice were inoculated intraperitoneally (i.p.) with 0.1 ml and other mice were inoculated intravenously (i.v.) with 0.5 ml of the suspension. Another portion of the suspension was plated directly on Sabouraud's dextrose agar medium containing cycloheximide. *B. dermatitidis* was recovered by both the *in vitro* and the *in vivo* method. Similarly, *B. dermatitidis* was recovered from the original potato material 200 days after inoculation. Additional attempts to isolate the fungus 3 years after establishing growth on the potato failed.

In other unpublished studies by the same authors, terraria were used for soil survival studies. In experimentally infected sterile soil samples, *B. dermatitidis* (strain FC-1) was recovered by *in vivo* methods for 21 months after inoculation. Using a similar terrarium, Smith and Furcolow reported that experimentally dry sterile soil inoculated with *B. dermatitidis* reduced the viable particles of the fungus by as much as 90% in 3 weeks.[16] They also showed that viable particles increased in number when the sterilized inoculated soil was kept at 100% humidity. They concluded that such a loss of viability with desiccation (72% in 3 days) may influence the recovery of this fungus from nature, which is probably a reasonable conclusion. Indeed, the longest period that elapsed from collection of a positive sample in Augusta, Georgia until it was inoculated into mice with recovery of *B. dermatitidis* was 18 days.[5] However, the first isolation of this pathogen from the environment was made from a dry sample collected in October 1958 and stored at room temperature until its inoculation in March 1960, an elapsed period of 18 months.[17]

4. GEOGRAPHIC DISTRIBUTION

The geographic distribution of blastomycosis has been determined primarily from a compilation of solitary case reports. Such presentations more often reflect the interest of clinicians, epidemiologists, and mycologists who are curious about the disease and publish their experiences rather than to a preponderance of the fungus. For the same reason, the limited number of investigated outbreaks and clusters of cases have occurred within the known areas of endemicity.

The endemic areas of histoplasmosis and coccidioidomycosis were defined in the 1940s and 1950s primarily through the isolation of the fungi from nature and the use of skin test surveys. The documentation of *H. capsulatum* and *C. immitis* as soil saprophytes in nature aided in defining the geographic distribution of these mycotic agents. Determination of the ecological niche of *B. dermatitidis* has been hindered by the lack of a sensitive method to isolate the organism from suspected sources of contamination. Development of a successful technique to isolate the organism from environmental samples is essential to define the geographic distribution of this fungus.

The skin test antigen for *B. dermatitidis* (blastomycin) was so unreliable that it was removed from the commercial market by the Food and Drug Administration (FDA) in 1972. If a specific antigen to detect delayed hypersensitivity becomes available, or some other technique to determine inapparent infection is developed, the geographic and demographic distribution of human cases of blastomycosis may be more accurately determined.

Blastomycosis was originally thought to occur only in the eastern United States and Canada. While there is no doubt that the preponderance of reports are from North America, it is by no means limited to this continent. Many early reports of "blastomycosis" were not actually cases of infection by *B. dermatitidis*. "Blastomycosis" (from blastospores) was a term used for many yeast infections. Some of these reports were infections due to *Candida* species and the expression "European blastomycosis" was a common synonym for cryptococcosis. Some reports used the more specific term "Gilchrist's disease," but careful examination of even these leaves doubt as to the accuracy of the diagnosis. Recently there have been sporadic reports of what appear to be authentic autochthonous cases of blastomycosis from other parts of the world. A substantial number of cases have occurred in eastern Canada and throughout Africa. Excluding cases in which a strong epidemiologic link between the patient and a fomite has been demonstrated, there appears to be evidence of cases from the Middle East and India.

4.1. North America

In North America, blastomycosis occurs primarily east of the 100th meridian (Fig. 1 of Chapter 5). This area appears to be a natural nidus for *B. dermatitidis* (or many microfoci) and conforms to Pavlovsky's theory on the natural nidality of disease.[18] Since it is not mandatory to report mycoses in the United States and Canada, the development of a more precise definition or quantitation of the endemic area has been further hindered. The distribution in the United States and Canada will be discussed separately.

4.1.1. United States

The first case of blastomycosis was mentioned by Gilchrist in 1894[19] and was fully described in 1896.[20] There was very little demographic history with the exception that the patient was referred to him from Philadelphia,

Pennsylvania. The second description of a patient with blastomycosis that appeared in the literature was reported by Gilchrist and Stokes. Again, there was little social history, but since the patient was referred to him by Dr. Halstead of the Johns Hopkins Hospital, he was presumably from the Baltimore, Maryland area.[21]

In the early 1900s, a large number of patients were reported from northern Illinois and southeastern Wisconsin and thus the name "Chicago disease" was applied to this mycosis. Subsequently, a wide distribution in the eastern United States was recognized. Today, the reported cases of blastomycosis in the United States occur as shown in Fig. 1. Many of the patients are from along the Mississippi River from Wisconsin to Louisiana and into the central Atlantic states. Random cases have been reported outside the apparent endemic area as early as 1908. Without reporting a residence history, Mullin presented a case from Nebraska.[22] Reports also document sporadic cases from Seattle, Washington,[23] and Colorado.[24]

A survey of blastomycosis in California was published by Casad *et al.* in 1967.[25] They reported 28 cases and concluded that all patients had resided or visited in the eastern part of the United States prior to the onset of their disease. Subsequently, Sorensen and Casad provided a detailed analysis of 37 cases (including those previously published) in a more extensive study.[26,27] They concluded that only one infection, a laboratory accident, was acquired in California.

A later study by Furcolow *et al.* of 1476 human and 385 canine cases showed the same distribution in the eastern states.[7] In this report, only two infected dogs resided west of the 100th meridian; both were in New Mexico. How much of this distribution pattern simply reflects clinician interest in this disease is unknown.

4.1.2. Canada

The distribution of *B. dermatitidis* in Canada appears to be similar to that in the United States, i.e., east of the 100th meridian (Fig. 1 of Chapter 5). The Canadian incidence data are compromised by the same deficiency as that of the United States: the reporting of blastomycosis, and other mycotic diseases, to national health authorities is not mandatory. Case reports and literature reviews by interested individuals provide the bulk of the data.

The first case of cutaneous blastomycosis in Canada was reported by Primrose in 1906 just 12 years after Gilchrist's original description of this mycosis.[28] The patient, from Toronto, Canada, had lived in Chicago, a known niche of *B. dermatitidis,* for 3 years and thus may have acquired his infection there. In 1948, Starrs and Klotz analyzed all the previously reported cases of blastomycosis in Canada and cast some doubt on most of

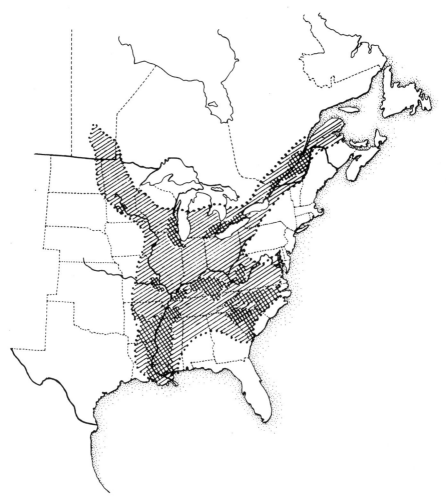

FIGURE 1. Distribution of blastomycosis in the United States. From Rippon JW: *Medical Mycology,* ed 3, 1988. W B Saunders, Co. Reprinted with permission.

them, accepting only two as conclusive.[29] They also reported a well-docu-mented case of a patient from Ottawa. Clinical data on 26 patients from the province of Manitoba were presented in 1972.[30] Most of these patients lived along the eastern border of the province.

Sekhon *et al.* reviewed the Canadian cases of blastomycosis in 1979.[31] These authors attempted to clarify reported cases, eliminate duplication of reports, and rely on laboratory diagnosis for confirmation. They reported that 115 of 119 cases occurred east of the 100th meridian. There were 59 patients from Quebec, 26 from Ontario, and 29 from Manitoba. In that review they also reported three new cases from Alberta and one from Saskatchewan. One of the three patients from Alberta had spent some years in Ontario, an endemic area for blastomycosis, and may have acquired his infection there. The endemicity in Ontario was confirmed by Kane *et al.* in 1983, who identified 38 patients from this province with blastomycosis.[32]

Saskatchewan was the site of two small outbreaks of blastomycosis in dogs between 1981 and 1986.[13] Seven dogs were from the community of Moose Jaw and eight were from a limited area (six by eight blocks) in the town of Regina, 70 km distant. Subsequently, the first autochthonous human case of blastomycosis from Alberta was reported by Sekhon *et al.* in 1982[33] followed by a canine case in 1988.[34]

In 1986, Dixon reported 142 cases of laboratory-proven blastomycosis that occurred between 1905 and 1986.[35] He added 23 patients to the 119 cases reported previously by Sekhon *et al.* He was of the opinion that Canada does ". . . not provide environmental conditions conducive to the multiplication and transmission of many of the fungal species that cause primary systemic disease in the otherwise healthy persons." However, it must also be noted here that the isolation of *B. dermatitidis* from the Canadian environment (Ontario) was reported in 1986 by Bakerspigel *et al.*[36] It was one of the few isolates of this organism from nature. The patient developed systemic blastomycosis and the fungus was isolated from his work environment.

Blastomycosis has now been diagnosed in five patients from British Columbia. All diagnoses are well documented, being proven either by culture or with histologic and serologic evidence of infection. However, this was a family who had lived in the known endemic area of Toronto prior to migrating to British Columbia and therefore does not prove endemicity of *B. dermatitidis* (A. S. Sekhon, personal communication).

Thus, in Canada, as in the United States, there are few cases of blastomycosis west of the 100th meridian.

4.1.3. Mexico

There appears to be only one well-documented case of autochthonous blastomycosis in North America south of the U.S. border; it occurred in Mexico. There are no unequivocal cases from Central or South America. Baez *et al.* reported the case of blastomycosis from Mexico in 1954.[37] The patient was a 34-year-old male from Penjamo, Guanajuato who left Mexico only briefly. Four years prior to the onset of illness, he spent 8 months in California. This would be an unlikely source of infection with *B. dermatitidis.* Guanajuato is located just on the 100th meridian.

A second report of blastomycosis from Mexico concerned a 22-year-old female from Colima, Mexico in 1974.[38] She had lived there since birth. Cultural evidence was not presented and the photomicrographs of yeasts were not conclusive for *B. dermatitidis.*

4.2. South America

In 1954, Montemayor reported a case of blastomycosis from Vene-zuela.[39] There is some doubt as to the accuracy of the identification of this organism. The yeasts shown in the tissue from the patient appear to have a narrow base and the usual double wall appearance of *B. dermatitidis* is not obvious. There was additional unpublished information that fails to support this report as an autochthonous case of blastomycosis (D. Borelli, personal communication). This patient may have been infected with *Paracoc-cidioides brasiliensis.*

A report entitled "The First Case of Blastomycosis Observed in Uruguay" was published in 1933.[40] The diagnosis was based on histologic examination of tissue. There was no culture of *B. dermatitidis.* Observation of the sections revealed yeasts with single buds. The tissue sections were reviewed many years later by one of the original authors, Dr. Juan Mackinnon, in 1950.[41] He determined that although the first diagnosis was based on the observation of only single budding cells, such findings were not uncommon with *P. brasiliensis.* He concluded that the patient was infected with *P. brasiliensis.*

A similar report of blastomycosis in Argentina was made by Niño in 1938.[42] He rejected six cases of previously reported blastomycosis and identified them as paracoccidioidomycosis. This reassessment was also based on morphology (thin cell wall, multiple buds) observed in histologic sections. He also reported four additional cases of blastomycosis from Argentina but *B. dermatitidis* was not isolated from any of the patients. Niño then retracted two cases and later stated that he was doubtful of the remaining cases.[41]

Fonseca stated that there were three cases of blastomycosis in Brazil, but also went on to say that there were no cultures from these patients, and that Gilchrist's disease was a syndrome and not a well-defined entity. He also admitted that the previously reported Brazilian cases were probably another disease.[43]

It is curious that more than 35 years has passed since these early reports and additional cases of unequivocal, autochthonous cases of blastomycosis have not been described. The lack of blastomycosis in Latin America can hardly be due to lack of recognition. There are many competent medical mycologists and physicians interested in mycotic diseases in Mexico and

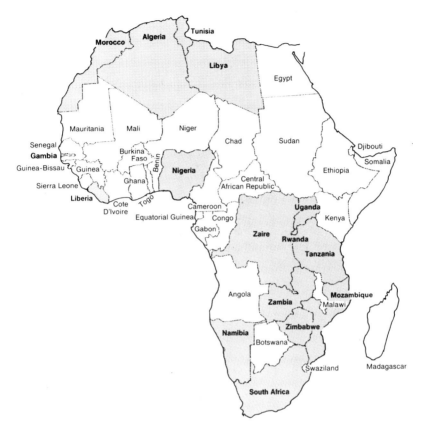

FIGURE 2. Distribution of reported cases of blastomycosis in Africa, based on information published in the review by Carman *et al.*[44] and Bianchi *et al.*[97,98]

Central and South America who are capable of diagnosing blastomycosis. This is substantiated by the prolific publications on *P. brasiliensis,* a morphologically similar, but distinct fungus that is common in that part of the world.

4.3. Africa

Blastomycosis seems to be ubiquitous in Africa. Authentic, autochthonous cases of blastomycosis have been reported in 16 African countries from Algeria to Zimbabwe (Fig. 2). Most cases have been well documented with descriptions of the isolates, reasonable photomicrographs, and the cultures have been sent to other mycologists or reference laboratories for confirmation. There is little doubt that these patients were actually infected with *B. dermatitidis.*

The most comprehensive study of this mycosis on that continent was that of Carman *et al.* who reviewed published and unpublished cases diagnosed between 1951 and 1987.[44] This paper is very thorough and the data presented have been utilized to construct the distribution map shown in Fig. 2. Geographically, the reported cases occurred from longitude 20°W through 40°E and from latitude 40°N to 40°S. It is apparent that *B. dermatitidis* is widely dispersed throughout the area and it appears that Africa is second only to North America in the extent of this disease.

There has been one arcane case of blastomycosis which may have been contracted in Ethiopia, Kenya, or Uganda. The reports by Bianchi *et al.* describe the patient as having been infected with a phycomycete.[97,98] Thus, this case has been obscured in the literature due to the misidentification of the causative agent. The patient, a 38-year-old white male at the time of the clinical onset, spent seven years in three African countries. His location at the time of exposure cannot be specifically determined. Drs. L. Ajello and F. W. Chandler examined the tissue sections in 1988 at the Centers for Disease Control. They are of the opinion that the etiologic agent is *B. dermatitidis.*[99] The figures in the original publication are also compatible with *B. dermatitidis.*[97]

The African strains of *B. dermatitidis* appear to be a different serotype from all other isolates. In 1970, McDonough stated that the African strains appeared to be the same species as the North American isolates by pairing isolates in mating studies.[45] He also showed that five of six African strains studied would not cross with the teleomorph, *Ajellomyces dermatitidis.* In 1971, Kwon-Chung reported that in mating experiments with this fungus, the four African strains she studied would not respond to the North American testor strains.[46]

In 1974, Sudman and Kaplan suggested that there may be antigenic differences between North American and African isolates of *B. dermatitidis.*[47] They prepared fluorescent antibody conjugates from antiglobulins to an American isolate and to an African isolate of the fungus. They concluded that the African isolates of *B. dermatitidis* were antigenically distinct from the American isolates.

Kaufman *et al.* studied 102 isolates of *B. dermatitidis* (88 from North America, 1 from Israel, 1 from India, and 12 from Africa).[48] All of the isolates except 11 African strains contained the A antigen. Only one African isolate, from an Algerian patient, contained the A antigen.

They also showed that the Algerian isolate containing the A antigen was of the − mating type when paired with the testor strains of *A. dermatitidis.* None of the other 11 African strains that were A antigen negative crossed with either the − or + testor strains. The Algerian strain had colonial and microscopic morphologic similarity with the North American strains which differed from the other non-A antigen African strains.

Vermeil *et al.* pointed out several characteristics of African isolates that differ from North American isolates.[49] The sexual states of the African strains were unknown (based on McDonough's work), the conidia of these isolates gathered in clusters, and the conversion of African strains from mycelial form to yeast form were more difficult.

Conversely, Summerbell *et al.* examined 18 North American and two African strains of *B. dermatitidis* by means of enzyme profiling.[50] Although this is not a proven technique for distinguishing biotypes of *B. dermatitidis,* this study did not show any distinction between the strains based on origin.

4.4. Europe

A report claiming to be the first case of blastomycosis from Europe was presented by Brody in 1947.[51] The patient was a United States serviceman. This American citizen (state of residence not given) was inducted into the Army in December 1942, sent to England in December 1943 and to France 9 months later in September 1944. He became ill with an atypical pneumonia in July 1944 and subsequently developed cutaneous disease. The description of the onset is similar to a primary illness although the patient had been out of the United States for over 18 months. This appears to be an authentic case of blastomycosis, confirmed by culture, but the geographic origin cannot be ascertained.

The first patient with blastomycosis described from Great Britain was reported in 1926.[52] While this appears to be a legitimate diagnosis of blastomycosis, and the 22-year-old patient was a lifelong resident of England, it probably is not an autochthonous infection. The patient's occupation was to chop wood packing cases that were used to ship automobiles from the United States to England, and this may have been the exposure to the fungus. However, this is another case that marks the association between wood and *B. dermatitidis* and is probably an illustration of fomite transmission.

Similarly, Symmers reported a presumptive case of blastomycosis in a 55-year-old male who never left Britain.[53] Although cultures were not obtained, histologic sections from both lungs contained organisms that are morphologically compatible with *B. dermatitidis.* The patient had daughters living in the United States who frequently sent their father glass ashtrays, which he collected. These were purchased in several states endemic for blastomycosis, including Illinois, North Carolina, and Mississippi. They were shipped to him in sawdust, wood shavings, and straw, substrates that are suspected of being associated with the ecological niche of *B. dermatitidis.*

Wegmann reported a case of blastomycosis from Switzerland in 1952.[54]

The diagnosis was based primarily on the clinical symptoms, a positive skin test reaction to blastomycin, a serum complement fixation titer of 1:8, and an isolate that was "yeast-like"—all compatible with, but not diagnostic of, blastomycosis. There were no further studies on the isolate and confirmation as *B. dermatitidis* remains uncertain.

In support of the diagnosis, the patient, a 50-year-old Swiss woman who never left Switzerland, worked in a cigarette factory in Zurich, and had been working with tobacco leaves prior to developing a bronchopneumonia. She worked alone sorting tobacco leaves in a dusty and poorly ventilated room. The leaves were imported from Durham, North Carolina, an endemic area for blastomycosis in the United States (T. Wegmann, personal communication). This could represent another instance of mechanical transmission of *B. dermatitidis.*

Kowalska *et al.* reported a case of blastomycosis from Poland in 1976.[55] The patient, a 51-year-old farmer, had never been abroad. This individual suffered from cutaneous lesions on the finger, wrist, and nose with what appeared to be bony involvement of the wrist. The photomicrographs in the paper show yeasts that appear to be compatible with *B. dermatitidis.* Tissue sections were examined at the Centers for Disease Control, Atlanta, Georgia by the fluorescent antibody technique and were compatible with *B. dermatitidis.*

The organism was isolated from this patient. The description of the cultures, the conversion from a yeast form to a mycelial form, and the photomicrograph of the mycelial form are convincing. Twenty-five years prior to his illness, in the post-World War II years, the patient helped in the distribution of clothes in his hometown. The clothing was contributed by families in the United States. The authors state that the temporal relationship makes this an unlikely source of infection. Present knowledge of the disease supports their interpretation. This may be a legitimate autochthonous case of blastomycosis from Poland.

4.5. Middle East

For the purposes of this discussion, the Middle East is defined as those countries bounded by the Mediterranean Sea, Red Sea, and Persian Gulf. The first report of blastomycosis in the Middle East was published in 1971.[56] The patient was a 46-year-old Lebanese farmer who was born in Brazil where he lived for 22 years before migrating to Lebanon. Although cultures of skin and exudate incubated at both 25 and 37°C did not yield the organism, the appearance of the cutaneous lesion and the histopathology were compatible with *B. dermatitidis.* The yeast cells had single buds and a thick wall. However, Kaplan and Ajello reviewed these tissue sections and believe the organisms are more compatible with *P. brasiliensis.*[57] This organism is the etiologic agent of paracoccidioidomycosis, a common mycosis in Brazil, the patient's home. This disease is known to have an incubation time that may be prolonged for many years.

In 1978 there were two reports of autochthonous cases of *B. dermatitidis* infection from the Middle East: Israel[57] and Lebanon.[58] The patient from Israel was originally from Poland but had not left Israel in almost 50 years. This patient's disease was confirmed first by fluorescent antibody studies of histological material and subsequently by culture. The second patient was a native Lebanese diagnosed in Lebanon, but who most likely became infected in Liberia where he resided for the previous 5 years. This infection was culturally confirmed. In 1980, the first case was reported from Saudi Arabia.[59] Three histological sections of biopsy material showed yeast forms compatible with *B. dermatitidis* and the organism was grown as a yeast at 37°C and in the mycelial form at 22°C. This appears to be a legitimate case although the authors did not respond to a request for the isolate.

A recent report of isolating *B. dermatitidis* from the hair of a rabbit captured on the West Bank of the Jordan River is not convincing.[60] There have been many studies to recover pathogenic fungi from soil samples by the hair-baiting technique, which was used by these authors. Although this method is successful for the recovery of keratinophilic fungi, there have been no reports of the isolation of *B. dermatitidis* or any other systemic pathogenic fungi. It should be pointed out that in 1934 Williams inoculated human hair with *B. dermatitidis* but did not obtain any growth of the fungus.[61] However, in 1935 he reported the successful growth of *B. dermatitidis* on human hair[62] but did not explain the discrepancy between the two accounts. Furthermore, from personal experience in studying the ecology of *B. dermatitidis,* it does not seem that this fungus is sufficiently resistant to xerophilic conditions such as the fur of a rabbit in the desert. In addition, there have been no reports of infected rabbits from the endemic areas of the United States or Canada, where rabbits are common. A culture of the isolate from the rabbit was not available from the authors. This report should be considered spurious unless supporting evidence is provided.

4.6. India

There were reports of at least 11 patients with blastomycosis in India between 1925 and 1961. In 1961, Randhawa *et al.* investigated four of these reports and rejected the authenticity of all of them.[63] In 1972, Mishra and Sandhu specifically reviewed and rejected six additional cases of blastomycosis previously reported from India.[64] Subsequently, in 1982, Khan *et al.* reported the isolation of *B. dermatitidis* from a bat collected in Old Delhi

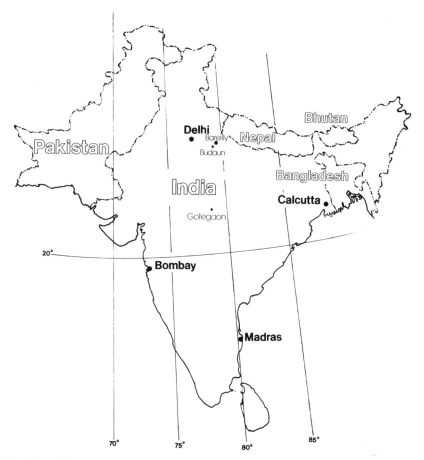

FIGURE 3. Distribution of reported cases of blastomycosis in India. Infected human beings were from Gotegaon and Rodhain (Budaun). The infected dog was found in Izatnagar, near Bareilly. Two positive bats were collected in Delhi (Old Delhi is a suburb of New Delhi).

(Fig. 3).[65] Only 1 of 155 bats examined yielded the fungus from lung tissue.

In 1983, Randhawa *et al.* reported the isolation of *B. dermatitidis* from a patient living in Rodhain, about 250 km southeast of Delhi, India (Budaun in Fig. 3).[66] The fungus was isolated from bronchial aspirate collected from a 40-year-old woman with respiratory illness. She had never traveled abroad. In this report, they also rejected the 11th previously reported case of blastomycosis. Isolates from the bat and from the patient were sent to the Centers for Disease Control, Atlanta, Georgia for confirmation. Both specimens were found to be legitimate strains of *B. dermatitidis* and have been deposited with the American Type Culture Collection.

In 1985, Randhawa *et al.* reported another isolation of *B. dermatitidis* from the same bat species collected in New Delhi.[67] On this occasion the isolate was obtained from liver tissue.

In 1988, Jambhekar *et al.* reported a case of disseminated blastomycosis in a 60-year-old Indian housewife.[68] The patient was from Gotegaon, Madhya Pradesh, 700 km south of Delhi. The histologic description of the biopsy material from a cutaneous lesion was compatible with *B. dermatitidis*. Although the photomicrographs in the report are not conclusive, tissue sections were submitted to the Centers for Disease Control. Confirmation was obtained by use of the direct fluorescent antibody conjugate for *B. dermatitidis*. Tissue sections were also examined by GMS, PAS, and with direct fluorescent antibody conjugate in our laboratory and we believe that the organisms are compatible with *B. dermatitidis*. Culture of the biopsy material was negative after 6 weeks. The patient responded to 2.0 g of amphotericin B and was still doing well 10 months later.

There is one report of blastomycosis in a mongrel dog from Izatnagar, India, 200 km east of Delhi (Fig. 3).[69] In 1983, Iyer reported the case that was diagnosed as *B. dermatitidis* infection based on histologic examination of lung lesions. The photomicrographs are convincing.

The evidence seems to indicate that *B. dermatitidis* does occur in Asia. Thus far, all the proven isolates of *B. dermatitidis* were from the central part of India, close to the 80th meridian (Fig. 3).

4.7. South Pacific

An outbreak of blastomycosis was reported among U.S. Army troops stationed in Okinawa.[70] The evidence to support the diagnosis of blastomycosis in the 23 servicemen affected was weak. Seventeen of the patients were considered to have subclinical infections based upon the organism being "identified incidentally on routine sputum and urine examinations." The isolation of *B. dermatitidis* from "routine" specimens is unusual. There were no additional clinical comments on these 17 patients. Six other cases were based on radiologic evidence plus the isolation of the organism from five (two patient isolates were from urine, one from sputum, and two from both urine and sputum). Two patients recovered in a few weeks with no treatment, one recovered with antibacterial treatment, one patient died before therapy could be initiated, and the outcome of one was not specified. Additional doubt about the etiology of these illnesses was raised by Schwarz and Baum.[71] They based their skepticism on the incomplete identification of the organism.

A report of blastomycosis in 1955 from Australia is dubious.[72] The patient, an 18-year-old female, was diagnosed with cutaneous blastomycosis by the clinical appearance of the lesions (large verrucous masses around both nares) and the histologic appearance of "yeast bodies" in deeper layers of the skin. The lesions finally resolved after 3 years of therapy with X rays, copper sulfate, cauterization, and oral and intravenous iodides. The etiology of this disease is questionable.

In summary, blastomycosis occurs in the eastern half of North America and throughout Africa. Sporadic infections have been reported from the Middle East and India. Isolated cases, which appear to be authentic human infections with *B. dermatitidis,* have been reported from England, Switzerland, and Poland, in which there is epidemiologic evidence of possible fomite transmission. There have been many worldwide reports of blastomycosis that have not withstood careful scrutiny (Fig. 4).

5. CONIDIA AS INFECTIOUS PARTICLES

It is assumed that conidia and mycelial fragments are the infectious form of *B. dermatitidis.* Particles that are between 0.5 and 5.0 μm will pass through the respiratory tract and enter the lung parenchyma. The conidia of *B. dermatitidis* range in size from 2 to 10 μm and thus may readily enter the alveoli. When the host defenses fail, an infection may be established.

Electron microscopic studies of mycelial fragments and conidia of *B. dermatitidis* that had been incubated at 37°C were reported by Garrison and Boyd in 1978.[73] They showed that the hyphal cells rapidly degenerated while the conidia underwent changes consistent with those seen when the mycelial form converts to the yeast form. Thus, it is reasonable to assume that the infective particles from nature are mainly conidia and, possibly, mycelial fragments.

The respiratory route of infection of *B. dermatitidis* was demonstrated in animal models in 1968.[74] Mammals (mice, rats, gerbils, hamsters, guinea pigs, and cats) were allowed to inhale infectious particles of *B. dermatitidis,* consisting of conidia and mycelial fragments, from sterile soil that had been seeded with the fungus. Pulmonary infections occurred in all species tested. Subsequently, other investigators have produced pulmonary blastomycosis in mice by the use of conidia.[75-77] In these studies both the acute[76] and chronic[75] forms of pulmonary blastomycosis were produced.

6. ISOLATION FROM NATURE

6.1. Reports

Unlike the other systemic fungi (*H. capsulatum, Coccidioides immitis,* and *Cryptococcus neoformans*), *B. dermatitidis* has been infrequently iso-

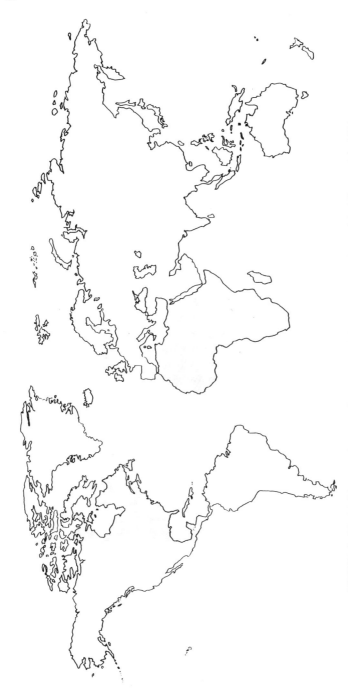

FIGURE 4. Worldwide endemic areas of blastomycosis from the authentic published literature in 1991.

TABLE 1
Isolations of *Blastomyces dermatitidis* from Natural Sites

Number of isolates	Type of substrate	State	Collection month	Moisture (rain)	pH	Year reported	ATTC no.	Ref. no.
1	Soil	Ky.	Oct.	N.R.[a]	5.8	1961	26198	17
10	Soil and organic debris	Ga.	Feb., Mar.	Yes	N.R.	1964	32090	5
1	Pigeon manure	Minn.	May	Yes	N.R.	1976	N.D.[b]	82
3	Soil and organic debris	Ga.	Dec., Feb.	Yes	N.R.	1979	N.D.	81
3	Soil and organic debris	Wisc.	Sept.	Yes	6.5	1986	60636	11
1	Soil and diatomaceous earth	Canada	N.R.	Yes	N.R.	1986	66136	36
1	Soil and organic debris	Wisc.	June	Yes	5.8	1987	60637	79

[a] N.R., not reported.
[b] N.D., not deposited.

lated from nature (Table 1). The first report of the recovery of this organism was made by Denton *et al.* in 1961.[17]

In the quest for the ecologic niche of *B. dermatitidis,* McDonough *et al.* collected 842 soil samples from Lexington, Kentucky, during a 16-month period.[78] This area was selected because of the high incidence of human and canine cases of blastomycosis. The samples were examined by *in vitro* and *in vivo* techniques but none yielded the fungus. As part of a cooperative agreement, every tenth specimen (a total of 54 samples) was submitted to Dr. J. Fred Denton at the Medical College of Georgia for examination by his technique. The primary novel aspect of this method was the intravenous (i.v.) inoculation of the soil suspension (tail vein technique) rather than the usual intraperitoneal (i.p.) injection. One sample, collected from a tobacco stripping shed, yielded *B. dermatitidis.* The success of this protocol has since been established.[11,79]

Thereupon, 101 samples were collected from the same tobacco barn but none of them were positive by the i.v. method.[80] Twelve of these samples were taken from the specific site where the positive sample was previously collected and 30 samples were from within a radius of 3 feet from the original positive site.

The Denton report and subsequent accounts of recovery of *B. dermatitidis* from environmental samples, collected in Georgia in 1964 and 1979, were received with question because neither the authors nor other investigators could consistently reproduce these results even from the same samples.[5,81]

In 1976, Sarosi and Serstock reported the isolation of *B. dermatitidis* from pigeon manure.[82] They observed yeast forms of the fungus by direct examination of the material which was the possible source of infection of a human being. The organism was cultured from the pigeon manure but these isolates were not confirmed by other investigators nor were either the patient isolate or the environmental isolate available for further studies. This skepticism about the recovery of *B. dermatitidis* remained until the report of Klein *et al.* in 1986.[11] They reported the isolation of *B. dermatitidis* from soil samples in association with an outbreak of acute pulmonary blastomycosis among 48 people at Eagle Creek, Wisconsin. In that study, environmental samples were examined in mice by both the i.v. tail vein technique and the i.p. method. *B. dermatitidis* was isolated from 2 of the 47 samples collected. The i.v. method was much more successful than the i.p. method for recovery. An attempt was made to repeat the isolations from the two positive samples but recovery was made from only one sample.

In the same year, Bakerspigel *et al.* reported the isolation of *B. dermatitidis* from a patient and the earthen floor of his workshop.[36] The samples were inoculated into mice using the i.v. tail vein technique. However, subsequent attempts to isolate the organism from the same samples failed, similar to previous experiences.

In 1987, another outbreak of human blastomycosis in Wisconsin led to the successful recovery of *B. dermatitidis* from the environment.[79] One of thirty-five specimens yielded *B. dermatitidis* by the mouse i.v. technique. A repeat isolation attempt from the positive sample after a short storage period using the same technique was also successful.

Two other isolations of *B. dermatitidis* from nature have been reported but neither could be substantiated by the authors.[60,83] The only common environmental elements of the various sites have been high organic content of the substrates and proximity to water or alluvial soil. However, each isolate of *B. dermatitidis* from nature contributes to a better understanding of the ecology of this organism.

Subsequent to the successful isolation of *B. dermatitidis* from naturally infected soil, many experiments were devised in an attempt to elucidate the reasons why the recovery of this fungus from nature was not readily repeated as it had been for the other terricolous pathogenic fungi. Unfavorable conditions for the propagation or recovery of *B. dermatitidis* that have been studied and reported include: drying,[16] lysis,[84] mycostatic and mycolytic factors on the mycelium[85] and on the yeast form,[86] and antagonism by other soil fungi.[87]

In 1967, Smith and Furcolow showed that drying had a deleterious effect on the survival of *B. dermatitidis* in sterilized soil that was seeded with the fungus.[16] In soil that was kept at room temperature with 100% relative humidity, the viable particles increased 100% while samples left to air dry or placed in a desiccator showed a decrease of 95% in viable particles in 5 to 10 days.

However, the conidia of *B. dermatitidis* seem to resist the effect of high temperature. Denton and DiSalvo reported that 100% of the conidia survived temperatures of 40°C but none were viable beyond 60°C.[88] In the same study, the conidium suspension that was stored at 0°C was thawed and refrozen several times during the next 3 months. There was a gradual increase in the number of conidia that germinated during this time.

The recovery of *B. dermatitidis* from nature may be related to the moisture content of the environment. As the humidity is increased, there is a greater liberation of infective particles. Such action could explain the successful isolations from nature. Recent rainfall was reported prior to the environmental recovery of *B. dermatitidis* in Augusta, Georgia[5,81] and the Tomorrow River in Nelsonville, Wisconsin.[79] It also rained prior to the outbreaks of blastomycosis in Eagle River, Wisconsin,[11] Tomorrow River, Wisconsin,[79] and Crystal River, Wisconsin.[79] McDonough *et al.* showed that it was difficult to liberate the conidia of *B. dermatitidis* from the mycelium. However, they demonstrated that moisture would cause the release of 99% of the conidia.[9] These findings are consistent with the association of *B. dermatitidis* infections and nearby sources of water.

6.2. Methods of Isolation

There are two means for isolating pathogenic fungi from soil, organic debris, or other inanimate substrates. These are *in vitro* and *in vivo*. The *in vitro* methods usually consist of dispensing the suspect inoculum on agar medium. The medium customarily contains sufficient nutrients to support the growth of the organism that is sought and some inhibitors (lower pH, dyes, antibiotics, and/or antifungal agents) to reduce the contaminants that are expected. Such a selective medium allows the more fastidious and slower-growing pathogens an opportunity to develop and be recovered. This method had been successful for some pathogenic fungi and is the method of choice for isolating *C. neoformans*.

The *in vivo* methods use a variety of laboratory animals including mice, gerbils, guinea pigs, dogs, and cats. Mice have been used in most studies. Experimental infections in mice have been established using i.p., i.v., intranasal (i.n.), and footpad inoculations. For the isolation of *B. dermatitidis* from environmental samples, the i.p. and i.v. methods have been used exclusively. The only successful recoveries have been with the i.v. procedure.

The method presently used to isolate *B. dermatitidis* from environmental samples is essentially a slight modification of the Denton technique.[5] Four weeks after inoculation of mice with the antibiotic-treated sample, the mice are sacrificed and the lungs, liver, and spleen are aseptically removed through a midline incision. The organs are minced and cultured on Sabouraud's dextrose agar plates containing 0.1 mg of streptomycin, 100 units of penicillin, and 1.0 mg of cycloheximide per ml. It is essential to note that the commercial preparations of inhibitory Sabouraud's dextrose agar do not contain the same amounts of antibiotics. Although the quantity of streptomycin and penicillin is adequate, the reduced amount of cycloheximide in the commercial media is detrimental. These media contain 0.5 mg cycloheximide per ml according to the recommendations of Georg *et al.;* however, their medium was developed for the isolation of fungal pathogens from clinical material.[89] The concentration of cycloheximide in the commercial medium is not sufficient to prohibit the overgrowth of contaminating fungi present in environmental samples before the pathogens appear. Therefore, the commercial medium must be supplemented with an additional 0.5 mg/ml of cycloheximide.

The plates are incubated at 25°C and observed weekly for 8 weeks.

Suspicious colonies are examined microscopically and transferred to fresh medium. It has been demonstrated that this extended period of observation will increase the yield of pathogenic fungi.[90]

Another unresolved variable in the attempt to isolate this fungus from the environment is the storage conditions for the samples prior to processing. The specimens have been stored for various periods of time at room temperature (25°C),[17] refrigerator temperature (5°C),[81] household freezer (−16°C),[5] food freezer (−23°C),[5] and in a hothouse.[82] There has been no correlation between the storage temperature of the environmental samples and the recovery of *B. dermatitidis.*

6.3. Environmental Characteristics

The composition of the natural substrates from which *B. dermatitidis* has been isolated has been described. Denton characterized the material from the tobacco barn where the first positive sample was obtained as brown clay loam containing fragments of tobacco with a pH of 5.8.[17] He also described the five sites where ten isolates were obtained.[5] There were many common characteristics of these sites. All five were located along 1.8 miles of road on an alluvium of the Savannah River at an elevation of 180 feet above mean sea level. The area was traversed by two creeks and was composed of clay soil over an underlying course of sand. Each of the specific samples was collected from a spot that was partially shaded from the sun but exposed to moisture from rain. The rainfall was 40 inches per year. The pH of these latter samples was not reported.

The cattle ramp specimen consisted of silt, mud, manure, rotted wood, and dried grass. Two samples were collected from the floor of a chicken house with minimal shelter from the elements. Chicken droppings, chicken feathers, straw, and rotted wood were abundant. The third site was similar to the latter. The fourth site, just above a creek bank, yielded three isolates. The specimens collected at this chicken house, abandoned for 4 years, contained similar material. The singular factor at this site was that all three samples were collected from chicken nests that were above the ground. It is of interest that this chicken house also yielded *H. capsulatum* and *C. neoformans.*[91] The fifth site also yielded three specimens that were positive for *B. dermatitidis* but they were from three separate structures: a rabbit pen containing droppings, silt, and rotted wood; the floor of a mule barn containing soil, manure, and rotting wood; and a shelf in a deteriorating shed. The shelf was 4 feet above the ground and the sample consisted of silt, lime whitewash, leaves, twigs, and other debris. Two samples collected from this shed 10 months later also were positive for *B. dermatitidis*. It had rained 2 days prior to obtaining these latter samples.[81]

An isolate reported by Sarosi and Serstock came from a bag of manure collected by a pigeon breeder.[82] With the exception of finding large numbers of yeast forms in a 10% KOH wet mount and that the pigeon manure was kept in a hothouse, there was no further description of the substrate. It is recognized, however, that pigeon excreta are acidic.

A sample collected in 1962 that yielded *B. dermatitidis* came from an urban dwelling.[81] The sample was taken from between the walls of an old house that was being razed. The debris contained dust, seeds, roach droppings and egg casings, and mouse droppings.

In reporting the first outbreak of blastomycosis that occurred at Grifton, North Carolina in 1955, Smith *et al.* noted that there had been an increase in rainfall during the period.[95] In the Eagle Creek, Wisconsin, outbreak, it had rained for 3 days prior to, and on the day of exposure.[11] The authors reported the isolation of *B. dermatitidis* from decomposed wood and two soil samples. These samples had an organic content of 64–70% and a pH range from 6.43 to 6.50.

Bakerspigel *et al.* isolated *B. dermatitidis* from the earthen floor of a wooden petroleum filtering shed.[36] The air and floor contained large amounts of diatomaceous earth and was watered down daily.

Klein *et al.* reported the isolation of *B. dermatitidis* from the banks of the Tomorrow River in Wisconsin.[79] It had rained 2 of the 3 days prior to the infection of their six patients and on each of the 3 days prior to the collection of the positive specimen. This sample was described as sandy loam soil containing dried leaves, twigs, stems, small roots, and other organic debris and the pH was 5.8.

The soil types where the fungus was recovered from nature in the United States are similar. The Lexington, Kentucky, and the Georgia isolates were all from an area of red and yellow podzolic soils and the Wisconsin isolates were from gray-brown podzolic soil. In an investigation of cases of canine blastomycosis in Wisconsin, 137 dogs lived along waterways where the soil was described as predominantly sandy with a pH ranging from 3.7 to 6.7.[92]

Denton and DiSalvo collected over 2300 samples during a 10-year period (1959–1968). They reported that the periodic appearance of *B. dermatitidis* may be a reflection of climatic conditions, noting that the positive samples were collected in February and March[5] (Table 1). Subsequent isolations in December and February led them to suggest that such conditions are favorable for the propagation and survival of *B. dermatitidis* during winter in the southeastern United States.[81] The clusters of human blastomycosis with a fairly accurate time of exposure occurred in December and January in North Carolina[93] and during March in Virginia.[94]

The isolations of *B. dermatitidis* from the Wisconsin outbreaks came from samples collected in September[11] and June.[79] In the outbreaks of human cases of blastomycosis in the northern United States, exposure, when possible to determine, also occurred during the summer months: one in May,[79] two in June,[11,79] and one in July.[12]

7. SUMMARY

The specific ecologic niche of *B. dermatitidis* remains unresolved but it is reasonable to assume that this fungus is a soil saprophyte as are many other pathogenic fungi. The literature contains reports of 20 isolates of *B. dermatitidis* from environmental samples (Table 1). Denton and DiSalvo observed that although there was not a specific ecologic association with certain species of animals as with *H. capsulatum* and *C. neoformans,* the substrates did come from animal habitats in general and that only 5 of 14 samples yielding *B. dermatitidis* actually contained soil.[5]

This association was also true in subsequent isolations of *B. dermatitidis.* The Eagle River, Wisconsin isolates were obtained from samples of decayed vegetation and organic debris collected at a beaver dam[11] and the Tomorrow River. Wisconsin samples were collected from a riverbank just below a groundhog burrow.[79] In addition to animal droppings, some common factors among the substrates from which *B. dermatitidis* has been isolated include acidic soil with a podzolic base, abundant organic debris, moisture, and shade from direct sunlight. Moisture (or rainfall) appears to be linked with the release of conidia, the presumed infective particles, from the mycelium or with the dispersal of solely conidia. The role of these factors eludes definite implication as essential for the survival or recovery of *B. dermatitidis* but one is impressed with these mutual elements of the positive sites.

Reasons for the paucity of isolation from nature offered by some investigators have been inhibition by other soil organisms[84] and the suggestion that *B. dermatitidis* goes through a life cycle with a dormant period.[4] Neither of these factors has been thoroughly investigated. The need for a more sensitive method of isolation is paramount.

The capacity of *B. dermatitidis* to survive in soil has been unequivocally demonstrated by the first recovery of this organism from a tobacco barn in Lexington, Kentucky.[17] A weimaraner dog with blastomycosis had been housed in the shed for 6 months prior to death from this disease and the positive sample was collected more than 2 years later. It could be reasoned that the soil seeded with the yeasts from the dog's lesions was free from antagonistic organisms because the dirt floors of tobacco barns are essentially sterilized when they are heated to 80°C for curing tobacco.

It is plausible that the ecologic niche, a small microfocus as described for *H. capsulatum,*[96] is composed largely of organic matter, slightly acidic, shaded but moist, close to but not necessarily in soil, and that man and animals are infected when they inhale aerosols of dust laden with conidia.[81]

REFERENCES

1. Schwarz J, Baum GL: Blastomycosis. *Am J Clin Pathol* 21:999–1029, 1951
2. Ricketts HT: Oidiomycosis of the skin and its fungi. *J Med Res* 6:374–554, 1901
3. Stober AM: Systemic blastomycosis: A report of its pathological, bacteriological and clinical features. *Arch Intern Med* 13:509–556, 1914
4. Greer AE: North American blastomycosis, in *Disseminating Diseases of the Lung.* Springfield, Ill, Charles C Thomas Co, 1962, pp 82–126
5. Denton JF, DiSalvo AF: Isolation of *Blastomyces dermatitidis* from natural sites at Augusta, Georgia. *Am J Trop Med* 13:716–722, 1964
6. Borelli D, Marcano C, Feo M: Actividades de la seccion de micologia medica, instituto de medicina tropical (Caracas), Durante el ano 1968. *Dermatol Venezolana* 8:887–904, 1969
7. Furcolow ML, Chick EW, Busey JF, et al: Prevalence and incidence studies of human and canine blastomycosis I. Cases in the U.S. *Am Rev Respir Dis* 102:60–67, 1970
8. McDonough ES, Kuzma JF: Epidemiological studies on blastomycosis in the state of Wisconsin. *Sabouraudia* 18:173–183, 1980
9. McDonough ES, Wisniewski TR, Penn LA, et al: Preliminary studies on conidial liberation of *Blastomyces dermatitidis* and *Histoplasma capsulatum. Sabouraudia* 14:199–204, 1976
10. Archer JR: Epidemiology of canine blastomycosis in Wisconsin. Master's thesis, University of Wisconsin, Stevens Point, 1985
11. Klein BS, Vergeront JM, Weeks RJ, et al: Isolation of *B. dermatitidis* in soil associated with a large outbreak of blastomycosis in Wisconsin. *N Engl J Med* 314:529–534, 1986
12. Cockerill FR III, Roberts GD, Rosenblatt JE, et al: Epidemic of pulmonary blastomycosis (Namekagon fever) in Wisconsin canoeists. *Chest* 86:688–692, 1984
13. Harasen GLG, Randall JW: Canine blastomycosis in southern Saskatchewan. *Can Vet J* 30:375–378, 1986
14. Dixon DM, Shadomy HJ, Shadomy S: In vitro growth and sporulation of *Blastomyces dermatitidis* on woody plant material. *Mycologia* 69:1193–1195, 1977
15. McDonough ES, Hierl DJ: Survival and growth of *Ajellomyces (Blastomyces) dermatitidis* on oak leaves coated with saliva. *Mycopathologia* 99:57–60, 1987
16. Smith CD, Furcolow ML: The susceptibility of *Blastomyces dermatitidis* to drying. *Proc Soc Exp Biol Med* 125:263–266, 1967
17. Denton JF, McDonough ES, Ajello L, et al: Isolation of *Blastomyces dermatitidis* from soil. *Science* 133:1126–1128, 1961
18. Pavlovsky EN: *Natural Nidality of Transmissible Diseases.* Urbana, University of Illinois Press, 1966
19. Gilchrist TC: Protozoan dermatitis. *J Cutan Vener Dis* 12:496, 1894
20. Gilchrist TC: A case of blastomycotic dermatitis in man. *Johns Hopkins Hosp Rep* 1:269–298, 1896

21. Gilchrist TC, Stokes WR: A case of pseudo-lupus vulgaris caused by a blastomyces. *J Exp Med* 3:53–83, 1898
22. Mullin CL: Report of a case of blastomycosis of the skin. *West Med Rev,* 1908, pp 482–486 (Read before the Nebraska State Medical Association in Lincoln, 5-19-21, 1908)
23. Scott MJ: Cutaneous blastomycosis. Report of case following dog bite. *Northwest Med* 54:255–257, 1955
24. Ehni W: Endogenous reactivation in blastomycosis. *Am J Med* 86:831, 1989
25. Casad RE, Waldmann WJ, Levan NE, et al: North American blastomycosis in California. *Calif Med* 106:20–27, 1967
26. Sorensen RH, Casad DE: Use of case survey technique to detect origin of blastomyces infections. *Public Health Rep* 84:514–520, 1969
27. Sorensen RH, Peterson ET, Waldmann WJ: Survey participation by practitioners: The key to establishing endemic boundaries of North American blastomycosis. *Clin Med* 79:19–23, 1972
28. Primrose A: Blastomycosis of the skin in man. *Edinburgh Med J* 20:215, 1906
29. Starrs RA, Klotz MO: North American blastomycosis (Gilchrist's disease) II. Analysis of Canadian reports and description of new case of the systemic type. *Arch Intern Med* 82:29–53, 1948
30. Kepron MW, Schoemperlin CB, Hershfield ES, et al: North American blastomycosis in central Canada. A review of 36 cases. *Can Med Assoc J* 106:243–246, 1972
31. Sekhon AS, Bogorus MS, Sims HV: Blastomycosis: Report of three cases from Alberta with a review of Canadian cases. *Mycopathologia* 68:53–63, 1979
32. Kane J, Righter J, Krajden S, et al: Blastomycosis: A new endemic focus in Canada. *Can Med Assoc J* 129:728–730, 1983
33. Sekhon AS, Jackson FL, Jacobs HJ: Blastomycosis: Report of the first case from Alberta, Canada. *Mycopathologia* 79:65–69, 1982
34. Sekhon AS, Marien GRJ, Eston B, et al: A canine case of North American blastomycosis in Alberta, Canada. *Mycoses* 31:454–458, 1988
35. Dixon JMS: Impact of the mycoses in Canada and strategies for their control, VI International Congress on the Mycoses, scientific publication 479. Pan American Health Organization, 1986
36. Bakerspigel A, Kane J, Schaus D: Isolation of *Blastomyces dermatitidis* from an earthen floor in southwestern Ontario, Canada. *J Clin Microbiol* 24:890–891, 1986
37. Baez MM, Mota AR, Ochoa AG: Blastomycosis Norteamericana en Mexico. *Rev Inst Salubr Enferm Trop Mexico City* 14:225–232, 1954
38. Bada del Morral MA, Medina de los Santos P, Barbosa M: Blastomicosis pulmonar, presentacion de un caso clinico. *Alergia* 21:81–91, 1974
39. Montemayor L: *Blastomyces dermatitidis*—Gilchrist and Stokes 1898 en Venezuela. *Gac Med Caracas* 62:675–689, 1954
40. Talice RV, Mackinnon JE: Primer caso de Blastomicosis (Tipo Gilchrist) observado en el Uruguay. *Arch Urug Med Cir Espec* 3:177–203, 1933
41. Mackinnon JE, Vinelli H: Caracteres Diferenciales—De *Paracoccidioides brasiliensis* y *Blastomyces dermatitidis* en Los Tejidos. *An Fac Med Montevideo* 35:299–310, 1950
42. Niño FL: Contribucion al estudio de las blastomicosis en la republica argentina: Capitulo V Granuloma criptococcico: estudio de un nuevo caso argentina. *Biol Inst Clin Quir (Buenos Aires)* 14:656–755, 1938
43. Fonseca O: *Parasitologia Medica,* vol I. Editora Guanabara. Rio de Janeiro, 1943
44. Carman WF, Frean JA, Crewe-Brown HH, et al: Blastomycosis in Africa (A review of new cases diagnosed between 1951 and 1987). *Mycopathologia* 107:25–32, 1989

45. McDonough ES: Blastomycosis—Epidemiology and biology of its etiologic agent *Ajellomyces dermatitidis. Mycopathol Mycol Appl* 41:195–201, 1970
46. Kwon-Chung KJ: Genetic analysis on the incompatibility system of *Ajellomyces dermatitidis. Sabouraudia* 9:231–238, 1971
47. Sudman MS, Kaplan W: Antigenic relationship between American and African isolates of *Blastomyces dermatitidis* as determined by immunofluorescence. *Appl Microbiol* 27:496–499, 1974
48. Kaufman L, Standard PG, Weeks RJ, et al: Detection of two *Blastomyces dermatitidis* serotypes by exoantigen analysis. *J Clin Microbiol* 18:110–114, 1983
49. Vermeil C, Bouillard C, Miegeville M, et al: The echinulate conidia of *Blastomyces dermatitidis* Gilchrist and Stokes and the taxonomic status of this species. *Mykosen* 25:251–253, 1982
50. Summerbell RC, Kane J, Pincus DH: Enzymatic activity profiling as a potential biotyping method for *Ajellomyces dermatitidis. J Clin Microbiol* 28:1054–1056, 1990
51. Brody M: Blastomycosis, North American type. *Arch Dermatol Syphilol* 56:529–531, 1947
52. Dowling GB, Elworthy RR: Case of blastomycetic dermatitidis (Gilchrist). *Proc Soc Med* 19:4–10, 1926
53. Symmers WSC: Deep-seated fungal infections currently seen in the histopathologic service of a medical school laboratory in Britain. *Am J Clin Pathol* 46:514–537, 1966
54. Wegmann T: Blastomycose und andere pilzerkrankungen der lunge. *Dtsch Arch Klinsche Med* 199:192–205, 1952
55. Kowalska M, Hanski W, Bielunska S, et al: North American blastomycosis and possibilities of its occurrence in Poland. *Przegl Dermatol* 63:641–647, 1976
56. Malak JA, Farah FS: Blastomycosis in the Middle East. Report of a suspected case of N.A. blastomycosis. *Br J Dermatol* 84:161–166, 1971
57. Kuttin ES, Beemer AM, Levig J, et al: Occurrence of *Blastomyces dermatitidis* in Israel. First autochthonous Middle Eastern case. *Am J Trop Med Hyg* 27:1203–1205, 1978
58. Hasan FM, Jarrah T, Nassar V: The association of adenocarcinoma of the lung and blastomycosis from an unusual geographical location. *Br J Dis Chest* 72:242–246, 1978
59. Kingston M, El-Mishad MM, Ashraf Ali M: Blastomycosis in Saudi Arabia. *Am J Trop Med Hyg* 29:464–466, 1980
60. Ali-Shtayeh MS, Arda HM, Hassouna M, et al: Keratinophilic fungi on the hair of cows, donkeys, rabbits, cats, and dogs from the West Bank of Jordan. *Mycopathologia* 104:109–121, 1988
61. Williams JW: Scalp products and hair as a culture medium for certain pathogenic fungi. *Proc Exp Biol Med* 31:586–588, 1934
62. Williams JW: Scalp products and hair of men and women as culture media for certain pathogenic fungi. *Proc Exp Biol Med* 32:624–625, 1935
63. Randhawa HS, Sandhu RS, Viswanathan R: Medical mycology in India: A review of the work done since 1910. *Indian J Chest Dis* 3:33–49, 1961
64. Mishra SD, Sandhu RS: Deep mycoses in India—A critical review. *Mycopathol Mycol Appl* 48:339–365, 1972
65. Khan ZU, Randhawa HS, Lulla M: Isolation of *Blastomyces dermatitidis* from the lungs of a bat, *Rhinopoma hardwickei* gray, in Delhi. *Sabouraudia* 20:137–144, 1982
66. Randhawa HS, Khan ZU, Gaur SN: *Blastomyces dermatitidis* in India: First report of its isolation from clinical material. *Sabouraudia* 21:215–221, 1983
67. Randhawa HS, Chaturvedi VP, Kini S, et al: *Blastomyces dermatitidis* in bats: First report of its isolation from the liver of *Rhinopoma hardwickei* Gray. *Sabouraudia* 23:69–76, 1985

68. Jambhekar NA, Shrikhande SS, Advani SH, et al: Disseminated blastomycosis—A case report. *Indian J Pathol Microbiol* 31:330–333, 1988
69. Iyer PKR: Pulmonary blastomycosis in a dog in India. *Indian J Vet Pathol* 7:60–62, 1983
70. Bonoff CP: Acute primary pulmonary blastomycosis. *Radiology* 54:157–164, 1950
71. Schwarz J, Baum GL: Acute primary pulmonary blastomycosis. Letter to the Editor. *Radiology* 61:818, 1953
72. Macmillan H: Report on a case of localized blastomycosis. *Aust J Dermatol* 3:38–41, 1955
73. Garrison RG, Boyd KS: Role of the conidium in dimorphism of *Blastomyces dermatitidis*. *Mycopathologia* 64:29–33, 1978
74. Denton JF, DiSalvo AF: Respiratory infection of laboratory animals with conidia of *Blastomyces dermatitidis*. *Mycopathol Mycol Appl* 36:129–136, 1968
75. Williams JE, Moser SA: Chronic murine pulmonary blastomycosis induced by intratracheally inoculated *Blastomyces dermatitidis* conidia. *Am Rev Respir Dis* 135:17–25, 1987
76. Sugar AM, Picard M: Experimental blastomycosis pneumonia in mice by infection with conidia. *J Med Vet Mycol* 26:321–326, 1988
77. Frey CL, DeMarch P, Drutz DJ: Divergent patterns of pulmonary blastomycosis induced by conidia and yeasts in athymic and euthymic mice. *Am Rev Respir Dis* 140:118–124, 1989
78. McDonough ES, Ajello L, Ausherman RJ, et al: Human pathogenic fungi recovered from soil in an area endemic for North American blastomycosis. *Am J Hyg* 73:75–83, 1961
79. Klein BS, Vergeront JM, DiSalvo AF, et al: Two outbreaks of blastomycosis along rivers in Wisconsin. *Am Rev Respir Dis* 136:1333–1338, 1987
80. McDonough ES: Studies on the growth and survival of *Blastomyces dermatitidis* in soil, in Gibbons NE (ed): *Recent Progress in Microbiology, 8th International Congress of Microbiology*. Toronto, University of Toronto Press, 1963, pp 656–661
81. Denton JF, DiSalvo AF: Additional isolations of *Blastomyces dermatitidis* from natural sites. *Am J Trop Med Hyg* 28:697–700, 1979
82. Sarosi GA, Serstock DS: Isolation of *Blastomyces dermatitidis* from pigeon manure. *Am Rev Respir Dis* 114:1179–1183, 1976
83. Abou-Gabal M: Isolation of systemic mycotic causing fungi from the soil of Iowa. 57th Conference of Research Workers in Animal Diseases, Chicago, 1976
84. McDonough ES, Dubats JJ, Wisniewski TR, et al: Soil streptomycetes and bacteria related to lysis of *Blastomyces dermatitidis*. *Sabouraudia* 11:244–250, 1973
85. McDonough ES: Effects of natural soils on *B. dermatitidis, H. capsulatum* and *Allescheria boydii*. *Am J Hyg* 77:66–72, 1963
86. McDonough ES, Van Prooien R, Lewis AL: Lysis of *Blastomyces dermatitidis* yeast-phase cells in natural soil. *Am J Epidemiol* 81:86–94, 1965
87. Chaturvedi VP, Randhawa HS, Chaturvedi S, et al: In vitro interactions between *Blastomyces dermatitidis* and other zoopathogenic fungi. *Can J Microbiol* 34:897–900, 1988
88. Denton JF, DiSalvo AF: Effects of temperature on soil conidia of *Blastomyces dermatitidis*. *J Bacteriol* 85:717–718, 1963
89. Georg LK, Ajello L, Papageorge C: Use of cycloheximide in the selective isolation of fungi pathogenic to man. *J Lab Clin Med* 44:422–428, 1954
90. DiSalvo AF, Bigler WJ, Ajello L: Bat and soil studies for sources of histoplasmosis in Florida. *Am J Epidemiol* 89:606–614, 1969
91. Denton JF, DiSalvo, AF: The isolation of *H. capsulatum, C. neoformans* and *B. dermatitidis* from the same natural site. *Sabouraudia* 17:193–195, 1979
92. Archer JR, Trainer DO, Schell RF: Epidemiologic study of canine blastomycosis in Wisconsin. *J Am Vet Med Assoc* 190:1292–1295, 1987

93. Centers for Disease Control: Blastomycosis—North Carolina. *MMWR* 25:205–206, 1976
94. Armstrong CW, Jenkins SR, Kaufman L, et al: Common-source outbreak of blastomycosis in hunters and their dogs. *J Infect Dis* 155:568–570, 1987
95. Smith JG Jr, Harris JS, Conant NF, et al: An epidemic of North American blastomycosis. *JAMA* 158:641–646, 1955
96. DiSalvo AF, Johnson EM: Histoplasmosis in South Carolina: Support for the microfocus concept. *Am J Epidemiol* 109:480–492, 1979
97. Bianchi L, Della Torre B: Rara forma di ficomicosi umana a decorso piemico. Minerva Medica 53:2426–2473, 1962.
98. Bianchi L, Della Torre B, Martinazzi M: Fatal pancreatic necrosis in human phycomycosis. Path Microbiol 30:15–26, 1967.
99. Ajello L, personal communication, Atlanta, Georgia, 1991.

5

The Epidemiology of Blastomycosis

Arthur F. DiSalvo

1. INTRODUCTION

The study of epidemiology is important to determine causal factors. Elucidation of causal factors leads to the avoidance of the ecological niche, hazardous activities, or other risk factors associated with the etiologic agent. Forewarned is forearmed. Thus, without knowledge of the ecological niche of *Blastomyces dermatitidis,* it is perplexing to determine the epidemiology of blastomycosis.

Without comprehension of the epidemiology of a disease, it is difficult to prevent recurrent illness or to apply appropriate control measures. Study of the association between the occurrence of a disease and certain other events frequently leads to the determination of cause and effect. With blastomycosis this has been difficult for several reasons. The infected patients usually occur as solitary events; there is frequently a delay between the presenting symptoms and a definitive diagnosis; there has been little evidence on which to establish the incubation time; and the acute episode of illness may

Blastomycosis, edited by Yousef Al-Doory and Arthur F. DiSalvo, Plenum Medical Book Company, New York, 1992.

be a trivial or asymptomatic event that is not sufficiently significant to designate as the onset of disease. Thus, day zero of the exposure is usually unknown and therefore it is difficult to specify an incident, an activity, or a geographic site with the exposure. Such temporal relationships can frequently be identified in other diseases but until recently there have been too few reports of multiple exposures to recognize such a pattern in blastomycosis. There have only been 12 well-documented outbreaks of the disease further limiting the readily identified event. A complete understanding of the epidemiology of blastomycosis is further hindered by the absence of two classic parameters of epidemiology—incidence and prevalence. The rate or frequency of this mycosis cannot be determined (or even reasonably estimated) as long as it remains a nonreportable disease.

2. TRANSMISSION

Blastomycosis is not contagious. Five methods of transmission have been described: (1) inhalation, (2) accidental inoculation, (3) dog bites (a form of inoculation), (4) conjugal, and (5) intrauterine transmission. Although it is generally agreed that there is no man-to-man or animal-to-man transmission, under some highly unusual conditions, such transfer of the infectious agent may occur. The associated occurrence of blastomycosis in man and animals may be explained by a common exposure to a point source of contamination. The outbreak in Emporia, Virginia[1] or the "Case of the Fumbled Fungus"[2] are examples.

The route of entry of *B. dermatitidis* was thought to be both respiratory and transcutaneous. The classic work of Schwarz and Baum demonstrated that the lungs were the ordinary portal of entry.[3] They unequivocally demonstrated that *B. dermatitidis* is inhaled from the environment and may result in a subsequent subclinical or mild respiratory infection. Cutaneous blastomycosis is the result of hematogenous dissemination to the skin as well as to many other organs.

Transcutaneous blastomycosis has been shown to occur by two methods: trauma and animal bites. Schwarz reviewed the reported laboratory accidents resulting in cutaneous blastomycosis in 1983.[4] He accepted eight cases as transcutaneous primary blastomycosis. Additional transcutaneous infections occurred in two pathologists,[5] a veterinarian performing an autopsy on an infected dog[6] and a landscape worker who received a trauma on the foot with a piece of bark.[7]

The earliest account of accidental inoculation was reported in 1903 and demonstrates that this is a rare form of transmission.[8] There has also been one report of homologous transmission by means of a transthoracic needle aspiration.[9] The patient underwent this diagnostic procedure to evaluate pulmonary disease, which was subsequently diagnosed as blastomycosis. Following the hospital discharge, the patient presented with pulmonary symptoms compatible with blastomycosis and a lesion at the site of the aspiration. Examination of the sputum and the lesion revealed *B. dermatitidis* by microscopy and culture.

Equally as rare are cases of blastomycosis transmitted by the bites of dogs. Dogs are the most common animals with this disease and the distribution of canine blastomycosis coincides with the distribution of blastomycosis in human beings (see Chapter 13). There have been three reports of the transmission of blastomycosis by dog bites. Two of these are well documented in that blastomycosis was diagnosed in both the dog as well as the patient.[10,11] In the third report the patient developed cutaneous blastomycosis within 6 months of a dog bite.[12] Although this disease in the patient was well documented, the infection in the dog was not. Evidence to support the assumption that there is sufficient organism in oral secretions to produce dog bite transmission was presented by Hiemenz *et al.* who demonstrated numerous budding yeasts in the bronchial secretions of a dog that died from blastomycosis.[13] There is one well-documented case of conjugal transmission of this mycosis.[14,15] The husband had blastomycosis of the testicle, epididymis, and prostate and the wife developed blastomycosis of the endometrium, fallopian tubes, and peritoneum.

There have been six reports of blastomycosis in seven pregnant women.[16–21] All seven were treated with amphotericin B without harmful effects on the mother or the infant. In only one pregnancy was there evidence of intrauterine transmission of the infection.[16]

Procknow provided some evidence to support man-to-man transmission of blastomycosis in 1966.[22] A 31-year-old and a 28-year-old male factory worker were hospitalized at the same time with a confirmed diagnosis of blastomycosis. There were no common activities of these men except their close proximity in the workplace. The temporal relationship of their symptoms, signs, and diagnoses of blastomycosis appears to support his suggestion of communicability. However, there have been no further reports of proposed human-to-human transmission to reinforce this observation during the last 25 years.

3. INCUBATION PERIOD

From the limited data available, it can be reliably estimated that the incubation period of blastomycosis acquired by inhalation is from 4 to 8 weeks and that of primary transcutaneous blastomycosis, 1 to 5 weeks.

Information on which to base the incubation time has been sparse. Silent initial infection of the lung after inhalation of the infectious particles is probably quite common. The greatest impediment to determine the incubation time is the inability to clearly define the time of exposure. The actual time of the event has been difficult to fix when the source of the infecting organism is unknown. This important factor could be determined more precisely if the natural habitat were ascertained and the association between the nidus and the exposure could be made.

In recent years, the ecological niche of *B. dermatitidis* is slowly being defined. From some outbreaks, the time of exposure was determined by patient contact with a most likely source[23] or the only known temporal association of a group of individuals who developed blastomycosis.[24] There are only limited numbers of cases in which a singular event could be absolutely identified as the date of exposure[25-27] or when there was an association of the victims at a putative point source.[28]

Table 1 presents those reported infections with *B. dermatitidis,* by the respiratory route, in which a date of exposure can be reliably fixed. The shortest incubation period was 13 days and the longest was 102 days.

Unlike natural inhalation blastomycosis, the time of exposure in traumatic transcutaneous inoculation with *B. dermatitidis* is usually unequivocal. Primary transcutaneous blastomycosis is uncommon. It appears that most reported cases of primary cutaneous blastomycosis are either laboratory accidents or due to dog bites—events that are memorable. In those cases where the date of exposure and the date of onset are reported, the incubation time for inoculation blastomycosis ranged from 1 to 5 weeks (Table 2). The shortest incubation time, 5 days, occurred in a laboratorian who was stuck with a needle while inoculating animals.[30]

An immunocompromised renal transplant patient was reported as a case of primary cutaneous blastomycosis with an incubation period of 2

TABLE 1
Incubation Period for Inhalation Blastomycosis

Source	Number of patients	Number of days	Year reported	Ref.
Laboratory culture	1	52	1967	25
Laboratory	1	33	1970	26
Log cabin	1	43–44	1974	23
Pigeon manure	1	34	1976	27
River campsite	5	30–50	1984	24
Beaver dam	48	33–44	1986	28
River bank	7	16–102	1987	29
Underground fort	7	13–78	1987	29

TABLE 2
Incubation Period for Transcutaneous Blastomycosis

Source	Form	Number of days	Activity	Year reported	Ref.
Needle	Tissue	7	Autopsy	1903	8
Scalpel	Tissue	35	Autopsy	1955	31
Needle	Tissue	7	Autopsy	1955	31
Broken glass	Yeast	14	Lab. acc.	1959	32
Needle	Mycelium	15	Inoc. animals	1971	33
Needle	Yeast	5	Inoc. animals	1977	30
Scalpel	Tissue	14	Autopsy	1982	6
Scalpel	Tissue	21	Autopsy	1983	5
Scalpel	Tissue	35	Autopsy	1983	5
Needle	Tissue	14	Lab. acc.	1984	34

weeks.[34] Although the patient was a veterinarian's assistant and a needlestick was documented at the site of the lesion, the authors state that there is no conclusive evidence that the needle was contaminated with *B. dermatitidis* or that the patient was not incubating the disease prior to the needlestick. A retrospective review of the chest roentgenogram did reveal possible interstitial infiltrates at the time of the hospital admission.

There have been three publications on blastomycosis of man due to dog bites but none of these reports present sufficient information to determine the incubation time.[10-12]

4. SKIN TESTING

Dermal reactivity to antigens of fungi has provided valuable epidemiologic data with respect to the geographic distribution of mycotic pathogens. The activity of these crude antigens is based on the host hypersensitivity reaction to the etiologic agent. The information gleaned from surveys has been extremely important in the delineation of the endemic areas for histoplasmosis and coccidioidomycosis. Without this knowledge it would have been difficult to specifically outline endemic areas of these mycoses or determine the magnitude of asymptomatic cases. Such a useful tool has not been developed for blastomycosis.

The skin test antigens for *B. dermatitidis* were made from either the yeast form or the mycelial form of the organism.[35] Both antigens were crude mixtures that varied in potency. These antigens lacked both sensitivity and specificity and, of course, were useless as diagnostic or epidemiologic means in immunocompromised patients. The commercial intradermal test, blastomycin, was prepared from the mycelial form. This antigen was originally marketed as a diagnostic reagent but results were so poor that the Food and Drug Administration (FDA) removed the product from the market in 1972. It never served as a diagnostic aid nor as an epidemiologic tool.

In lieu of the skin test, the lymphocyte response to antigens of *B. dermatitidis* may become an *in vitro* epidemiologic tool to detect subclinical infections of blastomycosis. Vaaler *et al.* studied two groups of forestry workers with daily exposure in endemic areas.[36] Thirty percent of forestry workers from northern Minnesota and northern Wisconsin, an endemic area for blastomycosis, demonstrated antigen-induced lymphocyte proliferation while none of 24 forestry workers from Washington, a nonendemic state, were positive. In a similar study in Arkansas, an endemic area for blastomycosis, all of seven co-workers of a patient with blastomycosis, and all of 18 patients treated for blastomycosis gave a positive test. All but one healthy control had a negative response.[37] The authors of both studies claim to be detecting subclinical cases of blastomycosis. Although more cumbersome than a skin test, this may be a useful tool in elucidating the epidemiology of this mycosis.

5. DEMOGRAPHIC ASPECTS

If one looks at the more recent reports of blastomycosis as the basis, where the diagnosis of infection with *B. dermatitidis* is more definitive, the age, race, and sex predilection that have previously been claimed appear to soften. Some reports of surveys in the literature from the last 35 years are shown in Table 3. Individual numbers do not always concur with totals because complete data were not always available to the original investigators. Although this list is meant to be representative and not complete, the variation of the demographic data in these reports is apparent.

5.1. Age

All age groups are susceptible to infection with *B. dermatitidis*. The youngest patient reported was 3 weeks of age[38] and the oldest patients were more than 90 years old[39] (Table 3). The age distribution varies with each series of cases published which is a reflection of the population examined. The paper by Furcolow *et al.* examined 1114 patients and represents the largest cohort studied.[39] They found that 87% of the patients were between 20 and 70 years of age. This finding is consistent with most demographic reports and is also consistent with the population engaged in occupations,

TABLE 3
Age, Race, and Sex Distribution in Patients with Blastomycosis

Age (years)		Sex	Race		State	Year	Ref.
Youngest	Oldest	(M/F)	B/W	Other	State	reported	Ref.
5 months	77	6/5	4/7	0	North Carolina	1955	41
10–19	80+	150/25	25/146	0	Kentucky	1966	42
0–9	70–90	111/16	52/75	0	Arkansas	1969	43
0–9	90–99	989/125	304/810	0	USA	1970	39
7	81	120ᵃ/10	40/90	0	USA	1977	44
2	75	24/4	—/—ᵇ	—	Canada	1983	45
6	77	32/4	0/27	9	Canada	1972	46
8	63	50/7	53/6	—	Africa	1989	47
19	75	34/6	13/27	1	USA	1968	48
19	69	197ᵃ/1	54/143	0	USA	1964	49
?	?	11ᵃ/5	2/14	—	Illinois	1970	50
0–9	80–89	89ᵃ/12	—/—	0	USA	1955	51
0–5	71+	75/11	59/27	0	Tennessee	1956	52
20–29	90+	33/7	—/—	—	West Virginia	1966	53
10	80	33/13	4/39	3	Wisconsin	1967	54
3 weeks	81	14/16	12/18	0	Louisiana	1989	38
—	—	16/32	5/43	0	Wisconsin	1986	28
3	30	1/4	5/0	0	North Carolina	1976	55
11	49	2/4	0/6	0	Wisconsin	1987	29
12	56	7/0	0/7	0	Wisconsin	1987	29

ᵃ Veterans Administration population.
ᵇ — not given.

avocations, and recreation that may bring the candidate in contact with the probable nidus of infection.

5.2. Sex

The literature discloses a variety of male/female ratios as shown in Table 3, but usually there are more male patients with blastomycosis. As noted in Table 3, several studies were performed on patients in Veterans Administration (V.A.) hospitals because complete records and clinical materials were available. Since, in the past, V.A. hospitals have traditionally seen primarily male patients, this bias is obvious.

Although Landay *et al.* have shown that female hamsters are more resistant to infection with *B. dermatitidis* than male hamsters,[40] the preponderance of male human beings with blastomycosis has likely been due to greater exposure to the etiologic agent and not to some innate susceptibility. This male/female ratio supports the concept that *B. dermatitidis* is probably a saprophyte in nature where more men than women are likely to be exposed. As the work force is now changing and more opportunities are open for women in construction, the armed services, and other outdoor activities in work and leisure, there will probably be more equality between men and women infected with *B. dermatitidis.*

It should be noted that where there were equal numbers of males and females exposed in clusters of blastomycosis, the attack rates did not vary significantly. In the Grifton, North Carolina, outbreak there were six males and five females infected[41]; in Bigfork, Minnesota there were 21 members of four families potentially exposed to the source of *B. dermatitidis.*[23] The paper does not reveal the number of males and females at the site but there were five females and seven males who developed acute pulmonary blastomycosis. In Namekegon, five men and three women were exposed; all but one female were infected.

5.3. Race

Unlike coccidioidomycosis, race susceptibility does not appear to be evident in blastomycosis. The number of blacks, whites, and others infected with *B. dermatitidis* is also shown in Table 3. This distribution sometimes reflects social groups: the white boys who lived and played together in the Crystal River outbreak[29]; the families in the Tomorrow River[29] and Bigfork outbreak[23]; and, of course, Africa is predominantly black. In Grifton, North Carolina, where the first outbreak of blastomycosis was reported, there were four black patients and seven white patients, which reflects the population of that small rural town.[41] The nine "others" from Canada,[46] the three "others" from Wisconsin,[54] and the one "other" from the V.A. hospitals[49] in Table 3 refer to American Indians.

It is generally assumed that the distribution of blastomycosis reflects the population in the community served by the institution reviewing their data.[56] The incidence in blacks and whites may vary when these data are analyzed as case rates. A difference was noted by Furcolow et al. when they reviewed their epidemiologic data.[39] They found 304 blacks and 810 whites with blastomycosis in their series. As case rates, this distribution was 1.6 cases per 100,000 for blacks and 0.5 case per 100,000 for whites. This difference between absolute numbers and rates was also observed in the report from Louisiana by Lowry et al.[38] In their small series of 30 cases, there were 12 blacks and 18 whites. As rates per 100,000, however, the incidence was 9.0 and 5.9 in blacks and whites, respectively. Until there is complete diagnosis of all patients with blastomycosis, including silent infections, accurate case rates will not be determined.

The age, sex, and race distribution of blastomycosis appear to be a matter of exposure and not susceptibility of the individual. Therefore, the clinician should consider blastomycosis in the differential diagnosis, when appropriate, in all patients. The real incidence will not be accurately determined until there is a means of detecting subclinical infection.

6. OUTBREAKS

There have now been at least 12 outbreaks or clusters of blastomycosis and all have occurred in the continental United States. Five clusters occurred in the mid-Atlantic states (North Carolina, Virginia, and Tennessee) and seven occurred in the north-central states (Wisconsin, Minnesota, and Illinois). The locations are shown in Fig. 1. The number of patients involved in each episode varied from 3 to 48. The etiologic agent was isolated from the point source in only two outbreaks.

Blastomycosis is not considered a contagious disease. It is assumed that, as in other mycotic infections, outbreaks occur when several persons or animals are exposed to a common nidus of the infectious particles. There is one report of the possible transmission of blastomycosis from a dog to man, but it is more likely that both were exposed to the same microfocus of *B. dermatitidis.*[57]

Pertinent features of the outbreaks are listed in Table 4. It should be noted that, with one exception, all outbreaks occurred in rural areas. The patients were engaged in anthropurgic activities associated with environmen-

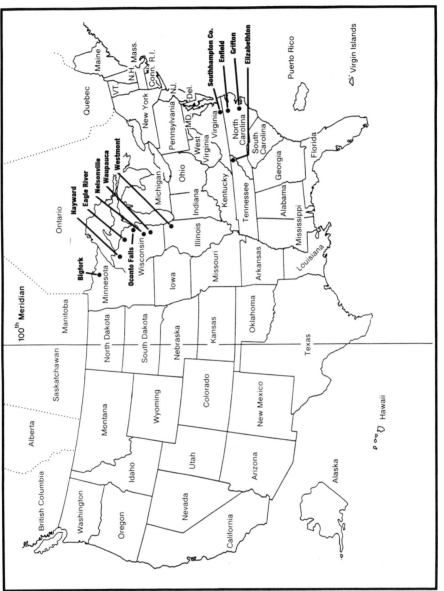

FIGURE 1. Distribution of outbreaks of blastomycosis. Note the grouping in the mid-Atlantic and north-central portion of the

TABLE 4
Some Features of Blastomycosis Outbreaks

Outbreak number	Year	Site	Number infected	Locale	Activity	Suspected environmental source	Onset of illness	Ref.
1	1954	North Carolina	11	Rural	Nonspecific	None	Oct.–Mar.	41
2	1972	Minnesota	12	Rural	Building log cabin	Wood, hay, sawdust	Oct.–Nov.	23
3	1975	Illinois	5	Urban	Road construction	Dust, soil	Aug.–Apr.	62
4	1975	North Carolina	5	Rural	Peanut harvest	Soil, vegetation	Nov.	55
5	1977	North Carolina	7	Rural	Nonspecific	?	July	—[a]
6	1979	Wisconsin	7	Rural	Camping	Rotted firewood	Aug.	24
7	1984	Wisconsin	48	Rural	Nature trail	Beaver dam[b]	July–Aug.	28
8	1984	Virginia	4	Rural	Raccoon hunting	Soil	Mar.	1
9	1985	Wisconsin	6	Rural	Underground	Soil, timber	May	29
10	1985	Wisconsin	7	Rural	Riverbank fishing	Soil, animal[b] burrow	June	29
11	1989	Tennessee	3	Rural	Nonspecific	Construction site?	May	63
12	1990	Wisconsin	10	Rural	Various anthropurgic activities	Swampy woodlands	Dec.–Feb.	—[a]

[a] Personal communication.
[b] *B. dermatitidis* isolated.

tal sources similar to the natural sites from which *B. dermatitidis* has been isolated. Decayed wood, organic matter, or animal droppings were usually present in the substrate.

The first reported outbreak of blastomycosis occurred in Grifton, Pitt County, North Carolina, a tobacco-growing area, in 1954.[41] From October 1953 through May 1955, 11 patients from a town of approximately 1000 people were diagnosed with blastomycosis at Duke University. Eight patients resided inside the town limits and three lived within 4 miles from the center of town. The soil is a sandy loam and the records showed excess rainfall for 5 of the 7 months of the epidemic. Many environmental samples were taken but *B. dermatitidis* was not isolated.

Subsequently, after the recovery of *B. dermatitidis* from a tobacco barn in Lexington, Kentucky, in 1960,[58] it was decided to sample the Grifton area again using the isolation technique that had been successful. Justification to support this investigation was: (1) Grifton is a tobacco-growing area, (2) *B. dermatitidis* was isolated from a tobacco barn, (3) one of the Grifton patients played in a tobacco barn, (4) two patients lived in houses constructed on former tobacco fields, (5) reports from McDonough that *B. dermatitidis* was suppressed by other soil organisms,[59] (6) *B. dermatitidis* conidia will survive above 40°C,[60] and (7) knowledge that the temperature in barns reached 80°C during curing of tobacco, thus effectively reducing the competition for *B. dermatitidis* to survive and multiply.

In 1962, 253 samples were collected in the town of Grifton; 220 were from inside tobacco-curing barns. *B. dermatitidis* was not isolated from any.[61] However, the abrupt onset and termination of this outbreak reinforces the concept that there may be periods when *B. dermatitidis* blooms in the environment much as *Coccidioides immitis* does in the desert.

The second outbreak took place in 1972. Four families, consisting of 21 persons, were involved in clearing trees and brush from a wooded area 15 miles from Bigfork, Itasca County, Minnesota, a town of 464 persons.[23] They constructed a cabin on a lakeside site. Activities began in the summer and the cabin was finished in October. The cabin was constructed from new lumber. *B. dermatitidis* was isolated from 4 of the 12 patients with definite or probable blastomycosis. The onset of illness in the 7 symptomatic patients occurred in a 4-week period during the last week of October and the first week of November.

Environmental samples were collected in December and March. These consisted of hay, rotten wood, sawdust, and soil. The Denton i.v. mouse tail technique[58] was used, but none of the samples yielded *B. dermatitidis*. It was later learned that a picnic was held on an island just off shore from the building site. This may have been the point source but samples had not been collected there (R. J. Weeks, personal communication, 1981).

The third outbreak occurred in Westmont, DuPage County, Illinois.[62] Five residents of this community had culturally proven blastomycosis cases during the 9 months from August 1974 through April 1975. The novel aspect of this cluster is that it occurred in an urban area 20 miles west of Chicago. These patients had minimal outdoor exposure with the exception of one who kept a compost pile. They all lived within a 1-mile radius and the only possible common exposure that could be determined was heavy dust in the area during road construction. Environmental samples, including dust, compost, garden soil, and soil from the construction area, were examined by the i.v. mouse tail technique. *B. dermatitidis* was not isolated.

The fourth cluster also occurred in North Carolina, 60 miles north of the first outbreak. Five culturally proven cases of blastomycosis occurred in Enfield, Halifax County, North Carolina, a town of 3200, in 1975.[55] All patients became ill in November 1975. The only common event that could be determined was proximity to peanut farms that had been harvested 6 weeks prior to the illnesses. Attempts were made to isolate the etiologic agent but they were unsuccessful.

An outbreak of seven cases of blastomycosis in human beings and seven in dogs occurred in Trenton, Jones County, North Carolina, during a 12-month period in 1976–1977 (R. C. Baron, Epidemiologic report, North Carolina Department of Human Resources, 1977). Trenton, population 500, is located 30 miles south of Grifton, the site of the first reported outbreak. The patients and the infected dogs with blastomycosis lived within an area of about one block. Environmental sampling was planned but the report does not disclose if this was done.

The sixth outbreak occurred in northwestern Wisconsin near the town of Hayward, Sawyer County, in July 1979.[24] This location is approximately 200 miles southeast of Bigfork, Minnesota. Seven of eight persons in the group developed blastomycosis and *B. dermatitidis* was isolated from five of the patients. The individuals were canoeing on the Namekekon River and the suspected site of exposure was a campsite where they stopped for lunch. A campfire was made from precut logs and sawdust at the site. It was claimed that some of the logs were decaying and clouds of dust were released when they were dropped.

Nineteen environmental samples were collected 30 days after the exposure. These were examined at the Mayo Clinic (G. D. Roberts, personal communication, 1981) and in our laboratory using the Denton i.v. mouse tail technique. *B. dermatitidis* was not isolated.

The melding of the ecology and epidemiology of blastomycosis finally occurred in the seventh outbreak, which happened in 1984 and was reported in 1986 by Klein *et al.*[28] Two different groups of schoolchildren and adults visited an environmental camp at Eagle River, Vilas County, Wisconsin.

Forty-eight of the ninety-five participants evaluated had blastomycosis. Epidemiologic investigation implicated a beaver pond at the camp. At this site a running stream was obstructed by a beaver dam forming a large pond. A beaver hut was located on the pond, but close enough to the shore to allow visitors an opportunity to walk directly on the abandoned lodge. Environmental samples were examined in two independent laboratories by the Denton i.v. technique [Division of Mycotic Diseases, Centers for Disease Control (CDC) and the Bureau of Laboratories, South Carolina Department of Health]. Of the 47 samples tested, two from the beaver lodge and one from the dam yielded *B. dermatitidis.* The two samples from the lodge were positive at both laboratories while the dam sample was positive only at the CDC laboratory. A beaver lodge isolate has been deposited with the American Type Culture Collection (ATCC) as shown in Table 1 of Chapter 4.

The substrate from the beaver dam and the beaver lodge were high in organic matter (soil, decaying wood, animal droppings) and the pH was 6.5. This material was similar to the environmental samples from which *B. dermatitidis* had been isolated in the past and the association with water is again demonstrated. These features are also shown in Table 1 of Chapter 4. Thus, the general description of the ecologic niche has been more narrowly defined.

The eighth outbreak of blastomycosis, in 1984, again occurred in the mid-Atlantic states.[1] Four raccoon hunters and four of their hunting dogs from Emporia, Southampton County, Virginia developed blastomycosis. The hunting, on a weekly basis, was the only common temporal characteristic among the men and the dogs. Seventeen environmental samples were examined for *B. dermatitidis* but the organism was not isolated.

The next two outbreaks occurred in small Wisconsin towns, 20 miles apart, during the summer of 1985.[29] The first cluster of cases were exposed on the Tomorrow River, Nelsonville, Portage County. A family group went fishing on the long, sloping, tree-lined banks of the river, which passed along the edge of their farm. The soil was high in organic matter, well shaded by the trees and vegetation, and a groundhog burrow was at the top of the bank. The slope is quite steep so that there was slipping and soil disruption in climbing or descending the bank. Seven of the twelve persons at the site on 2 days developed blastomycosis. Eight environmental samples were collected from the riverbank and tested by the Denton i.v. mouse tail inoculation technique. *B. dermatitidis* was isolated from one sample.

The second cluster in the vicinity occurred on the banks of the Crystal River in the town of Waupaca, Waupaca County, Wisconsin. Seven boys played for 4 days in an underground timber fort, which was visited on one occasion by an adult man. The fort contained deteriorating boards and rugs and was located in a heavily shaded, moist area 6 m from the bank. The burrow of an unidentified animal, 0.5 m wide, was located between the fort and the river. The boys dug in the animal burrow. Six boys and the adult were diagnosed with blastomycosis. Sixteen soil samples from this site were examined for *B. dermatitidis* by the Denton i.v. technique but the fungus was not isolated.

The 11th cluster of cases occurred among three individuals in Elizabethton, Carter County, Tennessee in 1989.[63] Three young adults were diagnosed with blastomycosis within 8 days. Two patients lived in Elizabethton and the third patient lived approximately 10 miles away but spent 3 days each week in Elizabethton. The only common event that could be identified among the three was the frequent driving past a construction site in town. No attempts were made to isolate *B. dermatitidis* from environmental samples.

The last outbreak, which is still under investigation, occurred in Oconto Falls, Oconto County, Wisconsin (M. L. Procter, personal communication, 1990). Ten patients became infected with *B. dermatitidis* during the first 7 months of 1990. All patients lived in a swampy, forested area along the Oconto River. Besides the residential proximity, several of the patients harvested trees on this property, participated in pheasant hunting in the immediate area, or engaged in other anthropurgic activities.

One individual was digging under his house in a dirt basement to install a furnace. Another patient razed an old garage and chicken coop to build a new garage and a 9-year-old boy had been digging an underground fort. Infection of other individuals occurred where there was an excavation for a large pond and a 3-year-old patient was known to play in a chicken coop. Thirty-three environmental samples (average pH 5.5) were collected from suspected sources and tested by the Denton i.v. technique. None were positive for *B. dermatitidis.*

There have been two additional outbreaks of blastomycosis that were reported only in anecdotal fashion. Chick *et al.* described two clusters they studied in the 1950s.[64] The first cluster involved four black males living on farms close to each other in Bolivar County, Mississippi. There was a detailed epidemiologic study of the cases but the only commonality that could be ascertained was that each had close contact with soil and soil products. Environmental samples were examined but *B. dermatitidis* was not isolated.

The second cluster Chick studied was in a rural community in southern Arkansas. A white male farmer and 12 of his dogs had blastomycosis. A confirmed diagnosis was made in the man and 2 of the dogs but the 10 other dogs had similar pulmonary infections. The common epidemiologic feature of this cohort was the habit of the dogs to remain under the house. During the 6 months prior to his illness, the farmer had been under the house to make repairs. Environmental samples from this site were also examined for *B. dermatitidis* but the fungus was not isolated.

Out of an analysis of these limited data, the epidemiology of this mycosis and the ecology of the causative agent are beginning to emerge.

7. POSSIBLE HOSTS

7.1. The Canine Surrogate

Dogs appear to be as susceptible to *B. dermatitidis* as man. For this reason there have been many epidemiologic studies of blastomycosis in dogs and canine blastomycosis has become a surrogate indicator of *B. dermatitidis* and human blastomycosis. The incidence and prevalence of canine blastomycosis have long been used to establish and supplement the geographic distribution of this disease. This concept was advanced and investigated by Menges. In 1965 Menges *et al.* reported a study of canine blastomycosis in Arkansas.[65] Their specific aim was to determine the role of animals in the epidemiology of human blastomycosis. They concluded that man and animals acquire their infections from the same point source and that there is no evidence of the transmission of *B. dermatitidis* from man to animals or animals to man. This perception is presently accepted by most investigators.

Another study by Menges *et al.* that demonstrated the relationship between the epidemiology of blastomycosis in man and dog was published in 1969.[43] This paper, although extensive in numbers of cases, was limited to the state of Arkansas. They studied the distribution of 127 human and 110 canine infections. Although there was no commonality between the human and canine infections, the geographic areas with a higher incidence of blastomycosis in dogs also had a higher incidence of blastomycosis in human beings. The canine blastomycosis distribution map by Menges *et al.* also illustrates that all cases of canine blastomycosis occurred east of the 100th meridian.[43]

In a broader study of the epidemiology of human and canine blastomycosis, Furcolow *et al.,* in 1970, attempted to review all the human and canine cases in the United States.[39] They presented a map of the United States depicting the occurrence of human and canine blastomycosis for each state. Although there was variation in the number of infected individuals in these two species, the authors concluded that the distribution of canine cases supports the distribution of human cases and that the ratio of human to canine cases offers an additional epidemiologic tool.

In 1979, Sarosi *et al.* reported six patients with blastomycosis who owned or had close contact with dogs that were infected with *B. dermatiti-*

dis.[66] The etiologic agent in all human and canine infections was confirmed and the temporal occurrence between each pair was consistent with a common exposure.

A subsequent study on the epidemiology of blastomycosis in Wisconsin by McDonough and Kuzma examined 73 canine and 182 human cases of blastomycosis.[67] In one instance both a dog and an infant from the same household were infected with *B. dermatitidis.* Similarly, Archer *et al.* reported 3 cases of blastomycosis occurring simultaneously in both human beings and dogs in the same household.[68] Their review demonstrated an increase in canine cases of blastomycosis in the same areas of Wisconsin where three outbreaks of human disease were to occur within 3 years (Eagle River, Crystal River, Tomorrow River).

In a humorous presentation of a not-so-humorous event, Lieberman presented "The Case of the Fumbled Fungus" in 1963.[2] The patient was a resident of New York City for the years during which his blastomycosis was progressing. He was born and raised in South Carolina and lived most of his adult life in Virginia and had always shared the outdoor (and indoor) life with his dogs. During the 10 years of disease progression, none of his physicians made this association between his medical and social history and the etiologic agent.

In Augusta, Georgia, the site of the first isolation of *B. dermatitidis* from naturally infected soils, but where there are few human cases, dogs were examined for evidence of infection with this organism (J. F. Denton and A. F. DiSalvo, unpublished data). Between 1958 and 1960, 101 healthy, stray mongrel dogs, obtained from the local dog pound, were examined. Each dog was necropsied and the peribronchial lymph nodes were excised. Portions of the nodes were ground in saline with antibiotics and inoculated i.p. into four mice. After 4 weeks the mice were sacrificed, autopsied, and the lung, liver, and spleen were inoculated on Sabouraud's dextrose agar plates and tubes of brain heart infusion blood agar. The plates were incubated at 25°C and the tubes at 37°C. All cultures were reviewed on a weekly basis for 4 weeks. None were positive for *B. dermatitidis* and only one yielded *Cryptococcus neoformans.* This differs from McDonough's findings in which he found a close relationship between blastomycosis in human beings and blastomycosis in dogs.[67] However, his studies were done in an area that is highly endemic for this disease.

Additional evidence to support the hypothesis that man and dog are exposed to the same unrecognized environmental source of *B. dermatitidis* is presented in the outbreak from Emporia, Virginia in 1987.[1] In that report, four human patients (raccoon hunters) and four of their hunting dogs developed blastomycosis. Men and dogs all hunted together on a weekly basis.

7.2. Bat

Could the bat play a role in the ecology and epidemiology of blastomycosis as it may in histoplasmosis? In 1967, Tesh and Schneidau reported that *Tadarida brasiliensis* (Mexican free-tailed bat) was susceptible to experimental infection with *B. dermatitidis*.[69] Seven of seventeen experimentally infected bats, inoculated i.p. with *B. dermatitidis,* died from blastomycosis. Five infected bats excreted *B. dermatitidis* prior to death. Only one of nine surviving bats excreted the fungus in feces and this excretion ceased after 4 weeks and did not recur in the remaining 5 weeks until the animals were sacrificed. Thus, it may be that, if bats become susceptible to *B. dermatitidis* and they survive infection, they shed the viable fungus for only a limited time.

Chaturvedi *et al.* orally infected bats, *Rhinopoma hardwickei hardwickei,* with yeasts and mycelial forms of *B. dermatitidis*.[70] They found that the fungus was excreted in the feces rapidly, in low numbers, and for only 24 h. The excretion was the same from bats infected with yeasts or molds.

In 1982, Khan *et al.* reported the isolation of *B. dermatitidis* from 1 of 155 *R. hardwickei hardwickei* collected near Delhi, India.[71] In 1985, Randhawa *et al.* investigated another 627 bats belonging to five species from a nearby area.[72] They reported the isolation of *B. dermatitidis* from the liver of another *R. hardwickei hardwickei*.

Denton examined 371 bats from 1960 to 1968 specifically for evidence of *B. dermatitidis* infection (J. F. Denton, unpublished data). These represented 11 species collected in Georgia. The protocol consisted of capturing live bats, sacrificing them, and culturing the lungs, liver, and spleen on Sabouraud's dextrose agar at 25°C. *B. dermatitidis* was not isolated from any culture.

The role of these flying mammals in the ecology and epidemiology of histoplasmosis was studied extensively during the 1950s and 1960s. The methods of isolation and identification of both pathogenic fungi are the same and the search for *Histoplasma capsulatum* would have revealed *B. dermatitidis,* if it were present. DiSalvo, in summarizing these findings in 1971, concluded that in the 7569 bats examined by several investigators, *B. dermatitidis* was never isolated.[73] This finding seems to indicate that bats are an unlikely vector for the dissemination of *B. dermatitidis*.

8. OCCUPATIONAL MYCOSIS

The occupational aspects of blastomycosis were reviewed in 1983.[76] As has been stated about the alleged racial susceptibility to *B. dermatitidis,* an occupational distribution is probably a reflection of the population served by a particular institution. Harrell and Curtis stated, "There is no apparent occupation which predisposes to the development of North American blastomycosis. The statement that this disease occurs most commonly in the agricultural worker is true only of those reports emanating from agricultural areas. In the Detroit, Michigan, area the disease is found to be most common in automobile workers."[32]

Although this disease does not present any specific occupational hazard, any individual with a vocation or avocation that is associated with outdoor activities is at risk to exposure to *B. dermatitidis*. This apparent association was recognized very early. In 1901, Ricketts commented on the number of patients who were farmers, carpenters, or individuals with comparable exposure. This susceptibility is probably consistent with the patient population seen in a medical school clinic in downtown Chicago where he practiced.[77] Stober, in his review in 1914, had a similar experience. His series of patients were exposed to wood and soil in their inferior housing rather than in the workplace.[78] This cohort also came from downtown Chicago.

Three professions appear to be at specific risk: microbiologists, pathologists, and veterinarians.[4] Although these professional victims are relatively few in number, their peril is great due to the magnitude of their exposure when manipulating large numbers of organisms in cultures or at autopsy. Schwarz reviewed the occurrence of blastomycosis in laboratory workers.[4] He reported eight investigators who developed cutaneous blastomycosis through accidental inoculation, one who developed a pulmonary infection and one with osteomyelitis. The latter case was a technician who assisted in the environmental investigations of the ecologic niche of *B. dermatitidis*.[25]

Larson *et al.* stated that primary cutaneous blastomycosis was an occupational hazard to pathologists.[5] Five of the eleven cases they reviewed occurred from minor lacerations during autopsies on patients with blastomycosis. They also reported that 2 of 15 pathologists in Duluth, Minnesota developed blastomycosis under these conditions. Similar to pathologists, veterinarians are exposed during the autopsies of dogs dying with blastomycosis. Evidence to support the exposure of veterinarians to blastomycosis from dog bites was presented earlier in this chapter under the discussion of transmission.[10-13]

Table 5 presents the occupations of 771 patients with blastomycosis. These examples were selected from ten papers reported since 1955 and do not represent all such studies published. There was no uniform definitions of the various occupations and the list presented is a composite that includes some interpretation and grouping by the author. If one combines the occupations of "agriculture, farmer, laborer, miner, heavy equipment operator, and other outdoor occupation," this represents 372 patients or 48% of these reported cases. Similarly, if one were to combine "sawmill operator, car-

TABLE 5
Occupation of 771 Patients with Blastomycosis

Study	1	2	3	4	5	6	7	8	9	10	
Ref.	51	52	53	54	43	75	46	48	49	74	Total
Year	1955	1956	1966	1967	1969	1969	1972	1968	1964	1988	
Number	82	86	40	46	127	63	36	40	224	27	771
Occupation											
Agriculture	—	15	—	1	—	—	1	1	8	—	26
Farmer	15	—	—	2	37	14	6	12	52	6	144
Laborer	14	29	6	2	21	—	—	2	23	—	97
Miner	5	—	15	—	—	4	—	3	5	—	32
Heavy equip operator	—	—	—	1	—	3	—	—	5	1	10
Other outdoor	—	—	—	4	13	2	7	—	37	—	63
Sawmill	—	—	—	—	—	2	—	—	8	2	12
Carpenter	6	—	—	1	—	2	—	—	8	—	17
Construction	6	—	—	1	—	—	7	6	5	6	31
Professional	—	—	—	—	2	2	—	—	11	—	15
White-collar	—	11	—	3	3	3	7	1	—	—	28
Other indoor	28	—	7	16	28	4	—	9	62	12	166
Student	—	—	—	3	—	14	—	—	—	—	23
Housewife	8	—	—	10	—	6	6	3	—	—	29
Unknown	—	31	12	—	23	7	—	3	—	—	53
None given	—	—	—	2	—	—	—	—	—	—	25

penter, and construction worker," these represent 60 or an additional 8% of the patients. The patients in the categories of "professional, white-collar, other indoor, student, and housewife" represent 261 or 34% of the total. Therefore, it appears that a preponderance of the victims of this disease have an outdoor exposure.

If one considers that many people who develop blastomycosis do so as an outdoor recreational activity, the obvious association of an exposure to *B. dermatitidis* in the environment is essential to acquire this disease. A brief review of Table 4 shows that eight of the outbreaks bear out the association between exposure to a likely ecologic niche of *B. dermatitidis* and the infection with this fungus. Bradsher reported that 25 of the 80 patients with blastomycosis that he has treated in Arkansas worked in the forestry industry.[79]

There are many additional single case reports of individuals with an environmental exposure to wood or soil who developed blastomycosis. A few selected cases will be presented as examples. A 31-year-old pregnant female from Ontario, Canada with a home on the site of a former lumber mill was clearing rotted wood 5 months prior to her illness.[80] A 19-year-old Texan was employed to open sacks of clay to mix with fertilizer. The clay was dry and dusty and the employee did not wear a mask. The clay was from Virginia.[81] A 52-year-old male resident of Eagle River, Wisconsin, site of the first isolation of *B. dermatitidis* in association with a cluster of cases, developed pulmonary blastomycosis. He was a bulldozer operator on a cranberry farm.[82] A 34-year-old male landscaper developed cutaneous blastomycosis after traumatizing the affected area with a piece of bark while planting a tree.[7] A 72-year-old male from Ontario, Canada developed pulmonary blastomycosis while working in the dusty atmosphere inside a shed.[83] *B. dermatitidis* was isolated from the patient and the environment.

Thus, it is not the specific occupation that renders one susceptible to infection with *B. dermatitidis,* but the exposure of an individual to the probable ecologic niche of the fungus. This exposure is just as likely to occur in recreational pursuits as in earning a living. As in all medical diagnoses, a careful history by a knowledgeable clinician can lead to an early diagnosis.

9. SEASONALITY

There does not appear to be a seasonal incidence of blastomycosis in animals or man. It is difficult to evaluate the seasonality of this mycosis with any certainty because of the lack of sufficient information about the ecology and epidemiology of the disease. When one considers this gap in knowledge, the prolonged incubation period, and the frequent time-lapse before a definitive diagnosis is established, it is apparent that all reports, single cases or clusters, can only date the time when the patient felt sufficient discomfort to seek medical attention. As in most illnesses, retroactively dating the onset is frequently not precise.

Klein *et al.* reviewed the seasonal occurrence of blastomycosis reported in ten studies.[84] They concluded that human illness occurred more frequently during the winter months and that canine disease peaked during the summer and fall. However, if one looks at the months of reported clinical illness in the outbreaks shown in Table 6, it is apparent that the clusters of blastomycosis have occurred in all months of the year.

McDonough, reporting the season of onset for 44 cases from Wisconsin, found a fairly even distribution of human patients with blastomycosis during the winter, spring, and fall, but only 7% during the summer.[54] In a comparable study in Arkansas, Menges *et al.* reported similar findings among 93 human cases.[43] These figures are shown in Table 7.

Two studies have reported the season of onset in canine blastomycosis. Menges *et al.*, in their report of 100 dogs from Arkansas, showed that the onset of blastomycosis occurred in all months of the year.[43] Archer's study claimed that, in Wisconsin, the cases of canine blastomycosis increased in late spring through early fall.[85] The season of onset for the 195 dogs he studied is shown in Table 7 and differs little from that of Menges *et al.*

In 1979, Denton and DiSalvo stated that, based on soil isolations of the fungus, environmental conditions appear to be more favorable for the propagation or survival of *B. dermatitidis* during winter in the southeastern United States.[86] However, when observing clinical data from outbreaks of disease, the seasonal pattern is not obvious.

10. STRAIN SYNONYMS

In recent years, molecular techniques have been applied to medical mycology. Although these techniques are still in their infancy, investigations are in progress to specifically identify various strains of *B. dermatitidis*. As this biotyping capability is developed, environmental isolates may be identified as the etiologic agent of disease in individual patients and, therefore, indicate the specific source of infection for that person. Such tools will enhance the understanding of the epidemiology of blastomycosis.

To assist in the retrospective evaluation of such techniques, it is essential to correlate future investigations with previous work. Recent studies employed a relatively few strains of *B. dermatitidis* from the American Type Culture Collection (ATCC). Some investigators have used different terminology to describe the same isolate. Table 8 is an attempt to clarify these syn-

TABLE 6
Onset of Symptoms during 12 Outbreaks of Blastomycosis[a]

Outbreak number	State	Month of onset											
		Jan.	Feb.	Mar.	Apr.	May	June	July	Aug.	Sep.	Oct.	Nov.	Dec.
Southern United States													
1	North Carolina	b	b			X					X		X
4	North Carolina											X	
5	North Carolina							X					
8	Virginia			X									
11	Tennessee					X							
Northern United States													
2	Minnesota										X	X	
3	Illinois	X			X				X			X	
6	Wisconsin								X	X			
7	Wisconsin							X	X				
9	Wisconsin						X						
10	Wisconsin					X							
12	Wisconsin	X	X										X

[a] Adapted from Table 4.
[b] 8/11 patients had onset of symptoms in January, February, and March.

TABLE 7
Seasonal Distribution of Blastomycosis in Humans and Dogs

	Seasons					
	Spring	Summer	Fall	Winter	Year	Ref.
Humans	27%	7%	27%	39%	1967	54
	20%	16%	24%	40%	1969	43
Canine	26%	26%	30%	18%	1969	43
	21%	30%	28%	21%	1985	85

onyms. Thus, strain SCB-2, which infected a laboratory worker,[30] is the same strain called ATCC 26199 by Morozumi *et al.* in their evaluation of mouse susceptibility to infection with *B. dermatitidis.*[97] It is also the same strain used by Cox and Larsh to develop an antigen to *B. dermatitidis*[95,96] and by Vaaler *et al.* to determine subclinical infections in forestry workers.[100]

11. SUMMARY

Until there are adequate data, the epidemiology of blastomycosis will remain ambiguous. The present state of knowledge has been derived from case reports, rare outbreaks, and occasional geographically or temporally limited surveys. A significant deficiency is the reluctance of the United States Public Health Service to require the reporting of mycotic diseases as part of the vital statistics recorded for other infectious diseases. Without such statistics, it is impossible to determine the prevalence and incidence of blastomycosis. Present information only reflects an investigator's experience with clinically apparent infections.

Additional limitations are the lack of a skin test or other means of detecting past exposure, the inability to diagnose subclinical infection with *B. dermatitidis,* and the lack of a sensitive means to identify the ecologic niche of *B. dermatitidis.*

Recent outbreaks and studies of individual cases have provided some insight into the epidemiology of blastomycosis. The respiratory route and direct inoculation of the organism have been well characterized as means of transmission. There are limited data on conjugal and intrauterine transmission although these are not significant methods of infection. There is no evidence to support human-to-human, animal-to-animal, or animal-to-human transmission.

The incubation time seems to be emerging. After inhalation of in-

TABLE 8
Source and Synonyms of Some Strains of *B. dermatitidis* Deposited with the American Type Culture Collection
and Commonly Used in Experimental Studies

ATCC no.	Source	Original report	Synonym	Other publications
26197	Human, cutaneous	Ga-1 (87)		91,93,94,98
26198	Environmental	KL-1 (58)	Den X (89)	60,87,90,91,92,94
26199	Human, cutaneous	SCB-2 (30)		91,93,95–98,100
32090	Environmental	MCG-1 (88)		
60636	Environmental	Eagle River (28)		
60637	Environmental	Tomorrow River (29)		
60915	Human, cutaneous	(99)		
62541	Human, pulmonary	(29)		
62583	Human, pulmonary	(29)		

fectious particles, symptoms occur within 4 to 8 weeks. With primary inoculation blastomycosis, the incubation period is 1 to 5 weeks.

There have been 12 documented outbreaks of blastomycosis in human beings involving from 3 to 48 patients. All patients have probably been exposed to a specific nidus of *B. dermatitidis,* but only twice has this source been unequivocally identified. These two isolations of the fungus from the milieu of the patients have confirmed the conjecture of the natural habitat of *B. dermatitidis,* which began with Stober in 1914 and which had been sought by investigators for many years. The outbreaks have provided a general idea of the geographic distribution of blastomycosis as well as a strong suggestion of the ecologic niche.

There does not appear to be any human susceptibility related to age, race, or sex. Although no special occupation is associated with the disease, accidental infection is more frequent in laboratorians, pathologists, and veterinarians who work with the organism. It appears that those with an exposure to the probable environmental source of *B. dermatitidis,* either by occupation or by avocation, are more apt to become infected.

Although various species of animals have been reported to be infected with *B. dermatitidis,* only dogs are infected in large number. It appears that dogs are probably exposed to the same exogenous saprophytic source of the fungus as man. There is no apparent seasonality of infection in man or dog.

Increased surveillance, better laboratory tests for diagnosis, and a more sensitive method for detecting the organism in nature would enhance our knowledge of the epidemiology of blastomycosis.

REFERENCES

1. Armstrong CW, Jenkins SR, Kaufman L, et al: Common-source outbreak of blastomycosis in hunters and their dogs. *J Infect Dis* 155:568–570, 1987
2. Lieberman A: The case of the fumbled fungus. *J Indiana Med Assoc* 56:1017–1022, 1963
3. Schwarz J, Baum GL: Blastomycosis. *Am J Clin Pathol* 21:999–1029, 1951
4. Schwarz J: Laboratory infections with fungi, in DiSalvo AF (ed): *Occupational Mycoses.* Philadelphia, Lea & Febiger, 1983, pp 215–227
5. Larson DM, Eckman MR, Alber RL, et al: Primary cutaneous (inoculation) blastomycosis: An occupational hazard to pathologists. *Am J Clin Pathol* 79:253–255, 1983
6. Graham WR Jr, Callaway JL: Primary inoculation blastomycosis in a veterinarian. *J Am Acad Dermatol* 7:785–786, 1982
7. Kantor GR, Roenigk RK, Bailin PL, et al: Cutaneous blastomycosis. Report of a case presumably acquired by direct inoculation and treated with carbon dioxide laser vaporization. *Cleveland Clin J Med* 54:121–124, 1987
8. Evans MA: Clinical report of a case of blastomycosis of the skin from accidental inoculation. *JAMA* 40:1772–1775, 1903

9. Carter RR III, Wilson JP, Turner HR, et al: Cutaneous blastomycosis as a complication of transthoracic needle aspiration. *Chest* 91:917–918, 1987

10. Gnann JW Jr, Bressler GS, Bodet CA III, et al: Human blastomycosis after a dog bite. *Ann Intern Med* 98:48–49, 1983

11. Jaspers RH: Transmission of blastomyces from animals to man. *J Am Vet Med Assoc* 164:8, 1974

12. Scott MJ: Cutaneous blastomycosis. Report of case following dog bite. *Northwest Med* 54:255–257, 1955

13. Hiemenz JW, Coccari PH, Macher AM: Human blastomycosis from dog bites. *Ann Intern Med* 98:1030–1031, 1983

14. Craig MW, Davey WN, Green RA: Conjugal blastomycosis. *Am Rev Respir Dis* 102:86–90, 1970

15. Farber ER, Leary MS, Meadows TR: Endometrial blastomycosis acquired by sexual contact. *Obstet Gynecol* 32:195–199, 1968

16. Watts EA, Gard PD Jr, Tuthill SW: First reported case of intrauterine transmission of blastomycosis. *Pediatr Infect Dis* 2:308–310, 1983

17. Neiberg AD, Mavromatis F, Duke J, et al: *Blastomyces dermatitidis* treated during pregnancy: Report of a case. *Am J Obstet Gynecol* 128:911–912, 1977

18. Ismail MA, Lerner SA: Disseminated blastomycosis in a pregnant woman. *Am Rev Respir Dis* 126:350–353, 1982

19. Daniel L, Salit IE: Blastomycosis during pregnancy. *Can Med Assoc J* 131:759–761, 1984

20. Cohen I: Absence of congenital infection and teratogenesis in three children born to mothers with blastomycosis and treated with amphotericin B during pregnancy. *Pediatr Infect Dis* 6:76–77, 1987

21. Hager H, Welt SI, Cardasis JP, et al: Disseminated blastomycosis in a pregnant woman successfully treated with amphotericin-B. A case report. *J Reprod Med* 33:485–488, 1988

22. Procknow JJ: Disseminated blastomycosis treated successfully with the polypeptide antifungal agent X-5079C. Evidence for human to human transmission. *Am Rev Respir Dis* 94:761–772, 1966

23. Tosh FE, Hammerman KJ, Weeks RJ, et al: A common source epidemic of North American blastomycosis. *Am Rev Respir Dis* 109:525–529, 1974

24. Cockerill FR III, Roberts GD, Rosenblatt JE, et al: Epidemic of pulmonary blastomycosis (Namekagon fever) in Wisconsin canoeists. *Chest* 86:688–692, 1984

25. Denton JF, DiSalvo AF, Hirsch ML: Laboratory acquired North American blastomycosis. *JAMA* 199:935–936, 1967

26. Baum GL, Lerner PI: Primary pulmonary blastomycosis: A laboratory acquired infection. *Ann Intern Med* 73:263–265, 1970

27. Sarosi GA, Serstock DS: Isolation of *Blastomyces dermatitidis* from pigeon manure. *Am Rev Respir Dis* 114:1179–1183, 1976

28. Klein BS, Vergeront JM, Weeks RJ, et al: Isolation of *B. dermatitidis* in soil associated with a large outbreak of blastomycosis in Wisconsin. *N Engl J Med* 314:529–534, 1986

29. Klein BS, Vergeront JM, DiSalvo AF, et al: Two outbreaks of blastomycosis along rivers in Wisconsin. *Am Rev Respir Dis* 136:1333–1338, 1987

30. Larsh HW, Schwarz J: Accidental inoculation blastomycosis. *Cutis* 19:334–335, 1977

31. Wilson JW, Cawley EP, Weidman FD, et al: Primary cutaneous North American blastomycosis. *Arch Dermatol* 71:39–45, 1955

32. Harrell ER, Curtis AC: The treatment of North American blastomycosis with amphotericin B. *Arch Dermatol Syphilol* 76:561–569, 1957

33. Landay ME, Schwarz J: Primary cutaneous blastomycosis. *Arch Dermatol* 104:408–411, 1971
34. Butka BJ, Bennett SR, Johnson AC: Disseminated inoculation blastomycosis in a renal transplant recipient. *Am Rev Respir Dis* 130:1180–1183, 1984
35. Conant NF, Smith DT, Baker RD, et al: *Manual of Clinical Mycology,* ed 3. Philadelphia Saunders Co, 1971
36. Vaaler AK, Bradsher RW, Davies SF: Evidence of subclinical blastomycosis in forestry workers in northern Minnesota and northern Wisconsin. Program abstract, American Thoracic Society, 1990
37. Taft EF, Bradsher RW: Subclinical blastomycosis detected by lymphocyte transformation to blastomyces antigen. *Am Rev Respir Dis* 136:A267, 1987
38. Lowry PW, Kelso KY, McFarland LM: Blastomycosis in Washington Parish, Louisiana, 1976–1985. *Am J Epidemiol* 130:151–159, 1989
39. Furcolow ML, Chick EW, Busey JF, et al: Prevalence and incidence studies of human and canine blastomycosis. I. Cases in the US, 1885–1968. *Am Rev Respir Dis* 102:60–67, 1970
40. Landay ME, Mitten J, Millar J: Disseminated blastomycosis in hamsters. II. Effect of sex on susceptibility. *Mycopathol Mycol Appl* 42:73–80, 1970
41. Smith JG, Harris JS, Conant NF, et al: An epidemic of North American blastomycosis. *JAMA* 158:641–646, 1955
42. Furcolow MD, Balows A, Menges RW, et al: Blastomycosis. *JAMA* 198:115, 1966
43. Menges RW, Doto IL, Weeks RJ: Epidemiologic studies of blastomycosis in Arkansas. *Arch Environ Health* 18:956–971, 1969
44. Schwarz J, Salfelder K: Blastomycosis. A review of 152 cases: *Current Topics in Pathology.* Berlin, Springer-Verlag, 1977, pp 165–200
45. Kane J, Righter J, Krajden S, et al: Blastomycosis: a new endemic focus in Canada. *Can Med Assoc J* 129:728–730, 1983
46. Kepron MW, Schoemperlen CB, Hershfield ES, et al: North American blastomycosis in central Canada. A review of 36 cases. *Can Med Assoc J* 106:243–246, 1972
47. Carman WF, Frean JA, Crewe-Brown HH, et al: Blastomycosis in Africa (A review of known cases diagnosed between 1951 and 1987). *Mycopathologia* 107:25–32, 1989
48. Witorsch P, Utz JP: North American blastomycosis: A study of 40 patients. *Medicine* 47:169–200, 1968
49. Busey JE: Blastomycosis: I. A review of 198 collected cases in the VA Hospital. *Am Rev Respir Dis* 89:659–672, 1964
50. Klapman MH, Superfon NP, Solomon LM: North American blastomycosis. *Arch Dermatol* 101:653–658, 1970
51. Schwarz J, Goldman L: Epidemiologic study of North American blastomycosis. *Arch Dermatol* 71:84–88, 1955
52. Chick EW, Sutliff WD, Rakich JH, et al: Epidemiological aspects of cases of blastomycosis admitted to Memphis, Tennessee, hospitals during the period 1922–1954; a review of 86 cases. *Am J Med Sci* 231:253–262, 1956
53. Pfister AK, Hamaty D: A survey of North American blastomycosis in West Virginia. *W Va Med J* 62:434–435, 1966
54. McDonough ES: Epidemiology of 46 Wisconsin cases of North American blastomycosis, 1960–1964. *Mycopathol Mycol Appl* 31:163–173, 1967
55. Centers for Disease Control: Blastomycosis—North Carolina. *MMWR* 25:205–206, 1976
56. Chick EW: The epidemiology of blastomycosis, in Al-Doory Y (ed): *The Epidemiology of Human Mycotic Diseases.* Springfield, Ill, Charles C Thomas, 1975, pp 103–116
57. Schwartzman RM, Fusaro RM, Orkin M: Transmission of North American blastomycosis. Possible case of transmission from dog to human. *JAMA* 171:2185–2189, 1959

58. Denton JF, McDonough ES, Ajello L, et al: Isolation of *Blastomyces dermatitidis* from soil. *Science* 133:1126–1128, 1961

59. McDonough ES: Studies on the growth and survival of *Blastomyces dermatitidis* in soil. Recent progress in microbiology. *Int Congr Microbiol* 8:656–661, 1963

60. Denton JF, DiSalvo AF: Effects of temperature on soil conidia of *Blastomyces dermatitidis*. *J Bacteriol* 85:717–718, 1963

61. Denton JF, DiSalvo AF: The prevalence of Cryptococcus neoformans in various natural habitat. *J Int Soc Hum Anim Mycol* 6:213, 1968

62. Kitchen MS, Reiber CD, Eastin GB: An urban epidemic of North American blastomycosis. *Am Rev Respir Dis* 115:1063–1066, 1977

63. Frye MD, Seifer FD: An outbreak of blastomycosis in eastern Tennessee. *Mycopathologia* 116:15–21, 1991

64. Chick EW, Peters HJ, Denton JF: *Die Nordamerikanische blastomykose: Ergebnisse der allgemeinen pathologic und pathologischen anatomie.* Berlin, Springer-Verlag, 1960, pp 34–98

65. Menges RW, Furcolow ML, Selby LA: Clinical and epidemiologic studies on 79 canine blastomycosis cases in Arkansas. *Am J Epidemiol* 81:164–179, 1965

66. Sarosi GA, Eckman MR, Davies SC, et al: Canine blastomycosis as a harbinger of human disease. *Ann Intern Med* 91:733–735, 1979

67. McDonough ES, Kuzma JF: Epidemiological studies on blastomycosis in the State of Wisconsin. *Sabouraudia* 18:173–183, 1980

68. Archer JR, Trainer DO, Schell RJ: Epidemiologic study of canine blastomycosis in Wisconsin. *J Am Vet Med Assoc* 190:1292–1295, 1987

69. Tesh RB, Schneidau JD Jr: Experimental infection of bats (Tadarida brasiliensis) with *Blastomyces dermatitidis*. *J Infect Dis* 117:188–192, 1967

70. Chaturvedi VP, Randhawa HS, Kini S, et al: Survival of *Blastomyces dermatitidis* in the gastrointestinal tract of an orally infected insectivorous bat, *Rhinopoma hardwickei* Gray. *J Med Vet Mycol* 24:349–352, 1986

71. Khan ZU, Randhawa HS, Lulla M: Isolation of *Blastomyces dermatitidis* from the lungs of a bat, Rhinopoma hardwickei gray, in Delhi. *Sabouraudia* 20:137–144, 1982

72. Randhawa HS, Chaturvedi VP, Kini S: *Blastomyces dermatitidis* in bats: First report of its isolation from the liver of *Rhinopoma hardwickei* Gray. *J Med Vet Mycol* 23:69–76, 1985

73. DiSalvo AF: The role of bats in the ecology of *Histoplasma capsulatum,* in Ajello L, Chick EW, Furcolow ML (eds): *Histoplasmosis.* Springfield, Ill, Charles C Thomas, 1971, pp 149–161

74. DiSalvo AF: Blastomycosis an environmental puzzle. Editorial, *JSCMA* 84:558–559, 1988

75. Duttera MJ Jr, Osterhout S: North American blastomycosis. A survey of 63 cases. *South Med J* 62:295–301, 1969

76. DiSalvo AF: Blastomycosis, in DiSalvo AF (ed): *Occupational Mycoses.* Philadelphia, Lea & Febiger, 1983, pp 79–94

77. Ricketts HT: Oidiomycosis of the skin and its fungi. *J Med Res* 6:374–554, 1901

78. Stober AM: Systemic blastomycosis: A report of its pathological, bacteriological and clinical features. *Arch Intern Med* 13:509–556, 1914

79. Bradsher RW: Water and blastomycosis: Don't blame beaver. An editorial. *Am Rev Respir Dis* 136:1324–1326, 1987

80. Daniel L, Salit IE: Blastomycosis during pregnancy. *Can Med Assoc J* 131:759–761, 1984

81. Lawrence RM: Acute pulmonary blastomycosis acquired in west Texas. *Tex Med* 77:50–51, 1981

82. Varkey B, Lohaus G, Rose HD, et al: Blastomycosis: Clinical and immunologic aspects. *Chest* 77:789–795, 1980

83. Bakerspigel A, Kane J, Schaus D: Isolation of *Blastomyces dermatitidis* from an earthen floor in southwestern Ontario, Canada. *J Clin Microbiol* 24:890–891, 1986

84. Klein BS, Vergeront JM, Davis JP: Epidemiologic aspects of blastomycosis, the enigmatic systemic mycosis. *Semin Respir Infect* 1:29–39, 1986

85. Archer JR: Epidemiology of canine blastomycosis in Wisconsin. A thesis submitted in partial fulfillment of the requirements for the degree Master of Science. University of Wisconsin, Stevens Point, 1985

86. Denton JF, DiSalvo AF: Additional isolations of *Blastomyces dermatitidis* from natural sites. *Am J Trop Med Hyg* 28:697–700, 1979

87. DiSalvo AF, Denton JF: Lipid content of four strains of *B. dermatitidis* of different mouse virulence. *J Bacteriol* 85:927–931, 1963

88. Denton JF, DiSalvo AF: Isolation of *Blastomyces dermatitidis* from natural sites at Augusta, GA. *Am J Trop Med* 13:716–722, 1964

89. McDonough ES, Wisniewski TR, Penn LA, et al: Preliminary studies on conidial liberation of *Blastomyces dermatitidis* and *Histoplasma capsulatum. Sabouraudia* 14:199–204, 1976

90. Frey CL, Demarsh PL, Drutz DJ: Divergent patterns of pulmonary blastomycosis induced by conidia and yeasts in athymic and euthymic mice. *Am Rev Respir Dis* 140:118, 1989

91. Drutz DJ, Frey CL: Intracellular and extracellular defenses of human phagocytes against *Blastomyces dermatitidis* conidia and yeasts. *J Lab Clin Med* 105:737–750, 1985

92. Denton JF, DiSalvo AF: Respiratory infection of laboratory animals with conidia of *Blastomyces dermatitidis. Mycopathol Mycol Appl* 36:129–136, 1968

93. Sugar AM, Field KG: Susceptibility of *Blastomyces dermatitidis* conidia to products of oxidative metabolism. *Exp Mycol* 12:84–89, 1988

94. Cox RA, Mills LR, Best GK, et al: Histologic reactions to cell walls of an avirulent and a virulent strain of *Blastomyces dermatitidis. J Infect Dis* 129:179–186, 1974

95. Cox RA, Larsh HW: Isolation of skin test-active preparations from yeast-phase cells of *B. dermatitidis. Infect Immun* 10:42–47, 1974

96. Cox RA, Larsh HW: Yeast and mycelial phase of *Blastomyces dermatitidis:* Comparison using disc gel electrophoresis. *Infect Immun* 10:48–53, 1974

97. Morozumi PA, Halpern JW, Stevens DA: Susceptibility differences in inbred strains of mice to blastomycosis. *Infect Immun* 32:160–168, 1981

98. Brummer E, Stevens DA: Enhancing effect of murine polymorphonuclear neutrophils (PMN) on the multiplication of *Blastomyces dermatitidis* in vitro and in vivo. *Clin Exp Immunol* 54:587–594, 1983

99. Brass C, Volkman CM, Philpott DE, et al. Spontaneous mutant of *B. dermatitidis* attenuated in virulence for mice. *Sabouraudia* 20:145–158, 1982

100. Vaaler AK, Bradsher RW, Davies SF: Evidence of subclinical blastomycosis in forestry workers in northern Minnesota and northern Wisconsin. *Am J Med* 89:470–476, 1990

6

Diagnosis of Blastomycosis

Norman L. Goodman

Blastomycosis has numerous clinical manifestations and is clinically indistinguishable from many other fungal and bacterial diseases; therefore, a definitive diagnosis can be made only in the laboratory. A successful laboratory
diagnosis depends upon a series of procedures usually performed by several
people. None of these procedures is more important than the initial steps of
selecting the site from which the specimen is to be collected and collecting
the specimen. Without a good specimen, containing an appropriate number
of viable organisms, the expertise of the laboratorian is compromised. All
personnel involved in specimen selection, collection, and processing should
keep in mind that a laboratory test is no better than the specimen and the
specimen no better than the manner in which it was collected.

1. SPECIMEN SELECTION

The choice of site from which a specimen is collected often influences
the outcome of the diagnosis. There are several factors to consider when
selecting clinical specimens. (1) Obviously, the site of infection is important.
The specimen should be collected from a site in which the fungus is actively

Blastomycosis, edited by Yousef Al-Doory and Arthur F. DiSalvo, Plenum Medical Book Company, New York, 1992.

growing—an active lesion. For example, needle aspirate material from the center of a caseous pulmonary lesion may contain few, if any, viable organisms or scrapings from the center of a spontaneously healing cutaneous lesion often will not contain viable *Blastomyces dermatitidis.* (2) The site of infection is related to the stage of disease: primary, chronic, or disseminated. In primary pulmonary disease, the disease is localized, thus the specimen must be collected from that site. In primary disease, the fungus is often present in small numbers, sequestered in a small area and not released into sputum or other secretions. Such conditions make biopsy of the infected organ necessary for obtaining a diagnosis. Serological testing is often a helpful adjunctive test in this form of the disease. In chronic pulmonary disease, however, there is usually considerable tissue damage, with profuse growth of the fungus allowing us to isolate and identify the fungus from sputum without difficulty.

In disseminated blastomycosis, we have the option of collecting specimens from multiple sites, e.g., the prostate is often infected, making urine a good specimen to examine and culture. Cutaneous and subcutaneous lesions are common manifestations of disseminated disease. The cutaneous lesions usually are grossly contaminated by skin flora, but closed, subcutaneous abscesses are ideal sources of uncontaminated specimens when collected by aspiration. Furthermore, an aspirated specimen from a closed lesion, or draining site, is preferable to a sputum specimen.

2. SPECIMEN COLLECTION

A major portion of the mycological evaluations in the clinical laboratory are performed on seven types of specimens: Lower respiratory (sputum and bronchial washes), exudate, tissue, blood, cerebrospinal fluid, and urine.[1-3]

2.1. Pulmonary Secretions

2.1.1. Sputum

Sputum is the specimen most frequently submitted to the laboratory for the diagnosis of blastomycosis. Because the upper respiratory tract and oral cavity are heavily colonized by bacteria and yeasts, and may harbor other transient fungi, sputum should be collected in a manner that will prevent gross contamination. The specimen must be lower respiratory secretions, not saliva or sinus discharge. Most patients are unaware of this distinction, and they must be taught how to properly raise the sputum specimen.

Sputum should be collected early in the morning soon after the patient awakens. The patient's teeth should be brushed, or dentures removed, and the mouth thoroughly rinsed with water immediately before collecting the specimen. Ten to fifteen milliliters of sputum should be collected. The specimen should be collected in a sterile, screw-capped container, properly labeled, and promptly delivered to the laboratory.

2.1.2. Bronchial Washings

Bronchial washings should be placed in a sterile, screw-capped container, completely sealed, properly labeled, and delivered immediately to the laboratory. Specimens collected with single-lumen bronchoscopes are usually contaminated with upper respiratory flora while those collected by double-lumen scopes are not.

2.2. Exudates and Pus

Blastomycosis often presents with cutaneous and subcutaneous lesions. It may also present as abscesses in internal organs, including brain, from which exudates or pus may be collected for examination and culture. Specimens from these sites are very good because they contain no contaminating organisms. When closed lesions or abscesses are present, the specimen *should always be aspirated.* Specimens from open, cutaneous lesions also should be aspirated, if possible. If only a very small amount of exudate is present, aspirate the material into a tuberculin syringe, then aspirate a small amount of sterile saline to wash the specimen from the needle and syringe hub. The aspirated specimen may be left in the syringe, with needle removed and cap in place, or, preferably, expel the specimen into a sterile, screw-capped container, tightly seal, properly label, and transport directly to the laboratory.

Collecting specimens by swab is an inferior procedure for fungal evaluation. If swabs must be used, use at least two, small, nonabsorbent swabs and collect as much specimen as possible. Place the swabs in a sterile tube, seal the tube, and immediately take it to the laboratory.

2.3. Tissue

Tissue obtained by biopsy taken in the operating room or in the clinic or office is an excellent specimen for fungal culture and histopathological study.

The specimen should be collected under aseptic conditions and placed into a sterile, screw-capped container containing a small amount of sterile saline (without preservative) or sterile distilled water. The container should be tightly sealed, properly labeled, and immediately taken to the laboratory for processing. Large pieces of tissue from surgery or autopsy should be placed in moist, sterile gauze; placed in a sterile container; sealed and taken directly to the laboratory. Care must be taken to prevent drying and contamination of the specimen. If the tissue specimen cannot be immediately processed, it may be refrigerated, *but should not be frozen.*

2.4. Urine

The kidneys and prostate are often involved when a patient has disseminated blastomycosis; urine is an appropriate specimen in that form of disease.

It is essential that urine specimens be properly collected to prevent contamination with bacteria and yeasts from the genitalia.

Urine specimens may be collected by the midstream, clean-catch technique or with a sterile needle and syringe from the soft rubber connector of an indwelling catheter. Specimens must not be collected from the urine bag. If clean-catch specimens are used, the genitalia must be thoroughly cleansed prior to collecting the specimen.

Urine specimens should be collected in a sterile, screw-capped container, sealed, properly labeled, and transported immediately to the laboratory. If the specimen cannot be examined immediately, it should be refrigerated.

2.5. Cerebrospinal Fluid (CSF)

Blastomyces dermatitidis rarely causes meningitis and is rarely isolated from CSF. Therefore, CSF is not a specimen of choice for diagnosing this disease. CSF should be collected aseptically and care should be taken to prevent contamination. The sterile collection tube should have a lid that completely seals; preferably a screw-capped tube. In most cases, three sterile tubes of CSF are collected; the third tube should be used for mycological examination and culture. The specimen should be immediately taken to the laboratory for processing. If it cannot be processed immediately, the specimen should be left at room temperature or, preferably, incubated at 30°C.

2.6. Blood

Blastomyces dermatitidis is very rarely isolated from the blood; however, this specimen is often collected in cases with disseminated disease.

Blood specimens should be collected aseptically at the patient's bedside and placed directly into the culture medium or container provided for the blood culture system used.

There are other types of specimens that may be received in the laboratory, or for which you will be asked to recommend methods of collection. The basic rule to follow in collecting specimens is to preserve the specimen in the state in which it exists in the host. In this state, any organism in the specimen should remain viable, giving you the optimal chance to observe the fungal elements in the specimen and culture it on the appropriate medium. Any action that alters the state of the specimen may also alter the morphological form and viability of the fungus and result in erroneous interpretation of laboratory information.

When the appropriately collected specimen arrives in the laboratory, it should be examined and processed in a manner that will preserve the morphological integrity and viability of the etiological agent. In some cases, e.g., urine and CSF, the specimen should be centrifuged or filtered to concentrate the fungus. Preparations for microscopic examination should be made from the processed specimen at the same time the specimen is cultured.

3. DIRECT MICROSCOPIC EXAMINATION

A culturally proved laboratory diagnosis of blastomycosis will take several days or weeks. Without at least a tentative laboratory diagnosis, the physician must manage the patient on the basis of clinical data and judgment.

Frequently, *B. dermatitidis* can be seen in a fresh clinical specimen, providing the clinician information to make a tentative diagnosis and appropriately manage the patient.[1-4] The procedure for direct microscopic examination is easy to perform and provides information within a few minutes after the specimen is collected. Of course, all specimens must also be appropriately cultured.

Mounts for microscopic examination may be made as wet preparations with or without stain; as fixed smears with stain, or fixed, stained tissue. Wet preparations are most rapid, but stained specimens are often easier to read but more time-consuming.

A direct wet mount is made as follows:

1. Place a drop of 10% KOH containing 10% glycerol on a clean microscope slide. Add a small amount of the specimen to be examined and
   mix the two.
2. Add a clean coverslip to the drop.
3. Gently heat the slide over a flame to facilitate clearing the specimen;
   do not allow to boil.
4. Let the mount stand at room temperature for approximately 10–15
   min, or until the specimen clears.
5. Examine microscopically for the presence of fungal elements.

Fungi in the specimen will be more visible if a phase microscope is used.
When a standard brightfield microscope is used, the light intensity should be
reduced by reducing the opening in the iris diaphragm. Do not lower the
condenser.

The visibility of fungi in a wet preparation may be greatly enhanced by
using the dye Calcofluor White.[5] Calcofluor White may be used alone to
stain wet preparations or it may be used with KOH by adding one drop of
KOH and one drop of Calcofluor White to the specimen, add the coverslip,
allow to clear, and examine microscopically. A fluorescence microscope is
required for using Calcofluor White and specific filters are necessary to obtain the proper staining. Consult with your fluorescence microscope representative for the proper filters. With proper filters in place, fungal elements
will fluoresce white to bright green. This stain is very helpful in detecting *B.
dermatitidis* in clinical specimens.

Clinical specimens may be smeared and fixed on microscope slides and
stained by several methods. The most commonly used are the periodic acid–
Schiff (PAS), Giemsa, and Wright stains. All are excellent stains for fungi,
but are more time-consuming than the wet preparation described above.
Fungal elements—especially *B. dermatitidis*—may also be seen in Papanicolaou's (PAP) stained cytological preparations.

The Gram stain is commonly used to detect fungi in clinical specimens;
however, if the smear is heat fixed, the fungal cell is often distorted and is not
easily recognizable. For this reason, I do not recommend the Gram stain for
detecting fungi in clinical specimens.

Permanent sections of tissue are usually prepared for histopathological
studies and examination for fungal elements. Hematoxylin and eosin (H &
E), PAS, and Gomori methenamine silver (GMS) stains are appropriate to
demonstrate *B. dermatitidis* in tissue sections[1-3] (see Chapter 10).

Blastomyces dermatitidis is morphologically the same in all of these

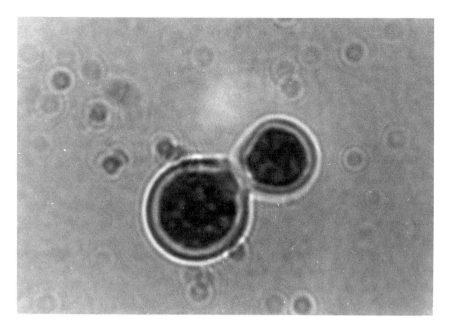

FIGURE 1. Potassium hydroxide wet preparation of sputum containing yeast of *B. dermatitidis*. 1000×.

preparations: a large single budding yeast, 8–15 μm in size, with a thick, toured" cell wall. Budding cells are connected by a broad base. Figure 1 is a KOH preparation of sputum containing *B. dermatitidis*. The fungus would appear morphologically similar in a Calcofluor White preparation, except the cell wall would fluoresce a brilliant apple-green when appropriate filters are used. The same morphological features are seen in permanent tissue sections stained with the accepted tissue stains (Fig. 2). These morphological features are unique to *B. dermatitidis* and when multiple yeasts with this characteristic are seen, a presumptive diagnosis can be made with confidence.

4. PROCESSING AND CULTURING CLINICAL SPECIMENS

When the correctly collected specimen is received in the laboratory, it should be processed as quickly as possible and in a manner that will preserve the etiologic agent(s) in their natural and viable form. Concentrating the organisms may increase the chance of recovering them.[1-3,6]

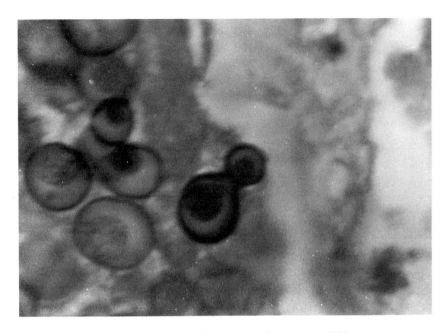

FIGURE 2. *B. dermatitidis* in section of lung tissue. 1000×.

4.1. Specimen Processing

The first step in "processing" a specimen is to determine the probability of the specimen containing only one organism—the etiologic agent—or multiple organisms—"contaminants." If only the etiologic agent is expected, minimal manipulation of the specimen is necessary.

4.1.1. Sputum

The recovery of *B. dermatitidis,* and other fungi, may be increased by selecting the mucopurulent portions for examination and culture. This material may be processed in two ways:

4.1.1.1. Unconcentrated. (a) Use two swabs, chopstick style, and retrieve the purulent material from the sputum.

(b) Spread approximately 0.5 ml of the specimen over the agar surface.

(c) Prepare wet mounts of the same specimen.

4.1.1.2. Concentrated. (a) Lyse the sputum by adding an equal volume of 0.5% *N*-acetyl-L-cysteine to the sputum. Thoroughly mix.

(b) Centrifuge the specimen to concentrate.

(c) Pipette 0.5 ml of the sediment to the surface of an agar plate and evenly spread the inoculum over the surface.

(d) Prepare a wet preparation for microscopic examination.

You should remember that the contaminating organisms in sputum will also be concentrated when the specimen is centrifuged and may overgrow nonselective media.

4.1.2. Bronchial Washings and Other Nonmucoid Respiratory Specimens

Pipette 0.5 ml to each plate and spread the inoculum evenly over the agar surface.

4.1.3. Exudates

(a) Aspirate from closed lesion. Treat as uncontaminated. Spread over the surface of nonselective media. Make a wet preparation for microscopic examination.

(b) Swab or aspirate from open lesion. Treat as contaminated. Spread the specimen over the surface of selective (inhibitory) and nonselective (noninhibitory) medium. Make a wet preparation for microscopic examination.

4.1.4. Tissue

(a) Place aseptically collected tissue into a sterile grinding vessel and homogenize the tissue. Spread 0.5 ml of the homogenate over the surface of each unit of nonselective media.

(b) Homogenize (grind) contaminated tissue as in (a) above and spread 0.5 ml over the surface of each plate of selective media.

4.1.5. Urine

Concentrate the urine by centrifugation and inoculate 0.5 ml of the sediment onto the surface of selective and nonselective media.

4.1.6. CSF

Spinal fluid may be processed by centrifugation or use of a 0.45-μm membrane filter.

(a) Centrifugation. Transfer the CSF specimen to a sterile, conical centrifuge tube. Centrifuge at 1500*g* for 15 min. Place four or five drops of the concentrated specimen onto the surface of a nonselective enriched medium.

(b) Filtration. Use a sterile syringe with a Swinnex adapter, fitted with a sterile 0.45-μm membrane filter. Pass the CSF through the filter. Aseptically remove the filter and place it, with side holding concentrate down, onto the surface of an enriched, nonselective medium. Each following day, lift the filter and place it onto a new site of the agar surface.

4.1.7. Blood

As stated earlier, *B. dermatitidis* is rarely isolated from blood, but blood is often cultured in disseminated fungal disease.

The DuPont Isolator appears to be the most effective system for isolating fungi from blood. Many commercial systems with biphasic media will grow fungi from blood more effectively than liquid bacterial blood culture systems. All systems require a specified volume of blood and each system has specific instructions for its correct use.

Many other specimen types may be processed for blastomycosis and other fungi. The primary rule in processing specimens is to treat the specimen in a way that will maintain the viability and morphological integrity of the etiologic agent.

4.2. Medium Selection

Selecting the proper medium for isolating *B. dermatitidis* from a clinical specimen is a critical step in diagnosing this fungal disease. The primary goal is to isolate the organism, then grow it in an identifiable form.

There are numerous media suitable for the recovery of *B. dermatitidis* from clinical specimens. If the specimen probably contains only one fungus, it is appropriate to use a single, enriched, medium with limited surface area to prevent drying, e.g., tubed media. If, however, the specimen contains multiple organisms, a battery of media, including a selective (inhibitory) agar medium, with a large surface area, e.g., petri dish, should be used to provide isolated colonies.[1]

Commonly used enriched media are:

(1) Brain heart infusion (BHI) agar
(2) BHI with 5% sheep blood
(3) Sabouraud brain heart infusion (SABHI) agar
(4) SABHI with 5% sheep blood

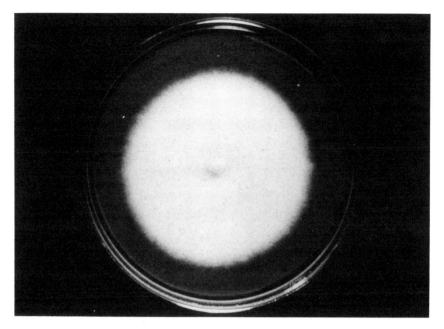

FIGURE 3. Mold culture of *B. dermatitidis* grown on modified Sabouraud agar at 30°C. (Reprinted by permission of ASM.)

Commonly used selective (inhibitory) media are:

(1) Sabouraud dextrose agar (SDA)
(2) SDA, BHI, and SABHI with 16 μg/ml chloramphenicol and 5 μg/ml gentamicin for inhibiting bacteria
(3) SDA, BHI, and SABHI with the above antibiotics and 500 μg/ml cycloheximide, for inhibiting bacteria and rapidly growing molds
(4) Inhibitory mold agar
(5) Yeast extract phosphate agar—a highly inhibitory medium for isolating *B. dermatitidis* and *Histoplasma capsulatum* from grossly contaminated specimens

The choice of media used in the laboratory should be made on the basis of the type of specimens received. Highly contaminated, mailed specimens received in a reference laboratory require different media than specimens from a pediatric hospital laboratory. In all cases, an enriched medium should be included in the battery of media.[1,2] At least one selective (inhibitory) medium should be included when multiple organisms may reside in the

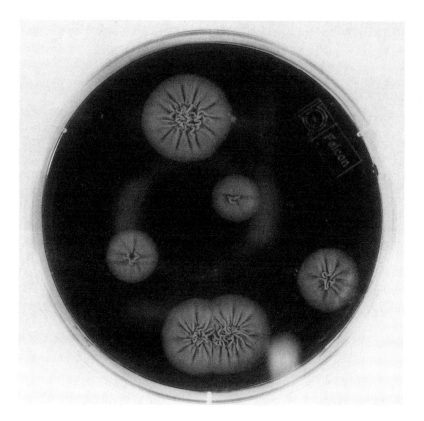

FIGURE 4. Mold culture of *B. dermatitidis* grown on brain heart infusion blood agar at 30°C.

specimen. Despite a long history of use, Sabouraud dextrose agar is not recommended for the primary isolation of *B. dermatitidis,* or other dimorphic fungi. It is acceptable to use in the battery of primary isolation media, provided another selective medium is also included.

4.3. Culture Procedure

The initial step in culturing the specimen is to determine if it is likely to contain multiple organisms, requiring the use of selective media. If the specimen is collected from a normally sterile site, e.g., pleural fluid, it can be

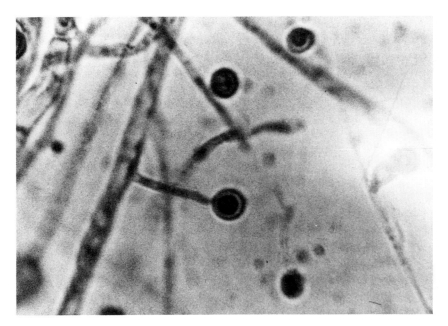

FIGURE 5. Microscopic morphology of mold form of *B. dermatitidis.* Note conidium on long conidiophore. 900×.

inoculated directly onto an enriched medium, such as BHI blood agar, which will provide an optimal environment for *B. dermatitidis,* or other fungi. However, if the specimen is expected to contain multiple organisms, selective media must be used. It is logical that since the isolation of colonies is necessary, a large surface area must be provided by using petri plates or bottles of agar.

Blastomyces dermatitidis and other disease-causing fungi are aerobic and generally grow optimally at 25 to 30°C. If logistically practical, cultures should be incubated at 30°C. Special procedures must be used for plated cultures incubated at 30°C: (1) the plate should contain 25–30 ml of medium (thick-pour), (2) the plate should be incubated in a humid environment, and (3) the plate lid should be secured to prevent it from falling from the plate. Rubber bands may be used or the opposite sides of the plate may be tabbed with tape. The plate should not be sealed with nondiffusible tape. A cabinet containing beakers of water is usually sufficient.

All cultures should be examined at least twice weekly for fungal growth and should be held at least 4 weeks before reporting them as negative.

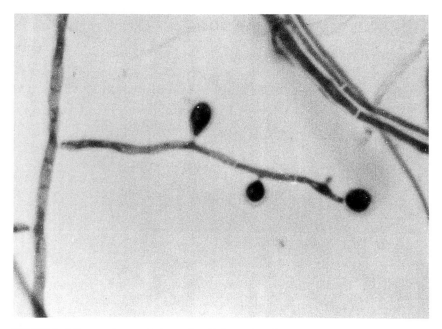

FIGURE 6. Microscopic morphology of mold form of *B. dermatitidis.* Note conidia on short conidiophores. 1100×.

5. IDENTIFICATION

5.1. Culture

The identification of *B. dermatitidis* is primarily dependent on recognized morphological characteristics of its yeast form, although it is commonly isolated in its mold form. Therefore, for a morphological identification, it must be converted from the mold form to the yeast form. In general, such conversion is easily accomplished on enriched media, such as BHI blood agar and cottonseed extract agar, incubated at 37°C. However, Middlebrook's 7H10 medium has been found to be the medium of choice for converting *B. dermatitidis.* Many isolates have produced identifiable yeasts on this medium in 24 h.[7]

Morphology. The mold (mycelial) form of *B. dermatitidis,* when grown on Sabouraud dextrose agar at 25–30°C, usually appears as a small, white, floccose colony in 7–10 days (Fig. 3), and will continue to enlarge and turn gray to tan with age. On enriched media, such as blood agar, incubated at 25–30°C, this mold grows as a glabrous or feltlike colony which is usually wrinkled and folded (Fig. 4). Conidium formation usually does not occur in

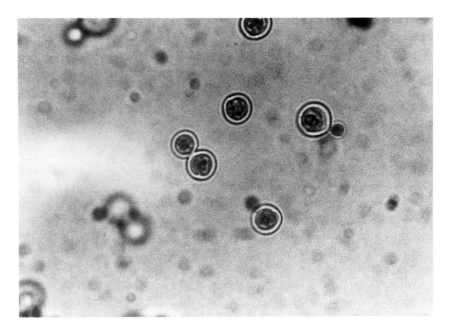

FIGURE 7. Microscopic morphology of yeast form of *B. dermatitidis.* 900×.

these colonies, so the culture should be transferred to modified Sabouraud dextrose agar to demonstrate the classical mold morphology. The conidia of *B. dermatitidis* are 2–10 μm in diameter, round to pyriform, and are borne on the tips of long or short conidiophores (Figs. 5 and 6). The conidia of *B. dermatitidis* must be differentiated from those of *Chrysosporium* spp., *Scedosporium apiospermium,* and *Trichophyton* spp.

The yeast form of *B. dermatitidis,* when grown on an enriched medium at 35–37°C, is a characteristically large, 8–15 μm in diameter, yeast. The yeasts are uniformly spherical, with a thick, refractile cell wall. A single bud is attached to the mother cell by a 4- to 5-μm-wide septum, which is a diagnostic characteristic (Fig. 7). Young, budding yeasts may occasionally produce narrow septa and thin-walled daughter cells.

The characteristic budding yeast form must be seen to make a definitive diagnosis of blastomycosis on the basis of culture morphology.

5.2. Exoantigen

Some isolates of *B. dermatitidis* grow slowly or pleomorphically and often do not sporulate well. Although, as previously stated, most isolates will readily convert to the yeast form, it is often advantageous to identify this fungus by another diagnostic procedure, the exoantigen technique. This procedure can be used to identify nonsporulating *B. dermatitidis,* and many other fungi.[8-11] DiSalvo has shown that this procedure may be used to identify mixed and nonviable mold cultures.[12,13]

The exoantigen procedure is easy to perform, is relatively inexpensive, and can be completed in 48 h. The test does, however, require a mature fungal colony.

The mold form of *B. dermatitidis* produce exoantigen (cell-free antigens) that are homologous to the diagnostic precipitins of the classical immunodiffusion test for antibody. The detection of specific exoantigen homologous to *B. dermatitidis* precipitin A, in an immunodiffusion test system, accurately identifies the fungus as *B. dermatitidis.* The procedure is performed as follows:

Cover a 10-day or older mold culture, growing on Sabouraud agar slant, with minimal growth area of 15×30 mm, with 8–10 ml of 1:5000 aqueous merthiolate solution. Leave the solution in place for 24–48 h, at room temperature. The soluble antigen diffuses into the solution. (Extraction may be enhanced if the agar slant is cut in two or three places to allow the extraction solution to penetrate more readily.[14]) Transfer the extract to an Amicon B-15 concentrator and concentrate it to $50\times$. Use the concentrated extract as the unknown (test) antigen in an immunodiffusion system. The extract (antigen) is tested against known, standardized, antiserum containing anti-*B. dermatitidis* A antibody. An immunodiffusion band of identity with this homologous antiserum is specific. Detailed procedures for performing the exoantigen test may be found in Refs. 10 and 11. It should be noted that a positive test is specific, but a negative test is not. Reagents and immunodiffusion plates are commercially available.

5.3. DNA Probes

Detection and identification of microorganisms, including fungi, is becoming more rapid with the development of DNA/RNA probes. The detection of small amounts of specific DNA or RNA of pathogenic fungi will allow the identification of fungi much faster than by morphology or exoantigen. Preliminary data on DNA probe assays for *B. dermatitidis* indicate that colonies of this fungus can be identified in the early stage of growth.[15]

This technology promises to greatly improve our ability to rapidly diagnose cases of blastomycosis and other mycoses.

REFERENCES

1. Koneman EW, Roberts GD: *Practical Laboratory Mycology,* ed 3. Baltimore, Williams & Wilkins, 1985
2. Larsh HW, Goodman NL: Fungi of systemic mycoses, in Lennette EH, Balows A, Hausler WJ, Shadomy JH (eds): *Manual of Clinical Microbiology,* ed 4. Washington, DC, American Society for Microbiology, 1985, pp 542–553
3. Rippon JW: *Medical Mycology: The Pathogenic Fungi and the Pathogenic Actinomycetes,* ed 3. Philadelphia, WB Saunders Co, 1988
4. Goodman NL: Direct microscopy in diagnosing fungal diseases. *Diagn Med* February 1985, pp 1–5
5. Hageage GT, Harrington BJ: Use of Calcofluor White in clinical mycology. *Lab Med* 15(2):109–112, 1984
6. Hariri AR, Hempel HO, Goodman NL: Effects of time lapse between sputum collection and culturing on isolation of clinically significant fungi. *J Clin Microbiol* 15(3):425–428, 1973
7. Hyden S, Goodman NL: Unpublished data
8. Kaufman L, Standard PG: Immunoidentification of cultures of fungi pathogenic to man. *Curr Microbiol* 1:135–140, 1973
9. Kaufman L, McLaughlin DW, Clark MJ, et al: Specific immunodiffusion test for blastomycosis. *Appl Microbiol* 26:244–247, 1973
10. Kaufman L, Reiss E: Serodiagnosis of fungal diseases, in Lennette EH, Balows A, Hausler WJ, Shadomy HJ (eds): *Manual of Clinical Microbiology,* ed 4. Washington, DC, American Society for Microbiology, 1985, pp 941–942
11. Standard PG, Kaufman L, Whaley SD: Exoantigen Test: Rapid Identification of Pathogenic Mould Isolates by Immunodiffusion. Immunology Series No. 11, Procedural Guide, US Department of Health and Human Services, PHS, CDC, Atlanta, 1985
12. DiSalvo AF, Terreni AA, Wooten AK: Use of the exoantigen test to identify *Blastomyces dermatitidis, Coccidioides immitis* and *Histoplasma capsulatum* in mixed cultures. *Am J Clin Pathol* 75(6):825–826, 1981
13. DiSalvo AF, Melonas J: Exoantigen identification of non-viable mycotic pathogens. Abstracts, X Congress of the International Society for Human and Animal Mycology, Barcelona, 1988
14. Standard PG: Personal communication
15. Rubin SM, Murphy-Clark KA, Bee GG, et al: Development of rapid non-isotopic DNA probe assays for fungi: *Blastomyces dermatitidis.* Abstracts of the 90th Annual Meeting of the ASM, 1990

7

Immunodiagnosis of Blastomycosis

Leo Kaufman

1. INTRODUCTION

Blastomycosis in its acute, chronic, or disseminated form does not present a distinct clinical picture. Its diagnosis is further complicated by the fact that the disease occurs in geographical areas where other mycotic diseases such as coccidioidomycosis and histoplasmosis, which cause similar clinical manifestations, are endemic. In addition, no reliable skin test is available to help identify cases. Differential diagnosis is difficult, and laboratory studies are essential for the diagnosis of blastomycosis.

Isolation of *Blastomyces dermatitidis* allows an unequivocal diagnosis. In many instances the fungus may be readily isolated and identified; however, in some situations, cultures from clinical specimens cannot be readily obtained, or isolation attempts are unsuccessful. In those circumstances, alternative laboratory procedures must be used to arrive at a diagnosis.

Immunologic tests are another means of diagnosing blastomycosis. Until 1973, such tests were considered ineffective because of their low sensitiv-

Blastomycosis, edited by Yousef Al-Doory and Arthur F. DiSalvo, Plenum Medical Book Company, New York, 1992.

ity and specificity. However, in 1973 Kaufman et al.[1] found that B. dermatitidis produces a specific antigen, which is designated A. This antigen subsequently was shown to be a glycoprotein constituent of the cell wall of the yeast form of B. dermatitidis.[2,3] Incorporation of the A antigen in complement fixation (CF),[2,4] immunodiffusion (ID),[1,2,4,5] enzyme immunosorbent assay (EIA),[6,7] Western blot,[8] and fluorescent antibody (FA)[2,9] tests led to the development of more sensitive and specific tests. These tests used alone or in combination have proven to be useful for the early diagnosis or monitoring of blastomycosis in humans,[1,6,10] canines,[10,11] dolphins,[12] and wolves.[13]

The intent in this chapter is to acquaint the reader with the currently available tests and to review their value in diagnosing blastomycosis.

2. DIAGNOSTIC TESTS

2.1. Complement Fixation Test

The CF test is time-consuming and complex. Properly controlled and performed, it provides reproducible results. It relies on the binding of complement by an antigen–antibody complex. This primary complex consists of B. dermatitidis antigen and homologous antibody from a patient's serum. An indicator system consisting of a second antigen–antibody complex, hemolysin, and sheep red blood cells is included to reveal whether complement has been bound by the primary complex. The fixation of complement indicates the presence of antibody as revealed by the absence of hemolysis. Human serum and cerebral spinal fluid (CSF) may readily be tested for evidence of B. dermatitidis antibodies. Titers of 1:8 are considered presumptive evidence of infection. The CF test is limited by the fact that canine and other lower animal specimens may be nontestable due to anticomplementary activity.

Serum CF tests with intact or ground yeast-form antigens of B. dermatitidis have historically been regarded as insensitive and nonspecific. The specificity of the test was substantially improved with the use of a diethylaminoethyl (DEAE) column-purified A antigen.[4,7] The CF test is capable of detecting acute and chronic disease but not as effectively as the EIA test.[6,10] Low sensitivity, ranging from 40% to 62%,[1,4,7,14] however, continues to hinder widespread use of the test. In a study using sera from 65 persons with proven blastomycosis and 168 controls,[7] the CF test (although completely specific) demonstrated only a 40% sensitivity. In spite of this low sensitivity, the test can be valuable in an epidemic since CF antibodies to the A antigen may be recognized as early as 1 month after the onset of illness.[10] Although CF reactions are helpful in establishing a diagnosis, they have limited value in determining prognosis. In established cases of blastomycosis, a decline in CF titer is evidence of a favorable prognosis. The serologic response, however, is often not as rapid as the clinical response.[1]

2.2. Immunodiffusion Test

The agar-gel ID test is easy to perform and read. It relies upon the interaction between a patient's serum that is positive for the A antibody and concentrated purified A antigen incubated at 37°C for 48 h. If homologous antibody is present, it will precipitate the antigen. The immune precipitate formed is checked for fusion with a reference precipitate to identify the A antibody. Only sera that form a distinct line of identity with the reference antigen–antibody precipitate are considered positive. Lines of nonidentity or lines of partial identity are considered suspicious. False-positive reactions have not been encountered. False-negative reactions may occur.

The test is moderately sensitive and it is particularly useful for assessing the significance of low CF and EIA titers, which may be nonspecific. The A precipitin has been detected in sera from humans,[1] canines,[5,10] dolphins,[12] polar bears,[15] and wolves.[13] It has also been detected in the CSF of patients with blastomycosis meningitis.[16] In some cases ID may provide the only means by which the disease is diagnosed.[1]

A review of the literature indicates that the ID test exhibits a sensitivity ranging from 26% to 79%, with a specificity of 100%.[1,4,6,14,17] In their study of 65 cases of blastomycosis and 168 controls, Turner et al.[7] reported that the test had a sensitivity of 65%, with a predictive value for a positive test of 100%. In many instances the test is more sensitive than the CF test.[1,7,14] It is capable of detecting the A precipitin in acutely ill patients within 1 month of the onset of illness.[10] Sensitivity, however, for detecting such patients varies from 30%[18] to 75%.[10] Sarosi and Davies[18] indicated that 70–80% of patients with chronic pulmonary and extrapulmonary blastomycosis may be positive by ID. With canine blastomycosis, the sensitivity of the ID test is greater than 90%.[5,11]

As with the CF test, the ID test appears to have limited value for monitoring patients. Recovery may occur without the concomitant disappearance of precipitins.[1] In confirmed cases of blastomycosis, however, it has been noted that the disappearance of precipitins offered evidence of a favorable prognosis.[1,7] This appears to be supported by data in two independent studies,[11,14] where the disappearance or reduction in intensity of the A precipitate following therapy was associated with clinical improvement. An additional study of canine specimens[5] showed that the A precipitin persisted in some clinically cured dogs. It is interesting to note that no recurrence of the A precipitin occurred in a dog that had relapsed.

2.3. Enzyme Immunosorbent Assay (EIA)

The indirect EIA has proven to be an important contribution toward development of a reliable method for diagnosing blastomycosis. In this test, antigen is coated on plastic wells, and varying dilutions of the patient's serum are added. If antibodies are present, they bind to the antigen and are then detected and measured by the addition of enzyme-conjugated anti-human or canine immunoglobulin G, followed by an appropriate enzyme substrate. The degree of substrate decomposition reflects the quantity of *B. dermatitidis* antibody reacting with the antigen.

Use of the EIA with purified A antigen resulted in improved sensitivity for blastomycosis antibody detection with minimal loss in specificity. In a series of applications with varied test formats and patient populations, the assay's sensitivity ranged from 77% to 100% and the specificity from 84% to 98%.[4,6,7,17,19] In a comparative evaluation, Turner and Kaufman,[19] using 1:16 as a minimal EIA titer, found the test to demonstrate a sensitivity of 80% and a specificity of 98%. Although the CF and ID tests were specific in this evaluation, they demonstrated sensitivities of only 40% and 65%, respectively. EIA titers ranging from 1:8 to 1:512 were noted in patients with acute pulmonary disease. To date, EIA tests with a variety of *B. dermatitidis* antigens, including purified A,[7,17] commercial yeast antigen,[20] yeast lysate antigen,[21] and commercial ID[22] antigens, have all demonstrated cross-reactivity, particularly with histoplasmosis case sera. In their study with the purified A antigen, Turner *et al.*[7] found no cross-reactivity at titers of 1:32 or greater. The EIA test with a 1:16 minimal titer demonstrated a predictive value of 94% for a positive reaction. Obviously, further antigen purification is needed to exclude moieties responsible for cross-reactivity.

The EIA is capable of detecting blastomycosis antibodies within a month of the onset of illness.[10,17] With acutely ill patients, however, the seroprevalence rate and antibody titers peak approximately 7 weeks after onset.[17] Accordingly, serial serologic testing should be considered in patients suspected of having acute disease who demonstrate negative serologic results soon after the onset of illness.

Since EIA titers of 1:16 or less are not always indicative of blastomycosis, it is recommended that sera from suspected cases of blastomycosis be tested concomitantly by EIA and ID tests. Any serum specimen with an A precipitin is considered positive for blastomycosis. EIA titers equal to or greater than 1:32, with or without an associated A precipitin, are considered diagnostic for blastomycosis. Specimens negative for the A precipitin that demonstrate EIA titers of 1:8 to 1:16 are considered suspicious for blastomycosis and must be followed up with studies of serial serum specimens to demonstrate the development of the specific A precipitin or higher EIA titers.

The study of serial specimens from a patient is useful for assessing the response of acute infections to antifungal therapy. Data suggest that fourfold or greater reductions in titer indicate a favorable prognosis.[7,17]

The sensitivity of the EIA test makes it suitable for testing and monitoring CSF specimens from patients with suspected blastomycotic meningitis. CSF from one proven case demonstrated a 1:8 CF titer, an A precipitin, and an EIA titer of 1:128. EIA has also proven reliable for diagnosing canine blastomycosis.[7] In a study of 6 canine cases and 31 controls, the test demonstrated excellent sensitivity (100%) and specificity (97%).

Recently, Lo and Notenboom[23] reported a highly specific EIA for blastomycosis based upon the principle of antigen capture. Commercial A antigen captured with rabbit anti-A IgG produced from immune precipitates was used to bind the A antibody in the sera of patients with blastomycosis. This test appears very promising and awaits further evaluation.

2.4. Western Blot

The Western blot technique involves the separation of antigens by SDS-PAGE, transferring the resolved antigens to a nitrocellulose sheet by electro-transfer blot, and identifying the reaction of antibodies in the patient's sera with the resolved antigens through EIA. The test, which takes approximately 6 h, is relatively easy to perform once nitrocellulose strips with antigen are available. Appropriate controls must be used. The results are qualitative in nature, although differences in intensity of antibody reactions can be recorded.

SDS-PAGE analysis of the purified yeast culture filtrate of *B. dermatitidis* by Hurst *et al.*[8] showed it to consist of a minimum of 30 bands. Five of these bands were reactive with blastomycosis case sera in the Western blot test. One of the bands, a 98-kilodalton (kDa) glycoprotein, demonstrated its potential as a diagnostic antigen, due to its high sensitivity and intense reactivity with blastomycosis case sera diluted 1:100. In comparative studies with the EIA, the Western blot test showed only slightly improved sensitivity and specificity. Western blot tests with the 98-kDa antigen showed a sensitivity of 91% with blastomycosis case sera, while the EIA demonstrated a sensitivity of 88%. The specificity of the Western blot was 95%, whereas that of the EIA was 93%. Cross-reactions with histoplasmosis case sera, although fewer in Western blot, continued to be the most important problem complicating both assays. Electroelution of the 98-kDa antigen and demonstration of its identity to the A antigen in blastomycosis ID tests indicated that the glycoprotein contains the diagnostically significant A antigen. Additional studies are needed to further purify the 98-kDa antigen and to assess the value of Western blot for diagnosing blastomycosis.

2.5. Immunofluorescence

FA techniques may be used for the demonstration of the yeast-form cells of *B. dermatitidis* in infected tissue. Specific FA reagents for *B. dermatitidis* are produced by adsorbing rabbit anti-yeast-form *B. dermatitidis* fluorescein isothiocyanate-labeled antiglobulins with the yeast-form cells of *Histoplasma capsulatum* and *Geotrichum candidum*,[24] or from antiglobulins produced against the purified A antigen.[9] These specific conjugates make possible the rapid and accurate identification of viable and nonviable yeast-form cells of *B. dermatitidis* in culture and in clinical materials, including paraffin sections of formalin-fixed tissue. The conjugates are directed against yeast-form somatic antigens and will not identify the mycelial form of the fungus. Culture in the latter form may, however, be rapidly and specifically identified by the exoantigen procedure (Chapter 6). The FA techniques are particularly reliable for obtaining confirmatory data when blastomycosis is suspected from histologic studies and cultures were obtained.[13,25] FA reagents should be used when the results of histopathologic studies are inconclusive due to the development of atypical forms of *B. dermatitidis*,[26] or to avoid false-positive histologic diagnoses with tissue forms of other fungi, such as atypical nonencapsulated cryptococci and nonendosporulating *Coccidioides immitis* spherules, which may resemble the yeast form of *B. dermatitidis* as seen in tissue. FA reagents are also useful for differentiating the small yeast-form cells of *B. dermatitidis* (2 to 4 μm) from those of *H. capsulatum.*

2.6. Radioimmunoassay

Studies with the radioimmunoassay (RIA) test indicate that the procedure offers no advantages over EIA. RIA, using ^{125}I-labeled *Staphylococcus aureus* protein A, has been adapted for the serodiagnosis of blastomycosis.[27] Using a commercial *B. dermatitidis* yeast antigen, the test exhibited limited value for diagnosing blastomycosis, since cross-reactivity was noted with sera from 76% of the patients with histoplasmosis, 30% of patients with nonmycotic lung disorders, and 13% of normal individuals. Although nonspecific, using 1:16 as a minimal positive titer, the RIA was 100% sensitive.

In a later study, the RIA was compared with the CF and ID tests.[28] Surprisingly, the RIA demonstrated a sensitivity similar to that of the CF test (CF = 67%, RIA = 70%), while the ID test showed less sensitivity (33%). In 1987, Lambert and George[20] compared the enzyme and radioimmunoassays using commercial yeast *B. dermatitidis* antigen and found the EIA to be slightly more sensitive (83%) than the RIA (75%). False-positive reactions were apparent with both tests.

In a more recent development, Klein and Jones[29] described a promising RIA test using a radiolabeled 120-kDa protein derived from the cell wall of *B. dermatitidis*. The test demonstrated a sensitivity of 85% and a specificity of 100% when a minimal serum titer of 1:100 was used.

2.7. Cell-Mediated Immunity

2.7.1. *In Vivo* Tests

No reliable, specific skin test for blastomycosis is available. Consequently, the prevalence of resolved clinical or subclinical cases of blastomycosis cannot be accurately determined. The lack of such a skin test antigen also contributes to the poor comprehension of the epidemiology of blastomycosis. Two antigens with potentials for developing a skin test antigen have been reported.[4,30] Using isotachophoresis, Lancaster and Sprouse[30] isolated a fraction from blastomycin that was specific and sensitive in sensitized guinea pigs. A positive reaction was obtained in 48 h with 5.4 μg of antigen. More recently, Green *et al.*,[4] using DEAE-purified A antigen, reported 100% sensitivity and specificity in sensitized guinea pigs. They obtained positive reactions 48 h after intradermal injection of 15 μg of antigen. Follow-up studies are needed to ascertain the reliability of these antigens to detect delayed hypersensitivity in humans with blastomycosis.

2.7.2. *In Vitro* Tests

Blastomyces dermatitidis alkali-soluble–water-soluble antigens (B-ASWS) have been used as indicators of cellular immunity in blastomycosis.[31,32] Lymphocytes from patients with blastomycosis show more transformation with B-ASWS than do cells from patients with histoplasmosis. Recent studies indicate B-ASWS to be a reliable indicator of cellular immunity.[33] Lymphocyte transformation with B-ASWS, however, does not appear to be sufficiently specific for the early diagnosis of pulmonary blastomycosis. The usefulness of B-ASWS as a diagnostic reagent is questionable.

3. SUMMARY

The inability to isolate totally specific *B. dermatitidis* antigens hampers the development of accurate and reliable immunodiagnostic procedures for blastomycosis. In spite of this limitation, the sensitivity and specificity of EIA, ID, and Western blot procedures have improved substantially as a result of increased purification of the *B. dermatitidis* A antigen. These tests with purified A antigen, used alone or in combination, in many cases permit early diagnosis of blastomycosis and contribute to proper disease management. Studies with EIA and Western blot techniques indicate that the use of purified A antigen minimizes (but does not eliminate) nonspecificity, particularly that due to cross-reacting *H. capsulatum* antibodies. Accordingly, EIA or Western blot tests should be run concomitantly with the less sensitive but totally specific ID test to minimize false-positive diagnoses. These procedures are useful for diagnosing acute, chronic, and disseminated blastomycosis in humans and lower animals. They may be applied to serum and CSF specimens. Whenever possible, serologic diagnosis should be supported by the histologic and/or cultural demonstration of *B. dermatitidis*. Specific FA reagents are reliable for such demonstrations. They are also useful for detecting and identifying the yeast form of *B. dermatitidis* in clinical specimens where blastomycosis is suspected from histologic studies and cultures were not obtained.

REFERENCES

1. Kaufman L, McLaughlin D, Clark M, et al: Specific immunodiffusion test for blastomycosis. *Appl Microbiol* 26:244–247, 1973
2. Green JH, Harrell WK, Johnson J, et al: Preparation of reference antisera for laboratory diagnosis of blastomycosis. *J Clin Microbiol* 10:1–7, 1979
3. Young KD, Larsh HW: Identification of the active precipitin components in a purified preparation of the A antigen of *Blastomyces dermatitidis*. *Infect Immun* 33:171–177, 1981
4. Green JH, Harrell WK, Johnson J, et al: Isolation of an antigen from *Blastomyces dermatitidis* that is specific for the diagnosis of blastomycosis. *Curr Microbiol* 4:293–296, 1980
5. Legendre AM, Becker PU: Evaluation of the agar-gel immunodiffusion test in the diagnosis of canine blastomycosis. *Am J Vet Res* 41:2109–2111, 1980
6. Klein BJ, Kuritsky JN, Chappel WA, et al: Comparison of the enzyme immunoassay, immunodiffusion, and complement fixation tests in detecting antibody in human sera to the A antigen of *Blastomyces dermatitidis*. *Am Rev Respir Dis* 133:144–148, 1986

7. Turner SH, Kaufman L, Jalbert M: Diagnostic assessment of an enzyme-linked immunosorbent assay for human and canine blastomycosis. *J Clin Microbiol* 23:294–297, 1986

8. Hurst S, Kaufman L, Jalbert M: Western blot analysis and characterization of a purified *Blastomyces dermatitidis* culture filtrate antigen. Abstracts of the 89th Annual Meeting of the American Society for Microbiology, 1989, p 463

9. Sudman MS, Kaplan W: Antigenic relationship between American and African isolates of *Blastomyces dermatitidis* as determined by immunofluorescence. *Appl Microbiol* 27:496–499, 1974

10. Armstrong CW, Jenkins SR, Kaufman L, et al: Common-source outbreak of blastomycosis in hunters and their dogs. *J Infect Dis* 155:568–570, 1987

11. Phillips WE Jr, Kaufman L: Cultural and histopathologic confirmation of canine blastomycosis diagnosed by an agar-gel immunodiffusion test. *Am J Vet Res* 41:1263–1265, 1980

12. Cates MB, Kaufman L, Grabau JH, et al: Blastomycosis in an Atlantic bottlenose dolphin. *J Am Vet Med Assoc* 189:1148–1150, 1986

13. Thiel RR, Mech LD, Ruth GR, et al: Blastomycosis in wild wolves. *J Wildl Dis* 23:321–323, 1987

14. Williams JE, Murphy R, Standard PG, et al: Serologic response in blastomycosis: Diagnostic value of double immunodiffusion assay. *Am Rev Respir Dis* 128:209–212, 1981

15. Morris PJ, Legendre AM, Bowersock TL, et al: Diagnosis and treatment of systemic blastomycosis in a polar bear (*Ursus maritimus*) with itraconazole. *J Zoo Wildl Med* 20:336–345, 1989

16. Kaufman L: Special Plenary Lecture. Mycoserology: Its vital role in diagnosing systemic mycotic infections. *Jpn J Med Mycol* 24:1–8, 1983

17. Klein BS, Vergeront JM, Kaufman L, et al: Serological tests for blastomycosis: Assessments during a large point-source outbreak in Wisconsin. *J Infect Dis* 155:262–268, 1987

18. Sarosi GA, Davies SF: *Blastomyces dermatitidis* pneumonia, in Pennington JE (ed): *Respiratory Infections: Diagnosis and Management,* ed 2. New York, Raven Press, 1988, pp 508–513

19. Turner S, Kaufman L: Immunodiagnosis of blastomycosis. *Semin Respir Infect* 1:22–28, 1986

20. Lambert RS, George RB: Evaluation of enzyme immunoassay as a rapid screening test for histoplasmosis and blastomycosis. *Am Rev Respir Dis* 136:316–319, 1987

21. Johnson SM, Scalarone GM: Preparation and ELISA evaluation of *Blastomyces dermatitidis* yeast phase antigens. *Diagn Microbiol Infect Dis* 11:81–86, 1988

22. Wheeler JW, Owens RD, Scalarone GM: Enzyme immunoassay detection of antibodies in North American blastomycosis: Comparison of three *Blastomyces dermatitidis* antigens. *Mycoses* 31:459–465, 1988

23. Lo CY, Notenboom RH: A new enzyme immunoassay specific for blastomycosis. *Am Rev Respir Dis* 141:84–88, 1990

24. Kaplan W, Kaufman L: Specific fluorescent antiglobulins for the detection and identification of *Blastomyces dermatitidis* yeast-form cells. *Mycopathologia* 19:173–180, 1963

25. Stroud RK, Coles BM: Blastomycosis in an African lion. *J Am Vet Med Assoc* 177:842–844, 1980

26. Tang TT, Marsik FJ, Harb JM, et al: Cerebral blastomycosis: An immunodiagnostic study. *Am J Clin Pathol* 82:243–246, 1984

27. George RB, Lambert RS, Bruce MJ, et al: Radio-immunoassay: Sensitive screening test for histoplasmosis and blastomycosis. *Am Rev Respir Dis* 124:407–410, 1981

28. Kinasewitz GT, Penn RL, George RB: The spectrum and significance of pleural disease in blastomycosis. *Chest* 86:580–584, 1984

29. Klein BS, Jones JM: Isolation, purification and radiolabeling of a novel 120-kD surface protein on *Blastomyces dermatitidis* yeasts to detect antibody in infected patients. *J Clin Invest* 85:152–161, 1990

30. Lancaster MV, Sprouse RF: Preparative isotachophoretic separation of skin test antigens from blastomycin purified derivative. *Infect Immun* 13:758–762, 1976

31. Bradsher RW: Development of specific immunity in patients with pulmonary or extrapulmonary blastomycosis. *Am Rev Respir Dis* 129:430–434, 1984

32. Bradsher RW, Alford RH: *Blastomyces dermatitidis* antigen-induced lymphocyte reactivity in human blastomycosis. *Infect Immun* 33:485–490, 1981

33. Klein BS, Bradsher RW, Vergeront JM, et al: Development of long-term specific cellular immunity after acute *Blastomyces dermatitidis* infection: Assessments following a large point-source outbreak in Wisconsin. *J Infect Dis* 161:97–101, 1990

8

Immunology of Blastomycosis

Bruce S. Klein

1. INTRODUCTION

Blastomycosis is a systemic disease with a wide variety of pulmonary and extrapulmonary manifestations. Following inhalation of conidia into the lungs, the acute primary pulmonary infection can be asymptomatic or can produce an influenza or atypical pneumonia syndrome.[1] Acute blastomycotic pneumonia may resolve spontaneously.[2] Many patients, however, develop chronic and progressive forms of disease involving the lungs, the extrapulmonary organs (usually the skin, bones, joints, or prostrate gland), or both.[3] Although opportunistic infection among immunocompromised patients is uncommon,[4] it remains possible that such patients, if exposed, are more susceptible to infection.

2. INFLAMMATORY RESPONSE TO *B. DERMATITIDIS*

Blastomyces dermatitidis evokes a characteristic admixture of suppuration and granuloma formation in the skin and visceral organs of infected humans, with budding yeast-form organisms seen inside of and attached to

Blastomycosis, edited by Yousef Al-Doory and Arthur F. DiSalvo, Plenum Medical Book Company, New York, 1992.

phagocytes.[5] Understanding of the evolution of the inflammatory response to *B. dermatitidis* in humans is incomplete, however, because the preponderance of histopathological information has been obtained from autopsy series or descriptions of isolated rather than serial biopsy specimens. Recent work in inbred C57BL/6 mice has helped characterize the sequence of events that take place in the inflammatory response after an intravenous injection of 10^6 *B. dermatitidis* yeasts.[6] The tissue response progressed from acute neutrophilic invasion during the first 7 days of infection to pyogranuloma formation by the fifth week of infection. The lungs, brains, superficial fascia, livers, and spleens of the mice were involved. By the fifth week, the greatest burden of infection and inflammation was found in the lungs and brains, other visceral organs were less involved, and only small granulomas containing few yeasts were seen in the liver parenchyma. The lymph nodes and spleens were relatively spared.

A histological picture including suppuration and granuloma formation has also been reported in the tissues of congenitally athymic nude mice inoculated intravenously with *B. dermatitidis* yeasts.[7] By day 12 of infection a pyogranulomatous reaction was evident in the brain, with lesions consisting of three zones: central necrosis, an intermediate region of intense suppuration, and an accumulation of mononuclear cells around the periphery of the lesion. Although much larger numbers of yeast cells were seen in the lesions of nude mice than in their immunologically intact littermates, this study supports the hypothesis that granuloma formation is not entirely under the control of mature T cells (which nude mice lack because they have no thymus).

At least two products of *B. dermatitidis* have been associated with the influx of inflammatory cells found in lesions of blastomycosis. The first is a serum-independent chemotactic factor, detectable in the culture filtrate of growing yeasts, which stimulates the migration of both human neutrophils and monocytes.[8] The factor resists heat treatment at 100°C for 60 min and alkaline conditions, but is inactivated below pH 7. The molecular size of the chemotactic factor is unknown; however, it is retained after dialysis using a size cutoff of 3500 daltons. The second product of the organism is cell wall material found in an alkali-soluble, water-soluble extract of virulent *B. dermatitidis*.[9] Intraperitoneal inoculation of this extract elicits formation of granulomas that are histologically indistinguishable from the lesions seen following inoculation of experimental animals with live yeasts. An identically prepared extract from the cell wall of an avirulent strain of *B. dermatitidis* elicited suppuration but no granuloma formation, leading investigators to postulate that since the most striking chemical difference between extracts of the two strains was the amount of covalently bound phospholipid,[10] lipid in the cell wall might be responsible for the granulomatous reaction.

3. ANTIGENS OF *B. DERMATITIDIS*

Blastomycin, a culture filtrate of the mycelial form of *B. dermatitidis,* is no longer commercially available for use as a skin test antigen because of its lack of sensitivity and specificity. In two large series of human cases of culture-proven blastomycosis,[11,12] only 41% of patients in one and none in the other had a positive skin test using blastomycin. It is unlikely that the principal reason for the insensitivity of the antigen relates to either timing of the skin testing or anergy during the course of infection. In a longitudinal study of 48 adults and children infected during an outbreak of blastomycosis, only 60% of the patients developed a positive blastomycin skin test during 2 years of follow-up, despite complete resolution of disease.[13,14] The lack of specificity of blastomycin is illustrated by a study in which guinea pigs were sensitized with killed yeasts of *B. dermatitidis* or *Histoplasma capsulatum* and subsequently skin-tested[15]: 66% of the blastomyces-sensitized animals and 74% of the histoplasma-sensitized animals reacted to blastomycin.

Blastomyces alkali- and water-soluble antigen (B-ASWS), a cell wall fraction of the yeast form described by Cox and Larsh,[15] is far more sensitive and specific for assessing correlates of specific cellular immunity in blastomycosis. As its name implies, the antigen is isolated by alkali (1 N NaOH) denaturation of *B. dermatitidis* yeast cell walls. Extraction is most active at the outer cell wall layer due to cleavage of α-1,3-glucan linkages. Not only is B-ASWS more sensitive and specific than the previously available mycelial filtrate antigens; its activity is nearly equivalent and can be standardized from batch to batch.[16] The considerable value of B-ASWS has been shown in studies in laboratory animals[17] and in humans with sporadic[18,19] or epidemic disease.[13,14] However, the antigen remains impure—a complex mixture of lipid, polysaccharide, and protein with a molecular weight range of 30,000 to 50,000.[20] Preparative polyacrylamide gel electrophoresis and isoelectric focusing have shown that B-ASWS contains three or possibly four active components.[21] One accounts for the high sensitivity and specificity, whereas the others appear to account for cross-reactivity with heterologous fungi, particularly *H. capsulatum.* Indeed, lymphocytes from histoplasmosis patients proliferate in response to B-ASWS, albeit to a significantly lesser degree than those from blastomycosis patients.[22] This situation, however, is similar to that seen with other relatively specific fungal antigens, such as *H. capsulatum* skin test antigen, histoplasmin.[22]

The A antigen of *B. dermatitidis* was described by Kaufman *et al.,*[23] who found its activity in yeast broth filtrates. A subsequent study outlined methods for extraction and purification of the antigen and its preliminary use in testing for antibody and delayed-type hypersensitivity in blastomycosis.[24] Crude antigen is first isolated from the filtrate of yeast cells allowed to remain for 2 weeks at room temperature in phosphate-buffered saline. This material is fractionated on DEAE columns equilibrated with 0.02 M Tris-HCl buffer, pH 8.6. Fraction 4 contains A antigen. The activity of this antigen is not affected by proteinases, is labile when boiled for 10 min, and is stable for months at 5°C in phosphate buffer. Although several studies have clearly demonstrated that A antigen is useful for serodiagnosis of blastomycosis,[14,24–27] further characterization and purification of the antigen are needed to reduce cross-reactivity. At present, purified A antigen contains at least 25 protein and glycoprotein bands by Coomassie blue, periodic acid–Schiff, and silver staining.[28] The activity of the antigen is associated with two components in this material,[28] but the molecular size of the components has not been described. The precise location of A antigen in the yeast cell also remains uncertain. Some investigators have demonstrated it to be a product of the cell wall,[24] whereas others have also found it in the cytosol.[28]

Most recently, a novel antigen of *B. dermatitidis* yeasts has been isolated, purified, and partially characterized.[29] The molecule (designated WI-1) comprises 5% of the cell wall extract obtained after freezing and thawing yeast cells. Its molecular weight is approximately 120,000, and it is expressed on all strains of the organism thus far tested. Figure 1 shows a 10% SDS-PAGE gel of the crude extract from −20°C frozen *B. dermatitidis* yeast strain compared with electrophoretically eluted, concentrated, and pooled samples of WI-1 taken from the extract. Figure 2 shows antigenic variations among extracts from various strains of *B. dermatitidis*. Variability in expression and molecular size of the 120-kDa component, WI-1, between strains and the major 70-kDa component that distinguishes ATCC 26199 from other strains is obvious. Approximately 0.93 pg or 4.7×10^6 molecules of the antigen are present on the surface of an individual yeast cell of ATCC strain 60636, but none was found on a strain of *H. capsulatum*. Figure 3 demonstrates surface location of WI-1 on *B. dermatitidis* by immunogold staining. Serum from a rabbit immunized with WI-1 was used to stain the yeasts (A), preimmune serum served as a control (B), and an immune serum was adsorbed with 5 μg of WI-1 and *B. dermatitidis* yeasts (C). Preliminary studies have shown that the antigen can be used reliably to detect antibody as well as *in vitro* correlates of specific cellular immunity in patients with blastomycosis.

4. GENETIC FACTORS IN RESISTANCE TO *B. DERMATITIDIS* INFECTION

Clinically apparent blastomycosis has been diagnosed more frequently in males than females. Among 1114 cases in humans occurring in the United States between 1885 and 1968, 89% of the patients were men.[30] Similarly,

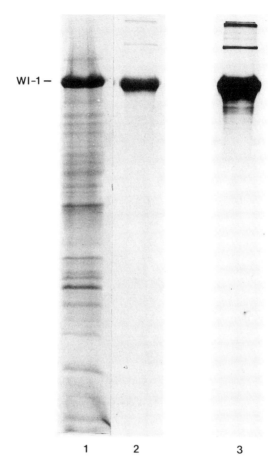

WI-1 —

1   2   3

FIGURE 1. Partially purified WI-1, a novel 120-kDa surface protein on *Blastomyces dermatitidis* yeasts. 1: gel of crude extract of strain 60636; 2–3: extract of WI-1. Coomassie brilliant blue used in 1 and 2, then silver nitrate on 3. (From Ref. 29.)

72% of the 47 clinical cases of canine blastomycosis reported in one series were in male dogs.[31] Male preponderance of disease could reflect hormone-related factors. This is consistent with laboratory studies in hamsters demonstrating that females were more resistant to the lethal effects of *B. dermatitidis* infection (52% survival versus 7%), and that ovariectomy increased the resistance of females (80% survival) and castration increased the resistance of males (40% survival).[32] Additionally, the improved survival that ovariectomy conferred on females was nullified by treatment with testosterone (47% survival).

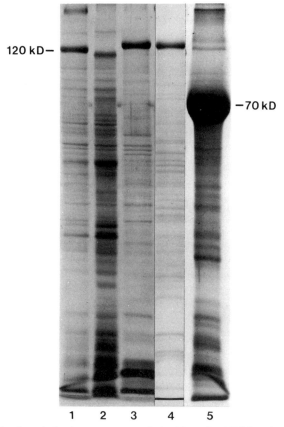

FIGURE 2. Antigenic variation between extracts derived from five ATCC strains of *B. dermatitidis* yeasts derived by freezing at −20°C: #60636 (1), 60637 (2), 26198 (3), 32090 (4), and 26199 (5).

Racial distribution of blastomycosis has inconsistently suggested a higher occurrence among blacks. Studies purporting this association were of early series of cases,[33,34] possibly reflecting the demographic features of populations seen in charity hospitals in rural and agricultural southern states or the predominant occupation of manual laborer among blacks in those states. This has not been confirmed in other large case series,[35] particularly those in the midwestern United States.

Inbred strains of mice show marked differences in susceptibility to experimental *B. dermatitidis* infection after pulmonary challenge with yeast-form organisms. Of eight strains with various *H-2* backgrounds evaluated in

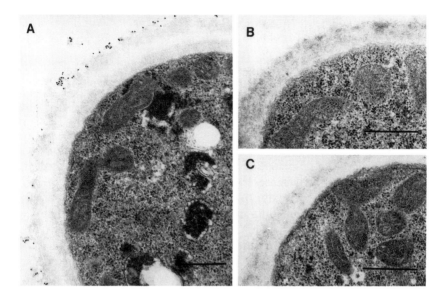

FIGURE 3. Immunogold staining of *B. dermatitidis* yeasts to demonstrate surface location of WI-1. Results are at a serum dilution of 1:100. Protein A gold containing 14-nm particles was used at a dilution of 1:15. Bar = 0.5 μm. (From Ref. 38.)

one study,[36] the C3H/HeJ strain had the highest mortality (88%) and the DBA/1J strain had the lowest (37%). The resistance of the C3H/HeN strain, which differs from the C3H/HeJ in that it exhibits sensitivity to lipopolysaccharide and lacks a defect in macrophage cytotoxicity, suggests that the susceptibility of C3H/HeJ mice is not related to the C3H background or *H-2* locus.

5. NATURAL RESISTANCE TO *B. DERMATITIDIS* INFECTION

The relatively low frequency of cases of clinically apparent blastomycosis might suggest that humans and animals are infrequently exposed to the habitat of *B. dermatitidis*. Alternatively, the high attack rates and large number of subclinical cases of infection that have been noted in some epidemic investigations[14,37] suggest that endemic exposure and infection are probably more common than is revealed using available diagnostic tests. This discrepancy between a low prevalence of disease and much higher prevalence of exposure suggests that natural or nonimmune mechanisms of resistance effectively limit disease caused by *B. dermatitidis*. The mechanisms, which include phagocytosis and intracellular and extracellular killing by polymorphonuclear leukocytes (PMNs) and mononuclear phagocytes and activation of complement, are discussed below.

5.1. Natural Cellular Resistance

5.1.1. PMNs

5.1.1.1. Phagocytosis and Killing of Conidia. In the setting of naturally acquired infection, inhalation of conidia of *B. dermatitidis* presents the initial challenge to host defense. Human PMNs phagocytize these infective particles rapidly and efficiently. *In vitro,* under conditions in which PMNs and conidia were cocultured at a ratio of 10:1, PMNs phagocytized 83% of the particles in 1 h and 90% in 2 h.[38] However, PMNs killed the conidia more slowly and incompletely, so that after 1 h only 18% of conidia were killed and after 3 h the maximum, 50%, were killed. The ingestion and killing of conidia were independent of fungal strain, whether avirulent or virulent. Optimal phagocytosis and killing required both complement and the divalent cations Ca^{2+} and Mg^{2+}. In the absence of these factors, PMNs phagocytized only 18% of conidia after 3 h, and killing of the particles was completely abrogated.

Upon interaction with pathogenic microorganisms, PMNs display enhanced oxidative metabolism involving increased oxygen consumption and production of chemically reactive oxygen metabolites such as hydrogen peroxide and superoxide anion (O_2^-).[39] Hydrogen peroxide and superoxide anion may react to yield reactive metabolites such as hydroxyl radical ($\cdot$ OH) and singlet oxygen ($^1O_2$). Hydrogen peroxide, upon exposure to halide and myeloperoxidase (an enzyme found in PMNs), may also produce halogenated oxidative anions, e.g., hypochlorous acid (HOCl). The reactive oxygen species generated by PMNs mediate much of the microbicidal activity of these cells,[39] although oxygen-independent killing mechanisms may also be involved.[40,41]

The phagocytosis and killing of *B. dermatitidis* conidia by PMNs is accomplished mainly by oxidative mechanisms. Coincubation of conidia with human PMNs elicits a rapid and pronounced oxidative burst, as measured by chemiluminescence response of the PMNs. By 20 min of exposure, PMNs have produced peak values that are approximately 70% of the positive control values produced by zymosan, a potent trigger of oxidative metabolism.[38] Inhibitors of the myeloperoxidase-mediated system of oxidative metabolism in PMNs (e.g., sodium azide) profoundly inhibit the killing of conidia by PMNs in a dose-dependent fashion. At a concentration of 2 mM, azide reduced PMN killing of conidia by 90% while having no significant effect on phagocytosis. Likewise, PMNs from a patient with chronic granulomatous disease (characterized by lack of a normal respiratory burst and concomitant abnormalities of oxidative metabolism) and PMNs in an anaerobic experimental environment exhibit a similarly profound defect in killing but not phagocytosis. Additional experiments have shown that blastomyces conidia are indeed exquisitely susceptible to the lethal effects of the chemical products of oxidative metabolism when they have been exposed to these products in a cell-free system.[42] Although some strain-related susceptibility was evident, virtually complete killing of conidia of all strains was achieved after 60 min of exposure to reactive oxygen metabolites.

5.1.1.2. Phagocytosis and Killing of Yeasts.

The yeasts of *B. dermatitidis* are considerably more difficult than conidia for PMNs to manage. The yeasts' large size may account for the limited amount of phagocytosis accomplished by PMNs. However, even relatively small yeasts of strain SCB-2 (ATCC 26199) may be inefficiently phagocytized. In one study, 87% of this strain and 97% of other strains remained extracellular after 2 h of coincubation at a ratio of 10 PMNs per yeast.[38] Sixbey *et al.*[43] probably studied an unusually small *B. dermatitidis* yeast strain—one that was 99% phagocytized in 30 min under comparable experimental conditions.

Blastomyces dermatitidis yeasts are also moderately resistant to killing by PMNs, regardless of strain size. Drutz and Frey[38] found that an average of only 18% of the yeasts of six strains were killed when PMNs and yeasts were coincubated for 2 h at the optimal ratio of 10 PMNs per yeast. Even replacing expended PMNs with fresh cells after 90 min boosted killing only from 18% to 30%. Sixbey *et al.*[43] found about 29% killing of yeasts (range 20–40%) in an assay using 10^5 or 10^6 yeasts plus 10^6 PMNs in 10% normal serum for 3 h, even though virtually all yeasts were ingested after 30 min. For most yeasts of *B. dermatitidis,* the mechanism of killing by PMNs may be similar to that described by Diamond *et al.*[44,45] for filamentous fungi: an extracellular process whereby the PMNs attach directly to yeast cells and empty granule contents into the extracellular space. It may also be possible that surrounding nonattached PMNs play a passive but important role by helping retain already discharged granule contents in the vicinity of the surrounded yeast, thus offering an extracellular envelope that facilitates yeast damage.

One group of investigators has obtained results with human PMNs that are strikingly different from those described above. After 72 h of coculture of PMNs and yeasts, the yeasts surprisingly showed more than a 60% enhancement of replication.[46] This enhancement was independent of yeast strain and PMN viability. Neutrophils killed by repeated freezing and thawing produced a similar effect. The same group reported similar results with murine PMNs obtained from the peritoneal cavities of BALB/c mice.[47] They also showed enhanced multiplication of the organism at a site of infection after yeasts and PMNs were inoculated together subcutaneously into the mice. The reasons for the discrepancy between the findings of this group and other groups are unclear. However, these findings raise the possibility that neutrophils at the site of a blastomycotic lesion may actually exacerbate the infection in its early stages.

Optimal PMN killing of yeasts, like that of conidia, requires complement and divalent cations and proceeds by predominantly oxidative mechanisms, although conidia are more sensitive to these mechanisms than yeasts. In the absence of complement, Ca^{2+}, and Mg^{2+}, PMN killing of yeasts is abrogated.[38] Upon exposure to *B. dermatitidis* yeasts, PMNs display a rapid and pronounced oxidative burst as measured by chemiluminescence response,[38,43,48] although this is smaller than the oxidative burst that follows exposure to conidia.[38] Studies with inhibitors of the respiratory burst, anaerobic conditions and PMNs from patients with chronic granulomatous disease yielded significantly reduced killing to 4 to 8% from 16% under control conditions.[38] Studies in a cell-free medium with an artificial myeloperoxidase-dependent oxidative killing system confirm the susceptibility of *B. dermatitidis* yeast to oxidative mechanisms of killing.[49,50] Of interest, however, is the observation that the yeasts are 50 times more resistant than conidia to the lethal effects of H_2O_2.[48] In addition, *B. dermatitidis* yeasts are approximately 20 times more resistant than opportunistic yeasts such as *Candida albicans* or *C. glabrata*. Nevertheless, the susceptibility to hypochlorite (ClO^-), which is probably an important oxidant of the myeloperoxidase system, or to a system comprised of H_2O_2–Fe^{2+}–iodide, in which Fe^{2+} replaces myeloperoxidase, does not discriminate between *B. dermatitidis* yeasts or opportunistic yeasts.[48]

5.1.1.3. Immune Activation of PMNs. The functional properties of PMNs may be modulated by cytokines, soluble factors elaborated by mononuclear cells, which enhance the phagocytic and microbicidal activities of the cells. In the mouse, PMNs elicited intraperitoneally (i.p.) with thioglycollate from normal and blastomyces-immune animals failed to kill *B. dermatitidis* yeasts in a 4-h *in vitro* assay.[51] In contrast, PMNs elicited from immune mice by an i.p. injection of nonviable *B. dermatitidis* yeasts effected a 60% reduction of the inoculum indicating markedly enhanced fungicidal activity of PMNs elicited by an immune reaction. Further work in this system has shown that peripheral blood PMNs from similarly immune-activated mice had comparably enhanced fungicidal activity,[52] and that the culture supernatants of spleen cells from immune mice stimulated with *B. dermatitidis* antigen *in vitro* conferred enhanced microbicidal activity to PMNs from nonimmune mice.[53] The activity in supernatants was dose-dependent, nondialyzable (molecular weight $\geq$ 14,000), and relatively heat labile. More recent work has shown that gamma-interferon (IFN-γ) can activate murine peritoneal PMNs from nonimmune animals to kill *B. dermatitidis in vitro*,[54] suggesting that this lymphokine may in part account for immunological activation of PMNs.

The mechanism whereby immunological activation confers enhanced fungicidal activity on murine PMNs involves an enhanced respiratory burst and production of reactive oxygen metabolites. Immunologically activated murine peritoneal PMNs produced a tenfold greater increase in respiratory burst activity than did nonactivated cells after incubation with *B. dermatitidis*.[55] Furthermore, both the enhanced killing and the respiratory burst were nearly eliminated or significantly impaired by inhibitors of oxidative metabolism such as superoxide dismutase (75% reduction), which removes O_2^-, sodium azide (64%), which inhibits myeloperoxidase and scavenges singlet oxygen, and catalase (52%), which cleaves H_2O_2.[56]

The *in vivo* relevance of these findings concerning immunological activation is unclear. However, one can imagine that PMNs that are otherwise weakly active against the formidable challenge of *B. dermatitidis* yeasts in the nonimmune host show considerably greater efficiency in clearing the pathogen from infected sites in the presence of lymphokines elaborated by specifically activated immune cells of the host.

5.1.2. Mononuclear Phagocytes

5.1.2.1. Alveolar Macrophages. Alveolar macrophages are the first line of defense against inhaled microbes, including *B. dermatitidis*. Under normal conditions, however, these cells are only modestly capable of ingesting *B. dermatitidis* yeasts. After 72 h of *in vitro* coincubation of yeasts with pulmonary alveolar macrophages from normal persons, only 12–18% of the cells had ingested the yeast, and the population of yeast had surprisingly increased by 52% over the starting inoculum.[57] Another group, however, working with murine alveolar macrophages under conditions involving coculture of cells from normal animals and yeasts, found that 0–5% of the organisms were killed after 4 h.[58,59] The reason for the discrepancy between findings of the two groups is unclear, but may relate to differences in assay conditions, size of inocula (ratio of macrophages to yeasts), and species origin of the alveolar cells. One explanation for the seemingly modest fungicidal activity of alveolar macrophages for *B. dermatitidis* might relate to the correspondingly modest respiratory burst the fungus triggers in alveolar macrophages. Under optimal conditions in which monolayers of murine alveolar macrophages are challenged with *B. dermatitidis* conidia, the particles elicit a respiratory burst (measured by O_2^- production) only 25–31% of that seen with the potent stimulus of zymosan, and the suboptimal response is independent of fungal strain.[60] Similar trends were found when *B. dermatitidis* yeast strains were evaluated in this assay system.[61]

Nonoxidative mechanisms may be important in alveolar macrophage clearance of *B. dermatitidis* conidia and yeasts, and efficient resistance to a respiratory challenge may require immunological activation of this first line of defense. Indeed, human alveolar macrophages of immune individuals ingest and inhibit the growth of *B. dermatitidis* yeasts significantly better than do cells of nonimmune persons. The fungicidal activity of nonimmune cells, however, can be enhanced by exposing the cells to culture supernatant of B-ASWS-activated lymphocytes from blastomyces-immune persons.[57] Similarly, the killing of yeasts by murine alveolar macrophages is augmented from 0 to 25% by coincubating the cells with the supernatant of concanavalin A-stimulated spleen cells or 1000 U/ml of IFN-γ.[58] Interestingly, antibody to IFN-γ abrogated the effect of the spleen cell supernatant. This suggests that IFN-γ accounts for most or all of the supernatant's immune augmentation. When mice were treated i.p. with 4×10^5 units of recombinant IFN-γ, their pulmonary macrophages showed enhanced killing of *B. dermatitidis* yeasts (38%, compared with 5% for cells of control mice).[59] Similar augmentation was found with a second dimorphic pathogen, *Paracoccidioides brasiliensis*. Inhibitors of oxidative metabolism (catalase, sodium azide, superoxide dismutase, and dimethylsulfoxide) were studied for their influence on immunologically augmented killing by murine pulmonary macrophages in this system. No agent had significant effects except dimethylsulfoxide, which reduced killing by a modest 21%. This finding supports the assertion that nonoxidative fungicidal mechanisms of activated macrophages, such as the cationic peptides in macrophage granules,[62] may constitute a major component of this defense system.

5.1.2.2. Murine Peritoneal Macrophages. Study of these cells provides an opportunity to evaluate the function of resident, tissue-based macrophages that would otherwise not be possible in humans because of the unavailability of specimens. Resident peritoneal macrophages or macrophages elicited by i.p. injection of thioglycolate are unable to kill *B. dermatitidis* yeasts *in vitro*. In contrast, immunological activation of mice by methods such as i.p. injection of Con A or *Mycobacterium bovis* BCG (which enhance spleen size and presumably lymphokine production),[63] or *in vitro* activation of the cells by coincubation with supernatants from Con A-stimulated spleen cells or recombinant IFN-γ, enables the macrophages to kill 21–26% of the yeasts.[63,64] Neither specific antibody nor complement enhances the killing by nonactivated or nonspecifically activated macrophages. Interestingly, *B. der-*

matitidis yeasts elicit a brisk oxidative burst and superoxide anion production in activated macrophages, although the responses as measured by enhanced chemiluminescence do not differ significantly from those of inactivated macrophages that are identically challenged.[64] Similarly, immunologically augmented killing mediated by these cells is not significantly impaired by inhibitors of oxidative metabolism (catalase, superoxide dismutase, dimethylsulfoxide, and azide). These results, like those with human alveolar macrophages, indicate that activated murine peritoneal macrophages kill *B. dermatitidis* by nonoxidative mechanisms.

5.1.2.3. Peripheral Blood Monocytes and Monocyte-Derived Macrophages. Monocytes and monocyte-derived macrophages from the blood of nonimmune persons are able to ingest and kill *B. dermatitidis* conidia. *In vitro,* at a ratio of 10 phagocytes per fungus, monocytes ingest 41% and kill 34% of conidia after 3 h of incubation. Macrophages exhibit even greater activity, ingesting 84% and killing 89% of conidia under the same conditions.[38] The differing fungicidal properties of these two cell types are magnified upon interaction with yeasts. Whereas monocytes ingest no yeasts and kill only 5% of the inoculum, macrophages ingest 18% and kill 41%. Morphological studies indicate that the killing of uningested yeasts by these cells is accomplished by extracellular mechanisms, in which there is membrane-to-membrane apposition of yeasts and macrophages. These observations provide additional support for the hypothesis that nonoxidative mechanisms, such as discharge of granular contents with antifungal effector molecules, contribute significantly to fungicidal activity of macrophages.

Monocyte-derived macrophages from the blood of immune individuals ingest and inhibit the growth of *B. dermatitidis* yeasts more avidly than do cells of nonimmune individuals, emphasizing the role of immune activation in augmenting function. By 72 h after coincubation of phagocytes and yeasts, 35% of macrophages from patients recovered from blastomycosis contain intracellular yeasts, as compared with 12% of cells from nonimmune persons.[65] Furthermore, growth of the yeasts is completely inhibited in the presence of immune macrophages, whereas the yeast population increased by 78% when incubated with cells of normal persons. This enhanced activity is explained by the fact that the macrophage monolayers are "contaminated" with 5–10% lymphocytes that, in persons who have recovered from disease, are responding specifically to the yeasts and secreting lymphokines. These findings are consistent with those with alveolar and murine peritoneal macrophages and underline the importance of immune augmentation for optimal function of peripheral blood monocyte-derived macrophages.

5.2. Complement

The role of complement in defense against *B. dermatitidis* infection has not been studied systematically. The studies previously discussed would indicate that complement is necessary for the PMNs' maximal phagocytosis and killing of *B. dermatitidis* conidia and their maximal killing of yeast. In contrast, the presence of murine serum (and by inference, complement) did not influence the killing of yeasts by murine alveolar and peritoneal macrophages. An accurate picture of the antifungal role of complement in defense against *B. dermatitidis* awaits future studies.

5.3. Summary

The relative ease with which nonspecific phagocytes dispense with *B. dermatitidis* conidia and, conversely, the relative difficulty that these cells have in ingesting and killing the yeasts in the absence of immune activation suggest that the dimorphism of *B. dermatitidis* confers a selective advantage in regard to pathogenicity. On the one hand, the extreme susceptibility of conidia to the gamut of nonspecific defense mechanisms may in part explain the relative rarity of blastomycosis as a clinically apparent problem. On the other, resistance of the yeast form explains why the organism is a primary fungal pathogen in the normal host, in contrast to opportunistic fungal pathogens that require compromised host defenses to establish infection and disease.

6. ACQUIRED RESISTANCE TO *B. DERMATITIDIS* INFECTION

Until recently, most of our understanding of acquired resistance to *B. dermatitidis* emerged from work with experimental animals, because suitable antigens were not available for study of human disease. Recently described antigens, including A antigen, WI-1, and B-ASWS, have now enabled investigators to begin to characterize features of acquired humoral and cellular immunity in human disease.

6.1. Humoral Immunity

6.1.1. Role of Antibody in Host Resistance

Although the role of antibody in host resistance to *B. dermatitidis* has not been systematically studied, the limited data indicate that specific antibody has no obvious role in defense against the infection. The adoptive transfer of immune serum, containing a titer of blastomyces-specific antibody of 1:80, offered no resistance to naive mice upon lethal challenge with *B. dermatitidis* yeasts.[66] In another study examining the passive transfer of delayed hypersensitivity, this immune function could not be transferred with immune serum from sensitized mice to naive mice.[67] Moreover, studies involving human PMNs,[43] and murine alveolar[68] and peritoneal[63] macrophages have shown that immune serum does not enhance the resistance mediated by these cells any more than nonimmune serum. This suggests that antibody plays no role in those defense mechanisms.

6.1.2. Serodiagnosis of Human Infection

Serodiagnosis of blastomycosis is the focus of a separate chapter in this book, and therefore only selected aspects will be discussed here. The identification and application of A antigen offer a major advance in serologic testing. Whereas the use of crude yeast-form antigens in the older complement fixation test yielded an assay with only 57% sensitivity and 30% specificity,[23] the use of A antigen in the complement fixation test increased these values to 62 and 100%.[24] The most recent immunodiffusion studies of A antigen have shown that it is highly specific (generally 100%) but still insensitive, yielding sensitivity values of 62 to 65% in studies of chronic disease[24–26] and 28% in a study of acute epidemic infection.[36] Conversely, use of A antigen in an enzyme immunoassay has improved the sensitivity to 77 to 100% in recent studies.[25–27] This, however, has been at the cost of specificity, with cross-reactivity occurring in a total of 17 (24%) of 72 control subjects who had other fungal infections. Purification of the active components in the heterogeneous material that characterizes A antigen and identification of the immunospecific determinants are necessary to resolve problems with cross-reactivity.

Preliminary work using the newly identified antigen WI-1 suggests that WI-1 may be more sensitive and specific than A antigen. In a radioimmunoassay using ^{125}I-labeled WI-1 as the antigen target, 185 sera were tested and antibody was detected in 58 (85%) of patients with blastomycosis. The geometric mean titer was quite high, 1:2981 (Fig. 4).[29] In contrast, only 2 (3%) of 73 patients with other fungal diseases and none of 44 healthy persons had detectable antibody to WI-1. No firm conclusions can be made about the relative value of A antigen and WI-1 for serodiagnosis because parallel assays incorporating the antigens were not compared. However, 76 sera from 38 patients with blastomycosis that had been tested in two previous studies for antibody to A antigen by EIA were tested for antibody to WI-1 by RIA. Only 58% had been considered seropositive when tested for antibody to A antigen

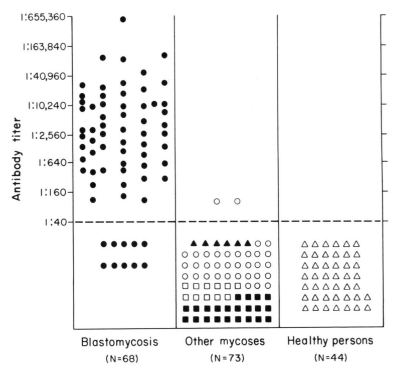

FIGURE 4. Detection of antibody to WI-1, a 120-kDa surface protein on *B. dermatitidis* yeasts in sera of patients with: blastomycosis (●); histoplasmosis (○); coccidioidomycosis (■); sporotrichosis (□); candidiasis (▲); healthy persons (△). Values above the dashed horizontal line are considered positive. (From Ref. 29.)

by EIA, whereas 82% were seropositive when tested for antibody to WI-1 by RIA (Fig. 5). The value of WI-1 for serodiagnosis of blastomycosis, or other immunologic studies of the disease, awaits additional confirmatory studies.

The development and clearance of antibody in blastomycosis follows a predictable time course. Peak titers are usually found between 50 and 70 days after onset of illness; titers wane between 116 and 200 days after onset; and the clearance of antibody is hastened by antifungal therapy (Fig. 6).[27] In a study of 27 patients, patients with disseminated infection were more likely to have detectable and significantly higher antibody titers to A antigen by EIA than those with localized pulmonary disease.[25] Other studies have found a wide range of antibody titers with the same assay independent of extent and severity of infection,[26,27] although it appears that falling antibody titers during a 4- to 8-month interval after therapy is instituted are associated with uncomplicated resolution of infection.

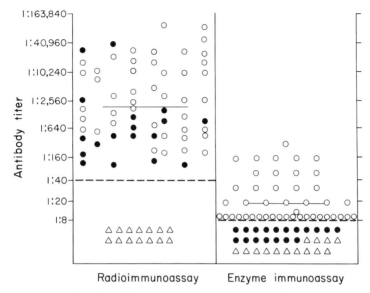

FIGURE 5. Comparison of radioimmunoassay (RIA) and enzyme immunoassay (EIA) for detection of antibody to *B. dermatitidis* in patients sera. Values above the dashed horizontal line are considered positive. O: RIA and EIA positive ($n = 44$); ●: RIA positive EIA negative ($n = 18$); △: RIA and EIA negative ($n = 14$). Solid horizontal line denotes the geometric mean titer of positive sera. (From Ref. 29.)

6.2. Cell-Mediated Immunity

6.2.1. Delayed-Type Hypersensitivity (DTH)

DTH has been studied in much greater depth in experimental animals than in humans because reliable skin test antigens for use in humans have been unavailable. After immunization in mice, the acquisition of DTH follows a somewhat predictable time course and is temporally correlated with the development of resistance to *B. dermatitidis* infection. Subcutaneous injection of C57BL/6J mice with low doses of viable *B. dermatitidis* yeasts produced a local infection that resolved, conferring DTH that peaked 15 days after immunization, as measured by footpad swelling response to antigen.[69] This functional capability could be transferred passively to naive mice by spleen cells of immunized mice, but not by serum.[67] Furthermore, mice immunized with either viable or merthiolate-killed yeasts demonstrated peak responses of DTH that coincided temporally with maximal resistance to a lethal challenge with live *B. dermatitidis* given intraperitoneally,[69] intra-

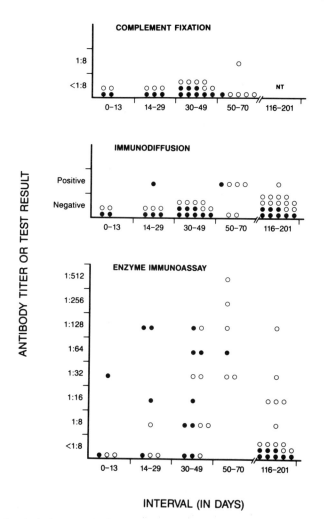

FIGURE 6. Serological test results for antibody to *B. dermatitidis* A antigen, by interval from onset of illness to testing, in serum specimens from 22 symptomatic patients in an outbreak of blastomycosis. ●, specimen from treated patient; ○, specimen from untreated patient; NT, not tested. (From Ref. 27.)

venously,[70] and intranasally.[71] These results indicate that the maturation of cell-mediated immunity is a vital aspect of host resistance to the infection.

DTH responses in experimental animals have been used to assess the reliability of blastomyces skin-test antigens such as B-ASWS and blastomy- cin. Positive responses to B-ASWS were found in 69% of blastomyces-sensitized guinea pigs but only 8% of histoplasma-sensitized guinea pigs.[15] The responses with two blastomycin antigens were less reliable. Commercial blastomycin yielded values of 37 and 40%, respectively, and blastomycin KCB-25 gave values of 66 and 74%. The activity of B-ASWS was enhanced by ultrafiltrate fractionation. The PM-10 residue yielded positive responses in 78 and 10% of the two groups, respectively. A 100 μg dose of this material produced an optimal response in the blastomyces-sensitized animals, and histological examination of the reactions confirmed that the cellular infiltration was principally mononuclear cells. Additional work has shown that the PM-10 residue can be further separated into four components by preparative disc electrophoresis.[21] Fraction number 4 yielded positive DTH responses in all blastomyces-infected guinea pigs but in none of the histoplasma-infected guinea pigs. The other three fractions and unfractionated B-ASWS showed less sensitivity and specificity.

Despite the large amount of convincing data on the value of B-ASWS for assessing DTH responses in experimental animals, the antigen has not been evaluated by skin testing in human infection. Application of these data should help clarify epidemiologic features of the disease.

6.2.2. In Vitro Correlates of DTH

6.2.2.1. Lymphocyte Proliferation. The subcutaneous administration of viable yeasts in BALB/cByJ mice elicits *in vitro* proliferative responses in spleen cells after 1 week and in contralateral lymph node cells after 3 weeks. These responses can be measured using B-ASWS, a blastomyces urea lysate antigen, or merthiolate-killed yeast cells.[71] Stimulating the cells with the urea lysate antigen yields the greatest proliferative responses, but they are not significantly greater than responses with the other antigens. The chronology of development of proliferative responses of the spleen cells in these animals is correlated with the development of DTH responses, so that both responses appear at 1 week and peak between 3 and 4 weeks after immunization.

In experimentally infected guinea pigs and infected humans, *in vitro* proliferative responses to B-ASWS have been studied as a marker of acquired cellular immunity and therefore of previous infection. B-ASWS elicited proliferation of lymph node cells from all 13 blastomyces-infected guinea pigs in one study, and the degree of response in these animals was significantly greater than that seen in histoplasma-infected or noninfected animals.[17] A linear response was obtained with increasing antigen concentrations; 100 μg was optimal. Bradsher and co-workers demonstrated that B-ASWS elicited lymphocyte proliferation in all 12 patients they evaluated who had recovered from blastomycosis between 2 months and 16 years be-

TABLE 1
Lymphocyte Proliferation to B-ASWS in Patients Infected during the 1984 Eagle River,
Wisconsin Epidemic of Blastomycosis[a]

Assay measure[b]	Interval from exposure to evaluation		
	3 months	7 months	21 months
Number of patients positive/tested	36/43 (84%)	27/45 (60%)	32/41 (78%)
Mean cpm ± S.E.M.			
E − C	16,852 ± 2664	9949 ± 1283	17,819 ± 3163
E/C	42.2 ± 5.3	10.7 ± 2.4	26.8 ± 3.7

[a] Modified from Klein BS et al., J Infect Dis 161:97–101, 1990.
[b] [³H]-Thymidine uptake by B-ASWS-stimulated [experimental (E)] and unstimulated [control (C)] lymphocytes was assessed by liquid scintillation counting. A positive assay was defined as E − C greater than 2000 and E/C greater than 5.

fore testing (median, 4.5 years).[19] The responses in these patients were significantly greater than responses in six normal adults with skin test reactivity to histoplasmin and 11 patients who had recovered from systemic histoplasmosis, although reactivity in the latter groups was also significantly greater than in the normal adults. These results showed that the assay can reliably identify previous *B. dermatitidis* infection in humans and discriminate it from infection with other dimorphic fungi, particularly *H. capsulatum*. A large epidemic of acute *B. dermatitidis* infection in 48 persons in Wisconsin allowed investigators to assess prospectively and longitudinally the acquisition of specific cellular immunity, as measured by a proliferative response to B-ASWS.[13,14] By 3 months after exposure to the fungus, 84% of infected persons had a proliferative response (Table 1). All 48 persons developed a response over the course of approximately 2 years following exposure, and 78% of the individuals tested at the end of this interval still had a proliferative response to B-ASWS. These studies suggest that a proliferative response to B-ASWS is a reliable marker of specific cellular immunity in blastomycosis and that the response persists in most patients for several years.

6.2.2.2. Lymphokines. T lymphocytes activated specifically by foreign antigen interact with other cells of the immune system by means of soluble mediators, or lymphokines. Lymphokines are water-soluble regulatory peptides that are produced by or act on lymphocytes.[72] The growing list of lymphokines includes interleukins, interferons, lymphotoxins, and tumor necrosis factors. IFN-γ is a very important regulator of the immune response. It is a 20- to 25-kDa glycosylated protein produced by T-helper cells following antigen stimulation, and interacts with a variety of cells within the lymphoid system. For example, it enhances the efficiency of foreign antigen presentation by macrophages by enhancing expression of MHC class II antigen. It enhances the phagocytic function of the cells by increasing the number of Fc receptors for IgG, and the microbicidal activity by increasing oxidative metabolism.

Lymphokines, and IFN-γ in particular, appear to be important in regulating the immune response to *B. dermatitidis*. Numerous studies discussed above have shown that lymphokine-containing supernatants endow macrophages of experimental animals and humans with enhanced fungicidal activity *in vitro* against *B. dermatitidis*. The availability of recombinant IFN-γ and anti-IFN-γ has made it possible to dissect the regulatory role of this peptide. Indeed, the enhanced killing of *B. dermatitidis* by murine alveolar[58] and peritoneal[73] macrophages treated with supernatants from Con A-stimulated spleen cell cultures could be largely neutralized by antibody to murine IFN-γ, suggesting that this peptide was the major activating factor in the supernatant. Additionally, if the cells were treated with IFN-γ alone, they exhibited greater killing of *B. dermatitidis*, comparable to that with Con A supernatants. The effect of IFN-γ is dose-dependent. A dose of 10,000 U/ml was optimal for enhanced killing of *B. dermatitidis*.[73] In contrast, only 10 U/ml was needed to enhance killing of *C. albicans* yeasts. These results indicate an important regulatory role for IFN-γ in macrophage-mediated killing of *B. dermatitidis*, and also underscore the relative resistance of the organism to this host defense mechanism when compared to other yeasts such as *C. albicans*.

Very little work has been done on involvement of other lymphokines in response to *B. dermatitidis*. Following stimulation with B-ASWS, mononuclear cells from patients recovered from blastomycosis and from blastomyces-infected guinea pigs produce migration inhibition factor. Presumably, this factor would serve to restrict or recruit effector cells to the site of an inflammatory lesion. However, its precise function in resistance to *B. dermatitidis* and molecular characteristics have not been explored.

6.2.3. T-Cell Subpopulations

One study examined the subpopulations of lymphocytes found in peripheral blood and alveolar lavage fluid of patients with pulmonary and extrapulmonary blastomycosis.[74] There was a significantly reduced number of T-helper cells and ratio of T-helper/suppressor cells in peripheral blood of patients with active disease in comparison to normal controls. Both defects resolved after 4 weeks of antifungal therapy. There was also a significant increase in the number and percentage of T-suppressor cells and a corre-

sponding decrease in the T-helper/suppressor ratio in bronchoalveolar lavage fluid of patients after treatment for 4 weeks, in comparison to normal
controls. These results suggest that there is compartmentalization of T-suppressor cells within the lungs of patients with blastomycosis. This observation is in contrast to findings in sarcoidosis, where there is compartmentalization of T-helper cells within the lungs.[75] The reasons for this difference and
the functional importance of these findings in blastomycosis are unclear, but
may reflect more efficient regulation of the immune response to the inciting
pathogen in blastomycosis.

6.3. Summary

In summary, there is no apparent relationship between development of
specific antiblastomyces antibody and resistance to infection, although the
availability of new antigens such as A antigen and WI-1 has led to more
reliable methods of antibody detection and serodiagnosis. Specific cellular
immunity has been demonstrated to be a principal component of acquired
resistance to *B. dermatitidis* in experimental animal models, and this functional capacity resides with antigen-specific T cells. Activated macrophages
are a principal effector cell of resistance. They acquire their microbicidal
activities after stimulation with lymphokines, particularly IFN-γ, released
from antigen-specific T cells. Studies of the cell-mediated immune response
in human blastomycosis have recently become possible with the availability
of B-ASWS. They have shown that virtually all patients infected with *B.
dermatitidis* develop specific cellular immunity, as measured by *in vitro*
lymphocyte proliferation to B-ASWS. This response correlates with enhanced *in vitro* phagocytosis and growth inhibition of *B. dermatitidis* by
peripheral blood monocyte-derived and alveolar macrophages. The results
further suggest that during the course of infection, activated T cells recognize
antigenic determinants in the yeast cell wall that can be liberated by alkali
hydrolysis and can elicit the various functional activities of these activated T
cells. The precise nature of these determinants and whether they can by
themselves induce resistance require further study.

7. IMMUNOMODULATION

7.1. Augmentation

7.1.1. Immunization

In the preceding sections, effective immunization against *B. dermatitidis* infection has been described in numerous murine model systems. DTH responses and resistance to infection are closely related, and the cells that confer immunity have been identified as Thy-1.2$^+$ T cells.[66] The identity of the responding T-cell subpopulation and the immunogenic determinants recognized on blastomyces have not been identified.

Virtually no work has been done to develop a vaccine for humans. This may relate to the perceived infrequency of blastomycosis as a clinical problem. Unfortunately, the actual prevalence and clinical importance of blastomycosis remain unknown in the absence of a reliable skin test, and may be underestimated. Before a histoplasmin skin test was developed, histoplasmosis was mistakenly believed to be a serious, infrequent, and often fatal disease.[76] However, skin testing proved that subclinical and mild forms of infection are common. Clarification of the epidemiology of blastomycosis may identify individuals or groups who by virtue of occupation or other activities are at high risk of severe infection. Such persons would be a target population for vaccination and other protective measures.

7.1.2. Immunotherapy

Approximately 80–90% of patients with blastomycosis respond to treatment. Of those who respond, 10–20% may relapse and require additional therapy. Patients with widely disseminated infection, especially involving progressive disease of the lungs, often die with blastomycosis. Newer forms of antifungal therapy, including immune enhancement, would clearly benefit patients who respond poorly to treatment. Immunotherapeutic agents that have been studied in blastomycosis are described below.

In vitro treatment of macrophages with IFN-γ endows them with enhanced fungicidal activity. A recent study extended this observation demonstrating that *in vivo* administration of IFN-γ to mice also activates these effector cells. BALB/cBy JIMR mice received 4×10^5 U IFN-γ i.p. Their pulmonary alveolar macrophages isolated 24 h later showed markedly enhanced killing of *B. dermatitidis* (38%) compared with cells of control mice (5%).[59] The effect of IFN-γ was dose dependent; 1×10^5 U also enhanced killing (29%), but less than the higher dose. This study demonstrates that systemic administration of IFN-γ acts in the pulmonary compartment, providing rationale for the use of IFN-γ therapeutically in refractory cases of pulmonary infection.

Thymosin, a hormone isolated from bovine thymus, augments cell-mediated immunity in immunodeficient animals[77] and humans.[78] Administration of thymosin to mice depleted of T cells restores their capacity to mount DTH responses to *B. dermatitidis*.[79] T-cell-depleted mice treated with thymosin before and after sensitization with *B. dermatitidis* showed DTH responses 62% greater than those in untreated immunodeficient mice. Thymosin treatment did not augment the normal DTH responses to *B.*

dermatitidis of immunocompetent mice. The influence of thymosin on the course of infection was not examined and needs further study.

N-Acetyl-muramyl-L-alanyl-D-isoglutamine, a synthetic muramyl dipeptide, is the minimum structure necessary for the adjuvant activity of cell wall preparations from mycobacteria.[80] When combined with oil and antigen, this compound has an adjuvant effect in stimulating cell-mediated and humoral immunity. Muramyl dipeptide and its desmethyl analogue afforded inconsistent protection and treatment benefits against pulmonary challenge with *B. dermatitidis* in several inbred strains of mice.[81] The most striking benefit was in BALB/c mice that received 400 mg of muramyl dipeptide or its desmethyl analogue on each of the 4 days before challenge. Mortality was reduced from 70% to 5% and 40% with the dipeptide and its analogue, respectively. Enhanced survival was barely significant in C3H/HeJ mice, and insignificant in DBA/2J mice. When the compounds were used for treatment beginning 4 days after challenge, the survival of BALB/c mice that received the desmethyl analogue improved to 70% from 40% in untreated controls. Neither C3H/HeJ or DBA/2J mice receiving these compounds survived longer than control animals. None of the mouse strains benefited when treatment was begun later than 4 days after challenge. Although these compounds enhanced resistance to *B. dermatitidis,* the strong genetic influence upon their effect would make them unsuitable for use in humans, given the extensive genetic diversity in the population.

7.2. Suppression

Immunoregulatory disturbances and suppression of immunity are common features following infection with the dimorphic fungi *H. capsulatum*[82] and *Coccidioides immitis*[83] and the yeasts *Cryptococcus neoformans*[84] and *Candida albicans.*[85] Suppression is generally seen with disseminated disease and has been ascribed to suppressor cells, soluble factors, immune complexes, or antibody, depending upon the pathogen. Despite the fact that *B. dermatitidis* infection disseminates frequently, immune suppression has been uncommon in blastomycosis.

Anergy has been described in some patients with disseminated blastomycosis. In one series of 40 patients, 20 had negative blastomycin skin tests and many were anergic.[86] Anergy was associated with disseminated, progressive infection and a very poor prognosis. Of 16 patients with negative skin tests and adequate follow-up, 10 (63%) died of infection. Another report described a previously healthy 13-year-old girl with disseminated blastomycosis that was refractory to treatment and associated with cutaneous anergy and greatly diminished lymphocyte responses to mitogens and antigens.[87]

Results from these reports suggest that *B. dermatitidis* may indeed produce immunoregulatory disturbances, leading to immune suppression and serious clinical consequences.

Diminished peripheral blood lymphocyte responses to mitogens and blastomyces or other antigens have been described in infected dogs and humans. Legendre *et al.*[88] reported depressed lymphocyte counts and *in vitro* proliferation to mitogens in ten dogs with severe clinical disease, but did not associate the defects with clinical outcome. Bradsher[19] followed the development of *in vitro* lymphocyte responses to B-ASWS, other soluble antigens, and mitogens in eight patients with pulmonary infection and eight patients with extrapulmonary infection. All patients with pulmonary disease had depressed responses to B-ASWS when they were initially diagnosed, whereas all eight patients with disseminated disease responded normally at that time. Both groups responded similarly to mitogens. After at least 2 weeks of antifungal therapy, all patients with localized disease showed a vigorous proliferative response to B-ASWS. The patients with extrapulmonary disease had a further increase in response, although the groups had similar responses to B-ASWS when subsequent assays were done. The initial unresponsiveness to B-ASWS in patients with localized disease may have been due to immune suppression or possibly compartmentalization of the immune response to the lung. However, given the extremely rapid correction of the defect and the unexplained and surprising finding that suppression was seen with localized rather than disseminated disease, a more plausible explanation may relate to the timing of patient testing with respect to the interval from onset. Patients with localized disease were initially tested a median of 4 weeks after onset, whereas those with disseminated disease were initially tested a median of 5 months after onset, giving the latter group more time to develop a specific cellular response.

Immunoregulatory disturbances following *B. dermatitidis* infection have been carefully examined in a murine model of disseminated blastomycosis.[6] Following inoculation of 10^6 yeasts intravenously into C57BL/6 mice, cellular immune responses become abnormal only late in the course of infection, i.e., the fifth week. At that time, mice demonstrate (1) depressed DTH responses to B-ASWS and nonspecific antigens, (2) impaired responses to the mitogens Con A and phytohemagglutinin, and (3) suppression by splenocytes from infected mice of the primary antibody response to sheep red blood cells by normal spleen cell cultures. These investigators postulated that the very late expression of suppressor cell activity in the mice could be explained by the fact that an insufficient amount of antigen accumulated in lymphoid organs to activate suppressor cells early in the infection. Indeed, the lymph nodes and spleens were remarkably spared of infection in the mice, a feature that this model shares with disseminated disease in man.

Given this observation, the hypothesis of these investigators may explain why suppressor cell activity and immune suppression have been observed only infrequently in human disease.

8. SUMMARY

Inhalation of *B. dermatitidis* conidia into the lung elicits a characteristic admixture of inflammatory cells including both neutrophils and mononuclear cells. Conidia are no match for these nonspecific phagocytes, which kill the infective particles efficiently through mechanisms of oxidative metabolism. However, conidia convert to yeasts in host tissue, offering the organism a selective advantage against these otherwise potent defense mechanisms. Yeasts are considerably more resistant to oxidative mechanisms of killing. The large size of yeasts also impedes phagocytosis by nonspecific phagocytes, leading to the requirement that most killing take place extracellularly, by membrane-to-membrane apposition. Antigen-specific T cells confer immunity upon the host and endow the phagocytes with enhanced fungicidal activity against the yeast. However, the precise nature of these T cells, what determinants they recognize in the cell wall of the yeast, and exactly how they regulate the immune response are unknown. Activation of phagocytes is mediated by lymphokines secreted by the T cells, especially IFN-γ. Activated macrophages from immune donors, for example, show markedly enhanced phagocytosis and growth inhibition of *B. dermatitidis,* when compared to the cells of nonimmune donors. Nonoxidative mechanisms appear to be important for killing of yeasts by these phagocytes, although the precise mechanism by which *B. dermatitidis* is eliminated is unknown. Answers to the questions raised here will help clarify our understanding of the immunopathogenesis of blastomycosis and may shed light on immune response mechanisms against other dimorphic fungi and yeasts.

ACKNOWLEDGMENTS. This work was supported in part by USPHS Grant AI00905. Carol Steinhart, Department of Veterans Affairs, Medical Research Service, William S. Middleton Memorial Veterans Hospital, provided editorial assistance. The secretarial center, Department of Medicine, University of Wisconsin Hospital and Clinics, prepared the manuscript.

REFERENCES

1. Sarosi GA, Hammerman KJ, Tosh FE, et al: Clinical features of acute pulmonary blastomycosis. *N Engl J Med* 290:540–543, 1974

2. Recht LD, Philips JR, Eckman MR, et al: Self-limited blastomycosis: A report of thirteen cases. *Am Rev Respir Dis* 120:1109–1112, 1979

3. Sarosi GA, Davies SF: Blastomycosis. *Am Rev Respir Dis* 120:911–938, 1979

4. Recht LD, Davies SF, Eckman MR, et al: Blastomycosis in immunocompromised patients. *Am Rev Respir Dis* 125:359–362, 1982

5. Schwartz J, Salfelder K: Blastomycosis. A review of 152 cases. *Curr Top Pathol* 65:165–200, 1977

6. Deepe GS Jr, Taylor CL, Bullock WE: Evolution of inflammatory response and cellular immune responses in a murine model of disseminated blastomycosis. *Infect Immun* 50:183–189, 1985

7. Miyaji M, Nishimura K: Granuloma formation and killing functions of granuloma in congenitally athymic nude mice infected with *Blastomyces dermatitidis* and *Paracoccidioides brasiliensis. Mycopathologia* 82:129–141, 1983

8. Thurmond LM, Mitchell TG: *Blastomyces dermatitidis* chemotactic factor: Kinetics of production and biological characterization evaluated by a modified neutrophil chemotaxis assay. *Infect Immun* 46:87–93, 1984

9. Cox RA, Mills LR, Best GK, et al: Histologic reaction to cell walls of an avirulent and a virulent strain of *Blastomyces dermatitidis. J Infect Dis* 129:179–186, 1974

10. Cox RA, Best GK: Cell wall composition of two strains of *Blastomyces dermatitidis* exhibiting differences in virulence for mice. *Infect Immun* 5:449–453, 1972

11. Blastomycosis Cooperative Study of the Veterans Administration: Blastomycosis I: A review of 198 collected cases in Veterans Administration hospitals. *Am Rev Respir Dis* 89:659–672, 1964

12. Witorsch P, Utz JP: North American blastomycosis: A study of 40 patients. *Medicine* 47:169–200, 1968

13. Klein BS, Bradsher RW, Vergeront JM, et al: The development of long-term specific cellular immunity after acute *Blastomyces dermatitidis* infection: Assessments following a large point-source outbreak in Wisconsin. *J Infect Dis* 161:97–101, 1990

14. Klein BS, Vergeront JM, Weeks RJ, et al: Isolation of *Blastomyces dermatitidis* in soil associated with a large outbreak of blastomycosis in Wisconsin. *N Engl J Med* 314:529–534, 1986

15. Cox RA, Larsh HW: Isolation of skin test active preparations from yeast-phase cells of Blastomyces dermatitidis. *Infect Immun* 10:42–47, 1974

16. Hall NK, Deighton F, Larsh HW: Use of an alkali-soluble water-soluble extract of *Blastomyces dermatitidis* yeast-phase cell walls and isoelectrically focused components in peripheral lymphocyte transformation. *Infect Immun* 19:411–415, 1978

17. Deighton F, Cox RA, Hall NK, et al: In vivo and in vitro cell-mediated immune responses to a cell wall antigen of *Blastomyces dermatitidis. Infect Immun* 15:429–435, 1977

18. Bradsher RW, Alford RH: *Blastomyces dermatitidis* antigen-induced lymphocyte reactivity in human blastomycosis. *Infect Immun* 33:485–490, 1981

19. Bradsher RW: Development of specific immunity in patients with pulmonary or extrapulmonary blastomycosis. *Am Rev Respir Dis* 129:430–434, 1984

20. Cox RA, Larsh HW: Yeast and mycelial-phase antigens of *Blastomyces dermatitidis:* Comparison using disc gel electrophoresis. *Infect Immun* 10:48–53, 1974

21. Lancaster MV, Sprouse RF: Isolation of a purified skin test antigen from *Blastomyces dermatitidis* yeast-phase cell wall. *Infect Immun* 14:623–625, 1976

22. Cox RA: Cross reactivity between antigens of *Coccidioides immitis, Histoplasma capsulatum* and *Blastomyces dermatitidis* in lymphocyte transformation assays. *Infect Immun* 25:932–938, 1979

23. Kaufman L, McLaughlin DW, Clark MJ, et al: Specific immunodiffusion test for blastomycosis. *Appl Microbiol* 26:244–247, 1973

24. Green JH, Harrell WK, Johnson JE, et al: Isolation of an antigen from *Blastomyces dermatitidis* that is specific for the diagnosis of blastomycosis. *Curr Microbiol* 4:293–296, 1980

25. Klein BS, Kuritsky HN, Chappel WA, et al: Comparison of the enzyme immunoassay, immunodiffusion and complement fixation tests in detecting antibody in human sera to the A antigen of *Blastomyces dermatitidis. Am Rev Respir Dis* 133:144–148, 1986

26. Turner SH, Kaufman L, Jalbert M: Diagnostic assessment of an enzyme-linked immunosorbent assay for human and canine blastomycosis. *J Clin Microbiol* 23:294–297, 1986

27. Klein BS, Vergeront JM, Kaufman L, et al: Serological tests for blastomycosis: Assessment during a large point-source outbreak in Wisconsin. *J Infect Dis* 155:262–268, 1987

28. Young KD, Larsh HW: Identification of the active precipitin components in a purified preparation of the A antigen of *Blastomyces dermatitidis. Infect Immun* 33:171–177, 1981

29. Klein BS, Jones JM: Isolation, purification and radiolabeling of a novel 120 kD surface protein on *Blastomyces dermatitidis* yeasts to detect antibody in infected patients. *J Clin Invest* 85:152–161, 1990

30. Furculow ML, Chick EW, Busey JD, et al: Prevalence and incidence studies of human and canine blastomycosis. I. Cases in the United States, 1885–1968. *Am Rev Respir Dis* 102:60–67, 1970

31. Legendre AM, Walker M, Buyukmihci N, et al: Canine blastomycosis: A review of 47 clinical cases. *J Am Vet Med Assoc* 178:1163–1168, 1981

32. Landay ME, Mitten J, Millar J: Disseminated blastomycosis in hamsters. II. Effect of sex on susceptibility. *Mycopathol Mycol Appl* 42:73–80, 1970

33. Abernathy RS: Clinical manifestations of pulmonary blastomycosis. *Ann Intern Med* 51:707–727, 1959

34. Kunkel WM, Weed LA, McDonald JR, et al: North American blastomycosis: Gilchrist's disease. A clinicopathologic study of 90 cases. *Surg Gynecol Obstet* 99:1–26, 1954

35. Chick EW, Sutliff WD, Rakish JH, et al: Epidemiological aspects of cases of blastomycosis admitted to Memphis, Tennessee hospitals during the period 1922–1954: A review of 86 cases. *Am J Med Sci* 231:253–262, 1956

36. Morozumi PA, Halpern JA, Stevens DA: Susceptibility differences of inbred strains of mice to blastomycosis. *Infect Immun* 32:160–168, 1981

37. Tosh FE, Hammerman KJ, Weeks RJ, et al: A common source epidemic of North American blastomycosis. *Am Rev Respir Dis* 109:525–529, 1974

38. Drutz DJ, Frey CL: Intracellular and extracellular defenses of human phagocytes against *Blastomyces dermatitidis* conidia and yeasts. *J Lab Clin Med* 105:737–750, 1985

39. Klebanoff SJ: Oxygen-dependent cytotoxic mechanisms of phagocytes, in Gallin JI, Fauci AS (eds): *Advances in Host Defense Mechanisms: Phagocytic Cells,* vol 1. New York, Raven Press, 1982, p 111

40. Lehrer RI, Ladra KM, Hake RB: Nonoxidative fungicidal mechanisms of mammalian granulocytes: Demonstration of components with candidacidal activity in human, rabbit, and guinea pig leukocytes. *Infect Immun* 11:1226–1234, 1975

41. Spitznagel JK, Shafer WM: Neutrophil killing of bacteria by oxygen-independent mechanisms: A historical summary. *Rev Infect Dis* 7:398–403, 1985

42. Sugar AM, Field KG: Susceptibility of *Blastomyces dermatitidis* (Bd) conidia to products of oxidative metabolism. *Abstr Annu Meet ASM* F10:390, 1987

43. Sixbey JW, Fields BT, Sun CN, et al: Interactions between human granulocytes and *Blastomyces dermatitidis. Infect Immun* 23:41–44, 1979

44. Diamond RD, Krzesicki R, Wellington J: Damage to pseudohyphae forms of *Candida albicans* by neutrophils in the absence of serum in vitro. *J Clin Invest* 61:349, 1978

45. Diamond RD, Krzesicki R: Mechanisms of attachment of neutrophils to *Candida albicans* pseudohyphae in the absence of serum, and subsequent damage to pseudohyphae by microbicidal processes of neutrophils in vitro. *J Clin Invest* 61:360–369, 1978

46. Brummer E, Stevens DA: Opposite effects of human monocytes, macrophages, and polymorphonuclear neutrophils on replication of *Blastomyces dermatitidis in vitro*. *Infect Immun* 36:297–303, 1982

47. Brummer E, Stevens DA: Enhancing effect of murine polymorphonuclear neutrophils (PMN) on the multiplication of *Blastomyces dermatitidis in vitro* and *in vivo*. *Clin Exp Immunol* 54:587–594, 1983

48. Schaffner A, Davis CE, Schaffner T, et al: *In vitro* susceptibility of fungi to killing by neutrophil granulocytes discriminates between primary pathogenicity and opportunism. *J Clin Invest* 78:511–524, 1986

49. Sugar AM, Chahal RS, Brummer E, et al: Susceptibility of *Blastomyces dermatitidis* strains to products of oxidative metabolism. *Infect Immun* 41:908–912, 1983

50. Sugar AM, Chahal RS, Brummer E, et al: The iron–hydrogen peroxide system in fungicidal activity against the yeast phase of *Blastomyces dermatitidis*. *J Leukocyte Biol* 36:545–548, 1984

51. Brummer E, Sugar AM, Stevens DA: Immunological activation of polymorphonuclear neutrophils for fungal killing: Studies with murine cells and *Blastomyces dermatitidis in vitro*. *J Leukocyte Biol* 36:505–520, 1984

52. Morrison CJ, Brummer E, Stevens DA: Effect of a local immune reaction on peripheral blood polymorphonuclear neutrophil microbicidal function: Studies with fungal targets. *Cell Immunol* 110:176–182, 1987

53. Brummer E, Stevens DA: Activation of murine polymorphonuclear neutrophils for fungicidal activity with supernatants from antigen-stimulated immune spleen cell cultures. *Infect Immun* 45:447–452, 1984

54. Morrison CJ, Brummer E, Isenberg RA, et al: Activation of murine polymorphonuclear neutrophils for fungicidal activity by recombinant gamma interferon. *J Leukocyte Biol* 41:434–440, 1987

55. Brummer E, Sugar AM, Stevens DA: Enhanced oxidative burst in immunologically activated but not elicited polymorphonuclear leukocytes correlates with fungicidal activity. *Infect Immun* 49:396–401, 1985

56. Morrison CJ, Isenberg RA, Stevens DA: Enhanced oxidative mechanisms in immunologically activated versus elicited polymorphonuclear neutrophils: Correlations with fungicidal activity. *J Med Microbiol* 25:115–121, 1988

57. Bradsher RW, Balk RA, Jacobs RF: Growth inhibition of *Blastomyces dermatitidis* in alveolar and peripheral macrophages from patients with blastomycosis. *Am Rev Respir Dis* 135:412–417, 1987

58. Brummer E, Stevens DA: Activation of pulmonary macrophages for fungicidal activity by gamma-interferon or lymphokines. *Clin Exp Immunol* 70:520–528, 1987

59. Brummer E, Hanson LH, Restrepo A, et al: In vivo and in vitro activation of pulmonary macrophages by IFN-γ for enhanced killing of *Paracoccidioides brasiliensis* or *Blastomyces dermatitidis*. *J Immunol* 140:2786–2789, 1988

60. Sugar AM, Field KG: Production of superoxide (O_2^-) by *Blastomyces dermatitidis* conidia and murine bronchoalveolar macrophages stimulated with conidia. *Clin Res* 35:493A, 1987

61. Sugar AM, Field KG: Production of superoxide (O_2^-) by *Blastomyces dermatitidis* (Bd) yeast forms and Bd challenged murine bronchoalveolar macrophages (BAM). *Abstr Annu Meet ASM* F45:396, 1987

62. Patterson-Delafield J, Martinez RJ, Lehrer RI: Microbicidal cationic proteins in rabbit

alveolar macrophages: A potential host-defense mechanism. *Infect Immun* 30:180–192, 1980

63. Brummer E, Sugar AM, Stevens DA: Activation of peritoneal macrophages by concanavalin A or *Mycobacterium bovis* BCG for fungicidal activity against *Blastomyces dermatitidis* and effect of specific antibody and complement. *Infect Immun* 39:817–822, 1983

64. Brummer E, Stevens DA: Fungicidal mechanisms of activated macrophages: Evidence for nonoxidative mechanisms for killing of *Blastomyces dermatitidis*. *Infect Immun* 55:3221–3224, 1987

65. Bradsher RW, Ulmer WC, Marmer DJ, et al: Intracellular growth and phagocytosis of *Blastomyces dermatitidis* by monocyte-derived macrophages from previously infected and normal subjects. *J Infect Dis* 151:57–64, 1985

66. Brummer E, Morozumi PA, Vo PT, et al: Protection against pulmonary blastomycosis: Adoptive transfer with T lymphocytes, but not serum, from resistant mice. *Cell Immunol* 73:349–359, 1982

67. Scillian JJ, Cozad GC, Spencer HD: Passive transfer of delayed hypersensitivity to *Blastomyces dermatitidis* between mice. *Infect Immun* 10:705–711, 1974

68. Sugar AM, Brummer E, Stevens DA: Fungicidal activity of murine bronchoalveolar macrophages against *Blastomyces dermatitidis*. *J Med Microbiol* 21:7–11, 1986

69. Spencer HD, Cozad GC: Role of delayed hypersensitivity in blastomycosis of mice. *Infect Immun* 7:329–334, 1973

70. Cozad GC, Chang CT: Cell-mediated immunoprotection in blastomycosis. *Infect Immun* 28:398–403, 1980

71. Morozumi PA, Brummer E, Stevens DA: Protection against pulmonary blastomycosis: Correlation with cellular and humoral immunity in mice after subcutaneous nonlethal infection. *Infect Immun* 37:670–678, 1982

72. Male D, Champion B, Cooke A (eds): *Lymphokines in Advanced Immunology.* Philadelphia, J B Lippincott Co, 1987

73. Brummer E, Morrisson CJ, Stevens DA: Recombinant and natural gamma-interferon activation of macrophages *in vitro:* Different dose requirements for induction of killing activity against phagocytizable and nonphagocytizable fungi. *Infect Immun* 49:724–730, 1985

74. Jacobs RF, Marmer DJ, Balk RA, et al: Lymphocyte subpopulations of blood and alveolar lavage in blastomycosis. *Chest* 88:579–585, 1985

75. Hunninghake GW, Crystal RG: Pulmonary sarcoidosis. A disorder mediated by excess helper T-lymphocyte activity at sites of disease activity. *N Engl J Med* 305:429–434, 1981

76. Parsons RJ, Zarafoanetis CJD: Histoplasmosis in man: Report of 7 cases and a review of 71 cases. *Arch Intern Med* 75:1–23, 1945

77. Law L, Goldstein AL, White A: Influence of thymosin in immunological competence of lymphoid cells from thymectomized mice. *Nature* 219:1391, 1968

78. Goldstein AL, Cohen GH, Rossio JL, et al: Use of thymosin in the treatment of primary immunodeficiency diseases and cancer. *Med Clin North Am* 60:591–606, 1976

79. Longley RE, Cozad GC: Thymosin restoration of cellular immunity to *Blastomyces dermatitidis* in T-cell-depleted mice. *Infect Immun* 26:187–192, 1979

80. Parant M: Biologic properties of a new synthetic adjuvant, muramyl dipeptide (MDP). *Semin Immunopathol* 2:101–118, 1979

81. Morozumi PA, Brummer E, Stevens DA: Immunostimulation with muramyl dipeptide and its desmethyl analogue: Studies of non-specific resistance to pulmonary blastomycosis in inbred mouse strains. *Mycopathologia* 81:35–39, 1983

82. Deepe GS Jr, Watson SR, Bullock WE: Generation of disparate immunoregulatory factors in two inbred strains of mice with disseminated histoplasmosis. *J Immunol* 129:2186–2191, 1982

83. Cantazaro A: Suppressor cells in coccidioidomycosis. *Cell Immunol* 64:235–245, 1981

84. Murphy JW, Moorhead JW: Regulation of cell mediated immunity in cryptococcosis. I. Induction of specific afferent T suppressor cells by cryptococcal antigen. *J Immunol* 128:276–283, 1982

85. Domer JE, Carrow EW: Candidiasis, in Cox RA (ed): *Immunology of the Fungal Diseases.* Boca Raton, CRC Press, 1989, pp 57–92

86. Smith DT: Immunologic types of blastomycosis: A report on 40 cases. *Ann Intern Med* 31:463–469, 1949

87. Fitzsimmons RB, Ferguson AC: Cellular immunity and nutrition in refractory disseminated blastomycosis. *Can Med Assoc J* 106:343–346, 1972

88. Legendre AM, Becker PU: Immunologic changes in acute canine blastomycosis. *Am J Vet Res* 43:2050–2053, 1982

9

Clinical Aspects of Blastomycosis

William A. Causey and Guy D. Campbell

1. INTRODUCTION

What is known of the spectrum of disease caused by *Blastomyces dermatitidis* comes from the study of published reports of sporadic cases, reviews of clinical experience of individual medical centers in endemic areas, from cooperative studies of investigators combining their experiences, and from studies of a few point-source outbreaks of blastomycosis. To this, the authors add their personal experience in diagnosis and treatment of patients with this disease.

Most infections with *B. dermatitidis* result from inhalation of fungal elements.[1] From an initial pulmonary focus, infection can spread by direct extension through the lung to the pleura, and across tissue boundaries to the chest wall, by endobronchial spread to other parts of the lung, and by lymphohematogenous deportation outside of the lung to virtually any extrapulmonary site. As a result, the clinical manifestation of both pulmonary blastomycosis and extrapulmonary blastomycosis may be extremely variable.

Our knowledge of the natural history of infection with this fungus is

Blastomycosis, edited by Yousef Al-Doory and Arthur F. DiSalvo, Plenum Medical Book Company, New York, 1992.

fragmentary at best. Acute, self-limited pulmonary infection has been observed in isolated sporadic cases, in accidental laboratory infection, and in patients described in several point-source outbreaks of blastomycosis. However, the frequency of asymptomatic infection and the frequency of spontaneous resolution of acute infection are unknown. Lack of availability of acceptable, sensitive, and specific serologic and skin tests has not permitted surveys of extended populations for evidence of unrecognized or asymptomatic infection. Thus, the actual prevalence of infection in endemic areas is unknown.

Additionally, the natural history of chronic forms of blastomycosis is not well established. It is not known, for instance, whether chronic pulmonary blastomycosis results from a progressive primary infection, from endogenous reactivation of a latent, healed pulmonary focus, or from exogenous reinfection in a patient sensitized from previous exposure to this fungus.

Nonetheless, it is apparent that blastomycosis is a systemic disease with a wide variety of pulmonary and extrapulmonary manifestations. The pulmonary disease can be acute, subacute, or chronic; it can mimic bacterial pneumonia, granulomatous diseases, other fungal infections, or bronchogenic carcinoma. Symptoms associated with pulmonary blastomycosis are likewise highly variable and nonspecific, and include cough, chest pain, chills, fever, sputum production, hemoptysis, weight loss, malaise, and myalgias.

Approximately two-thirds of patients in most series will have extrapulmonary manifestations,[1-4] often in more than one organ system. Recent experience suggests that metastasis[5] of infection outside the lung may be getting less common, and that the majority of patients are now presenting with single organ (lung) involvement. Skin, skeletal, and genitourinary systems are the most frequently involved extrapulmonary sites.

2. PULMONARY BLASTOMYCOSIS

2.1. Primary Infection

Since the studies of Schwarz and Baum,[1] it has been generally accepted that most blastomycosis occurs as a consequence of an initial pulmonary infection. Baum and Lerner later published a case report of a student technician who examined a culture of blastomycosis, and made smears without using a bacteriological hood. He subsequently developed symptoms, an abnormal X-ray, and positive sputum culture for *B. dermatitidis.*[6] Accidental inoculation (primary cutaneous) blastomycosis will be discussed later.

Most of what we know about acute primary pulmonary blastomycosis comes from the study of patients infected during the course of common source outbreaks,[7-14] but the total experience in this context amounts to fewer than 100 cases.[14] About half of infected individuals discovered during the course of these outbreaks are symptomatic, but their symptoms are highly nonspecific. They tend to mimic influenza or acute bacterial infection, and consist of abrupt onset of cough accompanied by fever, chills, myalgias, and arthralgias. The cough is usually nonproductive at first, but later may be associated with small amounts of purulent sputum. Chest pain, if present, is usually mild and transient. Chest X-ray findings in acute disease, whether the patient is symptomatic or asymptomatic, are likewise nonspecific, and usually consist of airspace disease in a lobar or segmental pattern, most commonly in the lower lobes. Pleural effusions and hilar adenopathy are uncommon, and a miliary pattern of infection has not been reported in association with acute primary infection. Spontaneous resolution may occur, and symptoms abate within 4 weeks. Radiographic changes may take longer to disappear.

Following inhalation of fungal elements, symptomatic or asymptomatic lung disease occurs with approximately half of the patients within 30–45 days. Thereafter, in those patients who do not spontaneously resolve, one of three courses may be taken: (1) Progression of the primary disease may evolve into either chronic pulmonary infection, extrapulmonary disease, or both. (2) After a period of apparent total resolution, endogenous reactivation may occur resulting in either chronic pulmonary disease or extrapulmonary infection, or both. (3) Finally, reexposure to an exogenous source of conidia following complete recovery may result in reinfection.

2.2. Chronic Blastomycosis

The vast majority of patients diagnosed with blastomycosis within an endemic area will have an indolent onset usually with slowly progressive disease best classified as chronic blastomycosis. The clinical manifestations are diverse: some patients with solely pulmonary, others with only extrapulmonary involvement, and some with both pulmonary and extrapulmonary infection.

2.2.1. Chronic Pulmonary Blastomycosis

Chronic pulmonary blastomycosis cannot be differentiated clinically from any other form of chronic lung disease. The symptoms may be particularly suggestive of chronic pulmonary tuberculosis or chronic histoplasmosis. Cough, sputum, weight loss, chest pain, night sweats, low-grade fever, skin lesions, and hemoptysis are the most common presenting complaints. A few patients will be asymptomatic despite a persistently abnormal X-ray.

There are no pathognomonic X-ray changes in pulmonary blastomycosis whether acute or chronic. Chronic disease is most often manifest in the upper lung fields.[4,15] Several different types of presentation are noted: alveolar disease with infiltrations containing air bronchograms in segmental and lobar fashion (Fig. 1), a masslike lesion at either the hilum or in the parenchyma (Fig. 2), interstitial disease sometimes with a nodular pattern (Fig. 3), and cavitary disease (Fig. 4). Calcification in blastomycosis is uncommon. Mild enlargement of hilar and mediastinal nodes is occasionally present. Miliary disease will be discussed later. Although pleural reaction is frequently noted on X-ray,[16–18] frank pulmonary effusion is uncommon but at times may be the only manifestation of the disease.[19] In the Veterans Administration Cooperative Study, only 4 of 198 patients with blastomycosis had a pleural effusion.[4]

Those patients presenting with a masslike lesion, especially in the area of the hilum, are often suspected of having bronchogenic carcinoma. This often leads to surgery which provides the correct diagnosis. Even if the lesion is completely removed surgically, our experience following patients who have had blastomycotic lesions excised at thoracotomy leads us to favor a course of therapy when the diagnosis is made. We have four patients who did not receive amphotericin B after such surgery: two subsequently developed miliary blastomycosis (one during the immediate postoperative period, and the other within the next 2–3 years), a third developed disease in the opposite lung field shortly after surgery, and the fourth patient returned a year and one-half later with paraplegia secondary to an epidural blastomycoma. Some clinicians have had a different experience and do not recommend antifungal treatment after apparent surgical removal of all diseased lung.[20]

2.2.2. Miliary Blastomycosis

Miliary blastomycosis resulting from a lymphohematogenous spread is rare and constitutes a medical emergency.[21–25] These patients are usually acutely and severely ill, dyspneic, and often progress to frank respiratory failure requiring ventilatory support (Fig. 5). Prompt diagnosis with immediate institution of amphotericin B therapy is mandatory as the disease carries a 50% mortality.[22] If sputum or nasotracheal suction is nondiagnostic, bronchoscopy with brushings, lavage, and transbronchial biopsy should provide the diagnosis.

3. EXTRAPULMONARY INFECTIONS

In most series, approximately two-thirds of the patients with chronic blastomycosis have extrapulmonary manifestations of disease with one or more organs involved.[1–4]

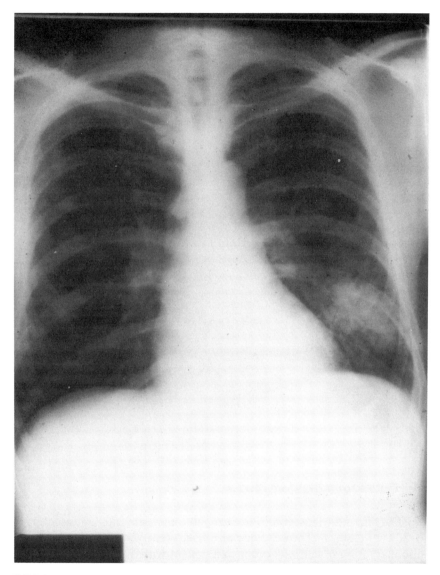

FIGURE 1. Pulmonary blastomycosis manifest as a segmental infiltrate with air bronchogram in the left lower lobe.

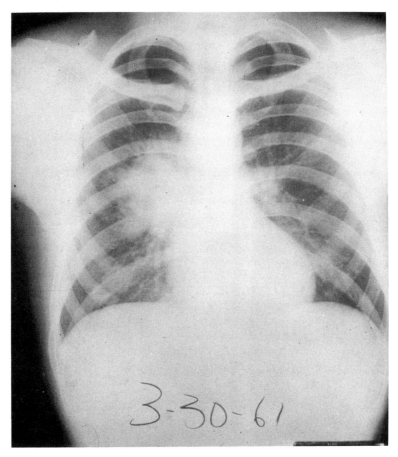

FIGURE 2. Pulmonary blastomycosis presenting as a large right hilar mass mimicking broncho-genic carcinoma.

3.1. Cutaneous Blastomycosis

The skin is the most common extrapulmonary site with lesions found in 40–80% of cases.[1-4] These lesions are most often accompanied by active pulmonary disease but may occur in a patient with a normal chest X-ray. The skin lesions begin as a small papulopustular lesion that increases in size. The central part of the lesion is often encrusted, but with time there is clearing in the central area with continual progression at the periphery with a 2- to 3-mm piling up at the margin with an abrupt change to normal skin distal to the elevation[26] (Fig. 6). This elevated portion contains numerous microabscesses and properly done and examined scrapings taken from this area al-

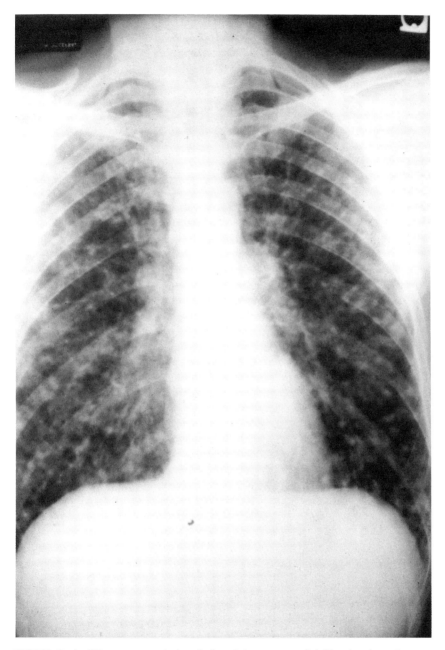

FIGURE 3. A diffuse, symmetrical reticulonodular pattern of infiltration in pulmonary blastomycosis.

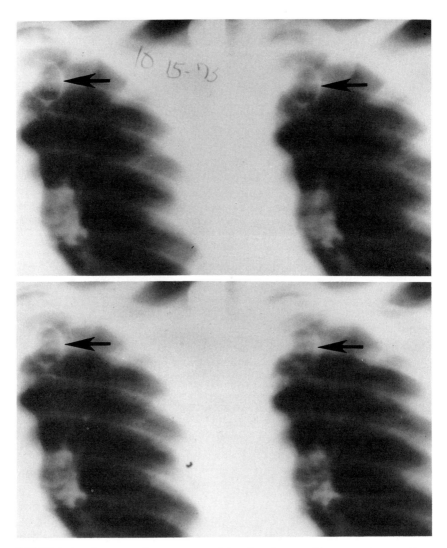

FIGURE 4. A rather unusual presentation of chronic pulmonary blastomycosis as a solitary thin-walled apical cavity as the only manifestation of disease.

most invariably reveal a positive smear and culture for *B. dermatitidis*. In other cases the papulopustular lesion ulcerates and appears as a classical ulcer with elevated margins (Fig. 7). Specimens of pus taken from the center of this lesion are almost always positive for *B. dermatitidis;* yeasts can be observed by wet preparation under the microscope using reduced light and

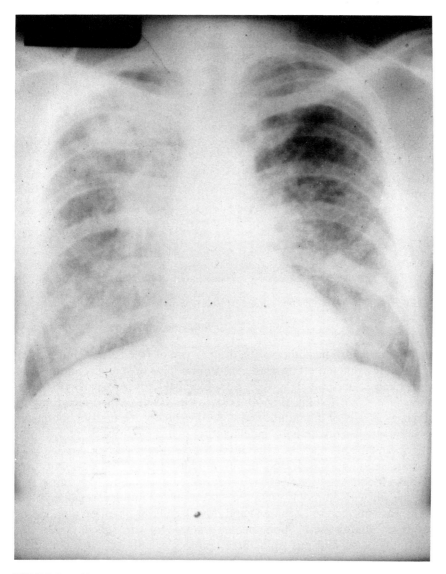

FIGURE 5. Miliary pulmonary blastomycosis resulting from lymphohematogenous spread within the lungs. This case developed 3 months after spontaneous clearing of an apparent primary infiltrate.

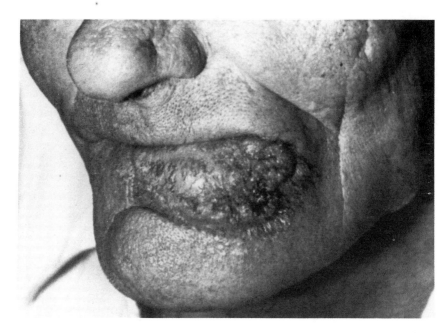

FIGURE 6. A typical blastomycotic skin lesion. Note heaped-up lesion and the sharp transition between the lesion and normal skin.

high-power field. The addition of a drop or two of 10% KOH solution may be helpful in differentiating yeast cells from cells of host origin. Lesions are more likely to occur in areas of the body exposed to the sun, particularly the brow, face, nose, and lips (Fig. 8). Lesions also occur in the mucous membrane, especially of the mouth and nose. The lesions are usually nontender and not associated with lymphadenopathy.

Subcutaneous nodules without involvement of overlying skin are cold abscesses and are considerably more ominous in their clinical implication than the lesions mentioned above. They are manifestations of systemic disease usually with dramatic pulmonary infection and multiple organ involvement. Patients tend to be quite ill and rapidly deteriorate unless amphotericin B is administered. Spontaneous drainage of the subcutaneous abscess may occur and pus from these lesions generally contains abundant yeast forms.

Primary inoculation blastomycosis usually results from laboratory accident.[27] Three cases followed dog bites.[28-30] The lesions resemble cutaneous sporotrichosis in their appearance and distribution. A chancroid ulcer appears at the site of inoculation and lymphangitis and lymphadenopathy are common, though systemic spread of infection has not been reported. Inoculation ulcers are generally painless and rarely require specific therapy,

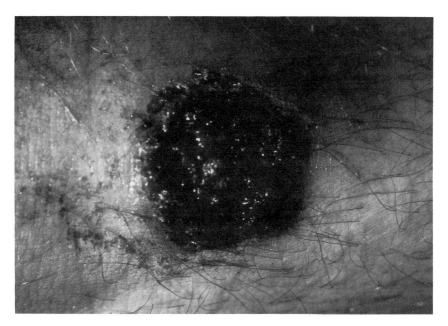

FIGURE 7. An indolent cutaneous ulcer of blastomycosis with typical moist base and elevated edges.

though lesions may take several months to resolve completely. (A special form of primary inoculation blastomycosis, that following sexual intercourse, will be discussed later.[31,32])

3.2. Bone and Joint

Bones and joints are involved in 10–40% of patients and usually lung disease is present.[1–4] As with other extrapulmonary manifestations of this disease, the lung lesions may have resolved before the bone and joint lesions develop. Long bones, ribs, and vertebrae are most frequently involved but almost any bone is vulnerable. The most common X-ray manifestation of skeletal blastomycosis is a well-circumscribed osteolytic lesion[4] (Fig. 9). Sometimes osteoblastic activity is evident around the border of the lesion. In chronic cases there is a moth-eaten appearance of the bone caused by widespread destruction. When the lesion is near the end of a bone it may extend into a joint, causing a purulent arthritis from which typical organisms may be smeared and cultured.[33] As long as the lesion consists only of a radiolucency without periosteal involvement, it is usually painless. If the patient

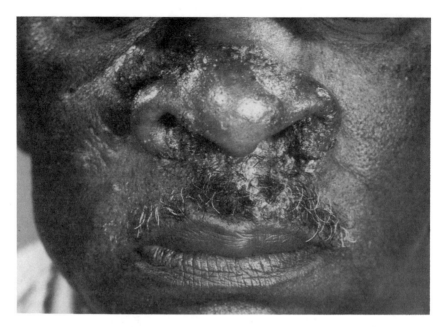

FIGURE 8. Dry, crusted blastomycotic lesions around the nostrils and on the nose.

develops swelling in the area of a bony lesion, pain occurs and draining sinuses may follow (Fig. 10). Joint infection may also occur without a bone lesion.[34,35]

Vertebral blastomycosis mimics vertebral tuberculosis. Both diseases involve the anterior portion of the vertebral bodies, destroy the interspace between adjacent vertebrae, and may produce paraspinal or psoas abscess.[36] The majority of patients will have active pulmonary disease.

3.3. Genitourinary

Genitourinary blastomycosis is seen mostly in men with different series reporting 10–30% incidence.[1-4] Although infection is limited to the prostate in 50% of patients, it also may invade the epididymis, seminal vesicle, testis, and kidney.[37] Prostatic symptoms consist of those associated with bladder outlet obstruction and may occasionally be severe enough to cause acute urinary retention. The prostate is usually tender and enlarged on palpation. Pain, swelling, and tenderness in the scrotum are common when scrotal contents are invaded. The prevailing opinion is that renal infection is pri-

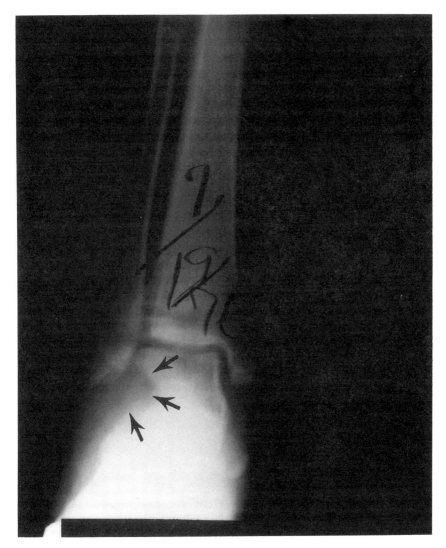

FIGURE 9. A large lytic lesion in the lateral aspect of the talus (arrows) and distal fibula.

marily hematogenous in origin and that the disease rarely progresses retrogradely to involve the kidney.[1,38] Bladder infection is uncommon. Smear and culture of urine and secretions following prostatic massage usually provides the diagnosis if the prostate is infected. At times, prostatic biopsy may be necessary not only to make a diagnosis but also to rule out possible carcinoma.

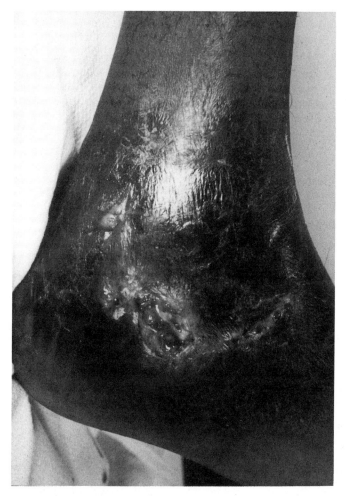

FIGURE 10. A chronic draining sinus overlying blastomycotic osteomyelitis (same patient as Fig. 9). Pus discharging from the sinus contained abundant *B. dermatitidis.*

Female urogenital blastomycosis is rare. Hamblen *et al.*[39] described a case of blastomycotic endometritis in 1935, the first case of urogenital blastomycosis reported in a female. In another case, intercourse with a male with blastomycosis of the right testis and prostate caused endometritis and bilateral salpingitis in the female.[31] In a similar case, cervical cytology in a female undergoing routine pelvic exam revealed organisms compatible with *B. dermatitidis,* and culture of the secretions was positive for blastomycosis. The husband had recently been treated with amphotericin B for pulmonary blastomycosis with a good response. Subsequent prostatic massage revealed organisms compatible with *B. dermatitidis*. Cervical cytology at 2 and 12 months was negative for blastomycosis.[32]

One case of tubo-ovarian and endometrial blastomycosis was diagnosed before surgery by cervical cytology and confirmed following excision of the lesion.[40] Faro and colleagues[41] admitted a patient for profuse vaginal bleeding. Endometrial biopsy revealed blastomycosis but the patient also had breast and thigh lesions due to the same infection.

3.4. Larynx

Hoarseness is the predominant symptom in patients with laryngeal blastomycosis.[42,43] This can result from unilateral vocal paralysis caused by recurrent laryngeal nerve dysfunction from pressure by hilar lung lesions. More commonly, nodular or ulcerative lesions may directly involve the larynx and produce hoarseness and upper airway obstruction (Fig. 11). Under direct

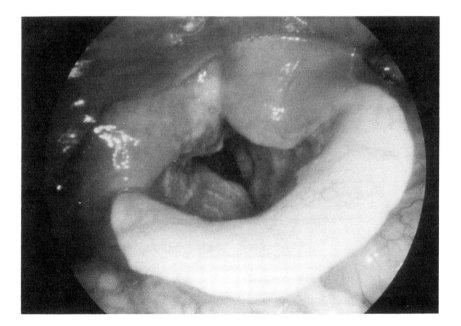

FIGURE 11. Endoscopic view through a rod lens telescope showing diffuse laryngeal blastomycosis. An erythematous, granulomatous lesion with irregular borders involves the posterior epiglottis, false vocal chords, true vocal chords, and arytenoids. Other laryngeal structures are edematous. The laryngeal airway is severely restricted.

vision the nodular or masslike lesions suggest laryngeal carcinoma, but biopsy provides a correct diagnosis. At times, patients develop respiratory distress secondary to laryngeal obstruction requiring emergency tracheostomy before the physician can proceed with the workup. Laryngeal blastomycosis usually occurs in association with overt pulmonary disease, but infection is considered secondary to hematogenous dissemination.[4] Rarely, patients with a long history of laryngeal symptoms will develop laryngocutaneous fistulas. Dumich and Neel[44] reported 6 patients with laryngeal disease in 107 patients with blastomycosis. Four of the six patients had no X-ray evidence of lung involvement.

Although hoarseness is the predominant symptom, patients may also complain of productive cough, weight loss, anorexia, or hemoptysis.

3.5. Central Nervous System (CNS)

CNS blastomycosis is quite uncommon. Buechner and Clawson[45] found 4.5% incidence of CNS disease in a retrospective study of 198 patients with blastomycosis.[3] With a long and special interest in a very highly endemic area, we have seen only 3 patients with CNS blastomycosis diagnosed during life. CNS involvement occurs in 3–10% of cases[1-4] as intracranial or epidural granuloma or abscess, meningitis, or a combination of these findings. Most CNS disease occurs late in the course of disseminated blastomycosis. Only a rare case has been reported with meningitis as the only identified source of infection.[46] Kravitz et al.[47] were able to find only 40 reported cases of blastomycosis meningitis in the world literature, but added 3 additional cases.

The predominant symptom of CNS blastomycosis is one of expanding mass lesion suggesting primary or metastatic tumor or abscess. Other symptoms are headache, altered consciousness, seizures, aphasia, or focal motor deficits. Predilection for involvement of posterior fossa structures often leads to gait disturbance, ataxia, and noncommunicating hydrocephalus.

Even when suspected, proving the diagnosis is quite difficult. When a patient with known blastomycosis develops symptoms or signs suggestive of meningitis or a focal mass lesion in the CNS, a CT scan should be obtained. If a focal lesion is present, it should be aspirated or biopsied. If hydrocephalus is present, ventricular fluid should be sampled for diagnosis. If the CT scan shows neither a mass lesion nor hydrocephalus, then lumbar cerebrospinal fluid (CSF) should be sampled. If repeat examination of lumbar CSF is nondiagnostic and CNS disease still suspected on the basis of an abnormal cell count or elevated protein level, then cisternal or ventricular fluid should be obtained for diagnosis. If a diagnosis is still not made, a meningeal biopsy should be considered. At least one diagnosis of meningeal blastomycosis was confirmed in CSF by immunodiffusion using blastomycin A antigen.[48] Usually other organs are involved and can provide the diagnosis, especially if aggressively sought.

Although CNS infection usually results from hematogenous spread, infection of the cranium or vertebral bodies may extend directly into the CNS as well.

3.6. Adrenal Gland

In 1962 Abernathy and Melby[49] reported a case of Addison's disease secondary to adrenal blastomycosis, stating that only two cases had been reported prior to 1962 with Addison's disease occurring $11\frac{1}{2}$ and 5 years respectively after the initial onset of blastomycosis.

Eberle et al.[50] reported a case of adrenal blastomycosis causing Addison's disease in a patient with prior disseminated blastomycosis. In 1977 Chandler[51] reported a single case of Addison's disease with the initial Addisonian crisis occurring with the first infusion of amphotericin B. Schwarz and Baum[1] found adrenal involvement in 4 of 58 cases of blastomycosis. The degree of destruction was described as moderate in 2 patients, focal in 1, with almost complete adrenal destruction in the fourth patient. Abernathy[49] found 2 of 8 fatal disseminated cases with adrenal involvement. Schwarz and Salfelder[38] in a review of 152 cases accumulated at the Armed Forces Institute of Pathology (AFIP) identified 18 cases of adrenal glands from patients with blastomycosis available for review. In 4 cases (2 of which were also reported by Schwarz and Baum in 1951[1]), the adrenal glands were involved. In a retrospective study of blastomycosis, Busey[3] reported adrenal involvement in 3 of 25 patients who had postmortem studies. Eberle et al.[50] estimated that approximately 10% of patients infected with blastomycosis had adrenal involvement but only a rare patient developed Addison's disease.

3.7. Other Manifestations of Blastomycosis

Other organ involvement includes breast,[41,57] esophagus,[52,55,56] eye,[60-62] heart,[1-3,52-54] middle ear cleft,[59] omentum,[3] pancreas,[3,52] pituitary,[1,2] skeletal muscle,[3] stomach,[3,4] thyroid,[2-4,38,52] and peritoneum.[3,40,52] Chapman[58] recently diagnosed a patient with peritoneal blastomycosis without other organ involvement.

Blastomycosis is rare in the gastrointestinal tract from the esophagogastric junction to the rectum, and oral and anal lesions are uncommon. Renal, hepatic, and splenic infection is not uncommon in disseminated disease but is rarely diagnosed because lesions in these organs uncommonly cause symptoms. A rare splenic abscess may be large enough to require drainage or excision. Involvement of unusual anatomic sites almost always indicates generalized systemic infection in a severely ill individual.

4. BLASTOMYCOSIS IN PREGNANCY

Although pregnancy has been shown to cause some decrease in immunity,[63] only a few cases of blastomycosis have been reported during pregnancy. Watts et al.[64] have reported one patient with undiagnosed skin lesions on her face 1 month before delivery. Two and one-half weeks after delivery, the mother's lesions had increased in size and number, and were described as "crusty." At 3 weeks of age, her infant was admitted to the Emergency Room because of rapid and "loud breathing." The baby sustained a cardiorespiratory arrest shortly after arrival at the hospital and resuscitation was unsuccessful. Autopsy of the infant revealed alveoli filled with the yeast form of *B. dermatitidis.* Examination of the mother at this time confirmed cutaneous blastomycosis. Although she had a normal urinalysis and no urinary symptoms, she did have a positive urine culture for blastomycosis. Whether infant infection occurred from transplacental transmission or from aspiration of infected maternal secretions during birth is uncertain. In a few other cases of blastomycosis occurring during pregnancy, whether treated or untreated before delivery, no evidence of blastomycosis was noted in the infant.[65,66] Ismail and Lerner[67] reported the successful treatment of a pregnant woman with blastomycosis with amphotericin B. They reviewed 20 cases of various fungal diseases in pregnant women treated with this drug during various trimesters of pregnancy. In no case did amphotericin B therapy appear to adversely affect the outcome of the pregnancy. Other reports confirm this, and patients so treated responded well to therapy.

5. COMBINED FUNGAL INFECTIONS

It is uncommon to find two or more fungi invading the same patient simultaneously. Salfelder et al.[68] collected eight cases from the literature with pulmonary blastomycosis and an additional fungal infection. Six of these cases had pulmonary histoplasmosis and an additional patient had pulmonary and cutaneous blastomycosis as well as pulmonary histoplasmosis. Another patient with blastomycosis grew *Cryptococcus neoformans* from the sputum but it was difficult to prove cryptococcal infection. We have had a similar patient with pulmonary blastomycosis with positive sputum cultures for *C. neoformans.*

Davidson and Sarosi[69] reported a patient with pulmonary blastomycosis and a lesion on the left ala nasi which was verrucose in appearance with black pustular satellites. Microscopic examination of tissue stained with hematoxylin and eosin (H&E) and periodic acid–Schiff (PAS) revealed the yeast form of *B. dermatitidis* and giant spherules of *Coccidioides immitis.* Eventually, both organisms were cultured from sputum and scrapings. At the time reported (1981), the authors stated that *C. immitis* and *B. dermatitidis* had never been reported simultaneously in the same patient. In 1983, Dismukes *et al.*[70] reporting their study using ketoconazole in a prospective study of systemic mycoses had one patient with disseminated blastomycosis and coccidioidomycosis. Following a course of therapy, the coccidioidomycosis relapsed 3 months later with positive skin culture for *C. immitis,* whereas the patient remained negative for *B. dermatitidis.* Pechan *et al.*[71] reported a renal transplant patient who rejected his kidney 28 days postoperatively despite large infusions of methylprednisolone. This patient subsequently developed bleeding at the esophagogastric junction from vomiting requiring a laparotomy and gastrotomy which ruled out ulceration of the stomach and duodenum. Thirty-six days after transplantation, pulmonary infiltrates developed. Sections from open lung biopsy revealed organisms of *Aspergillus* and another fungus that, on the basis of differential staining, the authors felt to be *B. dermatitidis.* Cultures were not obtained.

6. BLASTOMYCOSIS IN CHILDREN

In most reviews of the subject, 2–10% of patients with blastomycosis are less than 15 years of age at the time of diagnosis.[72] There has been no apparent sex or race predilection in pediatric cases. In recent common source outbreaks that involved predominantly children,[13,14] approximately half of those exposed were infected, and of those infected, approximately half were symptomatic. These findings are similar to those in previously reported common source outbreaks involving adults. Acute pulmonary blastomycosis in children appears to have a high tendency toward progression to chronic disease. If not treated, patients require very close and long-term follow-up.[73]

7. COMPROMISED HOST

Although invasive fungal infections are common in immunosuppressed patients, reports of blastomycosis in this setting are rare. This is in marked contradistinction to most deep fungal infections (cryptococcosis, histoplasmosis, coccidioidomycosis, candidiasis, and aspergillosis) which occur more frequently in immunosuppressed patients, are more likely to be disseminated, respond less favorably than in the normal host.

We had four patients who were receiving steroids at the time or shortly before presenting with the initial diagnosis of blastomycosis (one had emphysema, one had hepatitis, two had sarcoidosis). Three of these four patients developed miliary blastomycosis and one died. Recht et al.[74] noted that 3 of their 78 patients with blastomycosis were on corticosteroids at the time blastomycosis was diagnosed, and an additional 3 patients had a hematologic malignancy.

Witorsch and Utz[4] reported that 10 of their 28 patients with blastomycosis had an abnormal postprandial blood sugar at the time of diagnosis. After completion of therapy, 7 of these patients had an abnormal glucose tolerance. We also think there is increased risk of blastomycosis in diabetics.

Butka et al.[75] described a veterinary assistant who sustained an accidental contaminated needle inoculation of her thigh 2 years after renal transplantation. The patient was receiving 10 mg prednisone and 100 mg azathioprine once daily. Pseudomonas cellulitis developed at the puncture site 2 weeks later. The patient did not respond to incision and drainage or multiple intravenous antibiotics. Approximately 5 weeks after inoculation, progressive pulmonary infiltrates were noted. Open lung biopsy revealed B. dermatitidis as did biopsy of the thigh lesion. The patient responded to amphotericin B therapy. Their literature search revealed only 30 additional immunocompromised patients (some of whom they noted to be poorly documented) who developed blastomycosis.[75] The underlying conditions were renal and bone marrow transplantations, hematologic malignancies, and steroid-treated illnesses.

Winston et al.[76] found only one case of blastomycosis following bone marrow transplantation, but 37% of their transplant patients developed other fungal diseases. Recht et al.[74] reported no instance of blastomycosis in over 1000 renal transplant recipients, but during the same time interval they recognized 18 immunosuppressed patients with histoplasmosis and 3 with coccidioidomycosis.

The oncology service at the University of Mississippi School of Medicine has had only two immunosuppressed patients in the past 15 years who developed blastomycosis, and the hematology service has noted none despite being in one of the areas of high endemicity in the United States. Our experience in managing over 300 acquired immune deficiency syndrome (AIDS) patients in an endemic area for blastomycosis is noteworthy in that we have not yet recognized an infection with B. dermatitidis in a patient with HIV infection. We have had verbal reports of blastomycosis in four AIDS patients in other states. All four had rather typical clinical presentations and were apparently successfully treated with amphotericin B.

With the possible exception of an increased risk of miliary disease in steroid-treated patients, blastomycosis in immunosuppressed patients has similar manifestations as in immunocompetent patients. Response to treatment appears similar to that of an immunocompetent patient when the diagnosis is made prior to the terminal illness and amphotericin B is the antibiotic used.

REFERENCES

1. Schwarz J, Baum GL: Blastomycosis. *Am J Clin Pathol* 21:999–1029, 1951
2. Abernathy RS: Clinical manifestations of pulmonary blastomycosis. *Ann Intern Med* 51:707–727, 1959
3. Busey JF: Blastomycosis. 1. Review of 198 collected cases in Veterans Administration hospitals. *Am Rev Respir Dis* 89:659–672, 1964
4. Witorsch P, Utz JP: North American blastomycosis: A study of 40 patients. *Medicine* 47:169–200, 1968
5. Lin AC, Morris K, Hendricks K, et al: Epidemiologic and clinical study of endemic blastomycosis in MS (Abstract 270). Proceedings of the 29th Interscience Conference on Antimicrobial Agents and Chemotherapy, Houston, September 17–20, 1989
6. Baum GL, Lerner PL: Primary pulmonary blastomycosis: A laboratory-acquired infection. *Ann Intern Med* 73:263–265, 1970
7. Smith JG Jr, Harris JS, Conant NF, et al: An epidemic of North American blastomycosis. *JAMA* 158:641–646, 1955
8. Tosh FE, Hammerman KJ, Weeks RJ, et al: A common source epidemic of North American blastomycosis. *Am Rev Respir Dis* 109:525–529, 1974
9. Kitchen MS, Reiber CD, Eastin GB: An urban epidemic of North American blastomycosis. *Am Rev Respir Dis* 115:1063–1066, 1977
10. Blastomycosis—North Carolina. *MMWR* 25:205–206, 1976
11. Cockerill FR III, Roberts GD, Rosenblatt JE, et al: Epidemic of pulmonary blastomycosis (Namekagon fever) in Wisconsin canoeists. *Chest* 86:688–692, 1984
12. Armstrong CW, Jenkins SR, Kaufman L, et al: Common-source outbreak of blastomycosis in hunters and their dogs. *J Infect Dis* 155:568–570, 1987
13. Klein BS, Vergeront JM, Weeks RJ, et al: Isolation of *Blastomyces dermatitidis* in soil associated with a large outbreak of blastomycosis in Wisconsin. *N Engl J Med* 314:529–534, 1986
14. Klein BS, Vergeront JM, DiSalvo AF: Two outbreaks of blastomycosis along rivers in Wisconsin. Isolation of *Blastomyces dermatitidis* from riverbank soil and evidence of its transmission along waterways. *Am Rev Respir Dis* 136:1333–1338, 1987
15. Rabinowitz JG, Busch J, Buttram WR: Pulmonary manifestations of blastomycosis. Radiological support of a new concept. *Radiology* 120:25–32, 1976
16. Cush R, Light RW, George RB: Clinical and roentgenographic manifestations of acute and chronic blastomycosis. *Chest* 69:345–349, 1976
17. Kinasewitz GT, Penn RL, George RB: The spectrum and significance of pleural disease in blastomycosis. *Chest* 86:580–584, 1984

18. Arora NS, Oblinger MJ, Feldman PS: Chronic pleural blastomycosis with hyperprolactinemia, galactorrhea, and amenorrhea. *Am Rev Respir Dis* 120:451–455, 1979

19. Nelson O, Light RW: Granulomatous pleuritis secondary to blastomycosis. *Chest* 71:433–434, 1977

20. Edson RS, Keys TF: Treatment of primary pulmonary blastomycosis. Results of long-term follow-up. *Mayo Clin Proc* 56:683–685, 1981

21. Griffith JE, Campbell GD: Acute miliary blastomycosis presenting as fulminating respiratory failure. *Chest* 75:630–632, 1979

22. Shaw GB, Campbell GD, Busey JF: Miliary blastomycosis. *Am Rev Respir Dis* 113:81, 1976

23. George RB: Pulmonary mycoses. New concepts and new therapy. *Postgrad Med* 84:185–194, 1988

24. Stelling CB, Woodring JH, Rehm SR, et al: Miliary pulmonary blastomycosis. *Radiology* 150:7–13, 1984

25. Campbell G, Brunson JG: Clinicopathological conference: Miliary disease of the lung. *J Miss State Med Assoc* 14:196–201, 1973

26. Busey JF: North American blastomycosis. *Am Fam Physician/GP* 30:88–95, 1964

27. Larsh HW, Schwarz J: Accidental inoculation blastomycosis. *Cutis* 19:334–337, 1977

28. Scott MJ: Cutaneous blastomycosis. Report of case following dog bite. *Northwest Med* 54:255–257, 1955

29. Jaspers RH: Transmission of blastomyces from animals to man. *J Am Vet Med Assoc* 164:8, 1974

30. Gnann JW Jr, Bressler GS, Bodet CA III, et al: Human blastomycosis after a dog bite. *Ann Intern Med* 98:48–49, 1983

31. Farber ER, Leahy MS, Meadows TR: Endometrial blastomycosis acquired by sexual contact. *Obstet Gynecol* 32:195–199, 1968

32. Dyer ML, Young TL, Kattine AA, et al: Blastomycosis in a Papanicolaou smear. Report of a case with possible venereal transmission. *Acta Cytol* 27:285–287, 1983

33. Sanders LL: Blastomycosis arthritis. *Arthritis Rheum* 10:91–98, 1967

34. Fountain FF Jr: Acute blastomycotic arthritis. *Arch Intern Med* 132:684–688, 1973

35. George AL Jr, Hays JT, Graham BS: Blastomycosis presenting as monarticular arthritis. The role of synovial fluid cytology. *Arthritis Rheum* 28:516–521, 1985

36. Chapman SW: *Blastomyces dermatitidis,* in Mandell GL, Douglas RG Jr, Bennett JE (eds): *Principles and Practice of Infectious Diseases,* ed 3. Edinburgh, Churchill Livingstone, 1990, p 1999

37. Malin JM Jr, Anderson EE, Weber CH: North American blastomycosis of the urogenital tract. *J Urol* 102:754–757, 1969

38. Schwarz J, Salfelder K: Blastomycosis. A review of 152 cases. *Curr Top Pathol* 65:165–200, 1977

39. Hamblen EC, Baker RD, Martin DS: Blastomycosis of the female reproductive tract. With report of a case. *Am J Obstet Gynecol* 30:345–356, 1935

40. Murray JJ, Clark CA, Lands RH, et al: Reactivation blastomycosis presenting as a tubo-ovarian abscess. *Obstet Gynecol* 64:828–830, 1984

41. Faro S, Pastorek JG III, Collins J, et al: Severe uterine hemorrhage from blastomycosis of the endometrium. A case report. *J Reprod Med* 32:247–249, 1987

42. Ferguson GB: North American blastomycosis. A review of the literature and a report of two cases primary in the larynx. *Laryngoscope* 61:851–873, 1951

43. Payne J, Koopmann CF Jr: Laryngeal carcinoma—or is it laryngeal blastomycosis. *Laryngoscope* 94:608–611, 1984

44. Dumich PS, Neel HB III: Blastomycosis of the larynx. *Laryngoscope* 93:1266–1270, 1983

45. Buechner HA, Clawson CM: Blastomycosis of the central nervous system. II. A report of

nine cases from the Veterans Administration Cooperative Study. *Am Rev Respir Dis* 95:820–826, 1967

46. Gonyea EF: The spectrum of primary blastomycotic meningitis: A review of central nervous system blastomycosis. *Ann Neurol* 3:26–39, 1978

47. Kravitz GR, Davies SF, Eckman MR, et al: Chronic blastomycotic meningitis. *Am J Med* 71:501–505, 1981

48. Kaufman L: Mycoserology: Its vital role in diagnosing systemic mycotic infections. *Jpn J Med Mycol* 24:1–8, 1983

49. Abernathy RS, Melby JC: Addison's disease in North American blastomycosis. *N Engl J Med* 266:552–554, 1962

50. Eberle DE, Evans RB, Johnson RH: Disseminated North American blastomycosis. Occurrence with clinical manifestations of adrenal insufficiency. *JAMA* 238:2629–2630, 1977

51. Chandler PT: Addison's disease secondary to North American blastomycosis. *South Med J* 70:863–864, 1977

52. Martin DS, Smith DT: Blastomycosis (American blastomycosis, Gilchrist's disease); a review of the literature. *Am Rev Tuberc* 39:275–304, 1939

53. Pond NE, Humphreys RJ: Blastomycosis with cardiac involvement and peripheral embolization. *Am Heart J* 43:615–620, 1952

54. Merchant RK, Louria DB, Geisler PH, et al: Fungal endocarditis: Review of the literature and report of three cases. *Ann Intern Med* 48:242–266, 1958

55. Cherniss EI, Waisbren BA: North American blastomycosis: A clinical study of 40 cases. *Ann Intern Med* 44:105–123, 1956

56. McKenzie R, Khakoo R: Blastomycosis of the esophagus presenting with gastrointestinal bleeding. *Gastroenterology* 88:1271–1273, 1985

57. Seymour EQ: Blastomycosis of the breast. *AJR* 139:822–823, 1982

58. Chapman SW, University of Mississippi School of Medicine, Jackson MS, Personal communication, 1990

59. Louis T III, Lockey MW: Blastomycosis of the middle ear cleft. *South Med J* 67:1489–1491, 1974

60. Habte-Gabr E, Smith IM: North American blastomycosis in Iowa: Review of 34 cases. *J Chronic Dis* 26:585–594, 1973

61. Duttera MJ Jr, Osterhout S: North American blastomycosis: A survey of 63 cases. *South Med J* 62:295–301, 1969

62. Kunkel WM Jr, Weed LA, McDonald JR, et al: North American blastomycosis— Gilchrist's disease: A clinicopathologic study of ninety cases. *Int Abstr Surg* 99:1–25, 1954

63. Catanzaro A: Pulmonary mycosis in pregnant women. *Chest* Suppl 86:14S–18S, 1984

64. Watts EA, Gard PD Jr, Tuthill SW: First reported case of intrauterine transmission of blastomycosis. *Pediatr Infect Dis* 2:308–310, 1983

65. Daniel L, Salit IE: Blastomycosis during pregnancy. *Can Med Assoc J* 131:759–761, 1984

66. Hager H, Welt SI, Cardasis JP, et al: Disseminated blastomycosis in a pregnant woman successfully treated with amphotericin-B. A case report. *J Reprod Med* 33:485–488, 1988

67. Ismail MA, Lerner SA: Disseminated blastomycosis in a pregnant woman. Review of amphotericin B usage during pregnancy. *Am Rev Respir Dis* 126:350–353, 1982

68. Salfelder K, Mendelovici M, Schwarz J: Multiple deep fungus infections: Personal observations and a critical review of the world literature. *Curr Top Pathol* 57:123–177, 1973

69. Davidson W, Sarosi GA: Disseminated blastomycosis and cocciciodomycosis in the same patient. *Am Rev Respir Dis* 124:179, 1981

70. Dismukes WE, Stamm AM, Graybill JR, et al: Treatment of systemic mycoses with ketoconazole: Emphasis on toxicity and clinical response in 52 patients. *Ann Intern Med* 98:13–20, 1983

71. Pechan WB, Novick AC, Lalli A, et al: Pulmonary nodules in a renal transplant recipient. *J Urol* 124:111–114, 1980
72. Steele RW, Abernathy RS: Systemic blastomycosis in children. *Pediatr Infect Dis* 2:304–310, 1983
73. Powell DA, Schuit KE: Acute pulmonary blastomycosis in children: Clinical course and follow-up. *Pediatrics* 63:736–740, 1979
74. Recht LD, Davies SF, Eckman MR, et al: Blastomycosis in immunosuppressed patients. *Am Rev Respir Dis* 125:359–362, 1982
75. Butka BJ, Bennett SR, Johnson AC: Disseminated inoculation blastomycosis in a renal transplant recipient. *Am Rev Respir Dis* 130:1180–1183, 1984
76. Winston DJ, Gale RP, Meyer DV, et al: Infectious complications of human bone marrow transplantation. *Medicine* 58:1–31, 1979

10

Pathologic Features of Blastomycosis

Francis W. Chandler and John C. Watts

Blastomycosis is an acute or chronic systemic mycosis of humans and animals caused by the thermally dimorphic fungus *Blastomyces dermatitidis*.[1-4] The disease was long thought to be restricted to the North American continent, but in recent years autochthonous cases have been diagnosed in Africa, the Middle East, and Asia.[5-13] All available clinical and epidemiologic evidence indicates that humans and animals usually contract blastomycosis after inhalation of airborne infectious conidia of the mycelial form of the fungus growing as a saprophyte in nature, and that the primary focus of infection is in the lungs.[14,15] Primary cutaneous infection is rare, usually resulting from the accidental direct inoculation of the fungus into the skin and subcutaneous tissues.[16,17] This form of blastomycosis is an occupational hazard for medical technologists and pathologists, and it has also occurred following dog bites.[18-21] Laboratory-acquired primary pulmonary infection is exceedingly rare.[22] Blastomycosis is not contagious.

Blastomycosis, edited by Yousef Al-Doory and Arthur F. DiSalvo, Plenum Medical Book Company, New York, 1992.

1. CLINICOPATHOLOGIC FEATURES

The two major clinical forms of blastomycosis are systemic and cutaneous. Although both forms have a pulmonary inception, their clinical presentation, course, pathologic features, and prognosis differ.[23-31] Systemic blastomycosis is primarily a pulmonary infection that either remains confined to the lungs or disseminates hematogenously to other organs, particularly the skin, bones and joints, male genitourinary tract, mucosal surfaces, central nervous system, lymph nodes, heart, and adrenal glands. Untreated systemic infections are often severe, progressive, and fatal; the mortality is reported to be greater than 90%.[2,30] Patients with cutaneous blastomycosis present with papular, pustular, or indolent, ulcerative-nodular and verrucose skin lesions with crusted surfaces and raised, serpiginous, sharply slanted borders (Figs. 1 and 2). Lesions are usually painless, do not itch, and frequently occur on exposed parts of the body, particularly the face and hands. There is minimal erythema of adjacent skin, and regional lymphangitis and lymphadenopathy are uncommon. In this clinical form of the infection, primary pulmonary lesions are usually inapparent, systemic symptoms are absent or mild, and the general health of the patient is not impaired. Unless treated, the clinical course of cutaneous blastomycosis can run from months to years, with remissions and exacerbations and progressive increase in the size of lesions. As the skin lesions expand, they undergo central healing, leaving thin, atrophic, depigmented scars (Fig. 2). The rare primary cutaneous lesions of blastomycosis are localized, atypical, self-limited infections that are accompanied by regional lymphadenopathy and almost never disseminate.[16,17]

In the majority of patients, acute pulmonary infection by *B. dermatitidis* is an asymptomatic or a symptomatic but self-limited illness with nonspecific, influenza-like symptoms.[2,30,32-34] Nevertheless, chest radiographs usually reveal patchy areas of pulmonary consolidation that are often bilateral.[35-39] The posterior segments of the upper lung lobes are most often involved, but the middle and lower lobes may also be affected.[40] In the acute disease, pleural effusion and cavitation are uncommon, and fungemia does not occur as frequently as in histoplasmosis. Symptoms, when present, usually persist from a few days to 2 weeks, but radiographic abnormalities may not resolve for 6 months or longer. Some patients with self-limited pulmonary blastomycosis develop active lesions at distant sites, especially the skin and male genitourinary tract, up to 3 years after resolution of the primary infection. In a minority of patients, the acute blastomycotic pneumonia pursues a rapidly progressive clinical course characterized by widespread suppuration, necrosis, and cavitation of both lungs (Figs. 3 and 4).[41-43] Ulcerative bronchitis, found in about one-third of all cases, is thought to accelerate endobronchial spread of infection. Respiratory failure and hematogenous dissemination to many extrapulmonary sites result in fulminating disease and death, often in spite of aggressive therapy.[44-46]

Patients with clinically apparent blastomycosis usually present with chronic respiratory symptoms of insidious onset that have persisted for weeks to months. Symptoms include productive cough, pleuritic chest pain, dyspnea, low-grade fever, night sweats, weight loss, and, occasionally, hemoptysis. In addition to chronic pulmonary disease, about two-thirds of these patients also have skin lesions, one-third have bone lesions, and one-fifth of males have genitourinary tract lesions, especially of the prostate gland, epididymis, and testes.[2,26,30] Involvement of one or more of these organs along with typical chest radiographic findings is an important clue to the diagnosis. Chest radiographs often reveal mediastinal lymphadenopathy, diffuse reticulonodular or linear pulmonary infiltrates, and fibronodular densities with cavitation—findings that are indistinguishable from those seen in chronic active tuberculosis.[35-40] Fibrosis is frequent and often accompanied by cavitation; cavities are usually multiple and thin-walled. Pleural involvement also occurs frequently in chronic active pulmonary blastomycosis, and when severe, is associated with an unfavorable prognosis. In one series of 26 patients with biopsy- or culture-proven pulmonary blastomycosis, 88% had radiographic evidence of pleural lesions.[47] Solitary nodules or "coin lesions," frequently seen in histoplasmosis and coccidioidomycosis, are rare, and calcification of such lesions is even rarer. Late endogenous reactivation of residual pulmonary lesions seldom occurs.[48-50]

As with most other fungal infections, immunocompromised patients are at increased risk for the development of blastomycosis.[51,52] The clinical presentation of primary pulmonary blastomycosis in these patients is similar to that in immunocompetent individuals. However, the disease tends to

Color Figures

FIGURE 1. Cutaneous lesion of systemic blastomycosis. A solitary, sharply circumscribed nodular-ulcerative lesion is present on the left lower leg.

FIGURE 2. Cutaneous involvement in chronic systemic blastomycosis. A verrucose nodule with an expanding, serpiginous border and zone of central healing involves the right face and lower eyelid.

FIGURE 4. Pulmonary blastomycosis. Sectioned surface of right lung reveals multiple abscesses and granulomas. The pleura in this case is of normal thickness. (Courtesy of Dr. Norman L. Goodman.)

FIGURE 8. Pulmonary blastomycosis in a patient who had received long-term prednisone therapy for systemic lupus erythematosus. Note the persistent broad-based budding and variation in size of fungal cells. The single buds are often connected to parent cells by bud pores. (Gomori methenamine silver with hematoxylin and eosin counterstain, ×160.)

FIGURE 9. Microforms of *Blastomyces dermatitidis* in a cerebellar granuloma. Histiocytes contain numerous yeastlike cells, 2 to 4 μm in diameter, that have centrally retracted cytoplasm, poorly stained walls, and resemble the yeast forms of *Histoplasma capsulatum* var. *capsulatum*. (Hematoxylin and eosin, ×160.)

FIGURE 10. Rapidly proliferating microforms of *Blastomyces dermatitidis* in a pulmonary granuloma. Although unusually small, the yeast cells bud by a broad base, have thick walls, and are morphologically similar to typical blastomyces cells. (Gomori methenamine silver with hematoxylin and eosin counterstain, ×100.)

FIGURE 11. Microforms of *Blastomyces dermatitidis*. Unusually small but morphologically typical yeast forms are mixed with larger, conventional yeast forms of this fungus. The mixture of unusually small and typical forms of *B. dermatitidis* should not be mistaken for coexisting mycoses. (Gomori methenamine silver with hematoxylin and eosin counterstain, ×250.)

FIGURE 17. Detail of *Blastomyces dermatitidis* cells in acute blastomycotic pneumonia. Typical yeast forms with "doubly contoured" walls and broad-based buds are scattered throughout the suppurative alveolar exudate. One bud is connected to the parent cell by a large bud pore. (Hematoxylin and eosin, ×250.)

FIGURE 18. Acute pulmonary blastomycosis. The alveolar spaces are filled with neutrophils, necrotic debris, and proliferating *Blastomyces dermatitidis* cells that are predominantly extracellular. (Gomori methenamine silver with hematoxylin and eosin counterstain, ×100.)

FIGURE 23. Blastomycotic lymphadenitis. The wall of a large granuloma contains single and budding yeast forms of *Blastomyces dermatitidis* that are predominantly intracellular. Note the diagnostic broad-based budding of the fungal cells. (Gomori methenamine silver, ×160.)

FIGURE 27. Detail of *Blastomyces dermatitidis* cells within alveolar exudate. The rapidly dividing yeast forms are spherical, thick-walled, 8 to 15 μm in diameter, and have prominent cytoplasmic vacuoles. (Hematoxylin and eosin, ×160.)

FIGURE 29. Detail of *Blastomyces dermatitidis* cells illustrated in Fig. 28. Note the variation in size and shape of fungal cells, and in the thickness of their walls. Several blastomyces cells have fragmented walls. (Gomori methenamine silver, ×160.)

FIGURE 30. Systemic blastomycosis. Numerous single and budding *Blastomyces dermatitidis* cells occupy the lumen of a pulmonary artery, providing evidence of fungemia. (Gomori methenamine silver with hematoxylin and eosin counterstain, ×160.)

FIGURE 33. Direct immunofluorescence of *Blastomyces dermatitidis* in acute blastomycotic pneumonia. Single and budding intraalveolar yeast forms are brightly fluorescent. The immunofluorescence conjugate is species-specific and can be applied to deparaffinized sections of formalin-fixed tissue (×160).

FIGURE 34. Microforms of *Blastomyces dermatitidis* in a pulmonary granuloma. The sparse and unusually small blastomyces cells are decorated by direct immunofluorescence using a specific conjugate directed against the cell wall polysaccharide antigens of this fungus (×160).

FIGURE 35. Systemic blastomycosis in an African. The thick walls of the blastomyces cells react positively with mucin stains. Note the typical broad-based budding. (Alcian blue, ×250.)

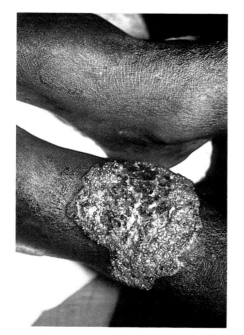

FIGURE 1.

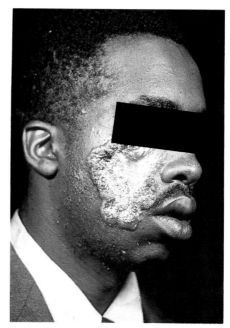

FIGURE 2.

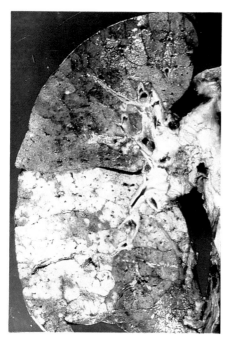

FIGURE 4.

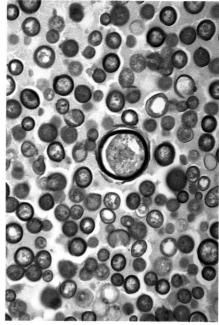

FIGURE 8.

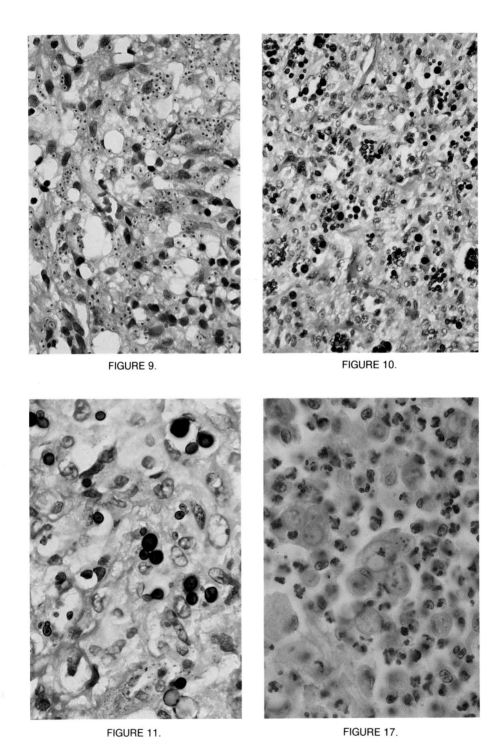

FIGURE 9.

FIGURE 10.

FIGURE 11.

FIGURE 17.

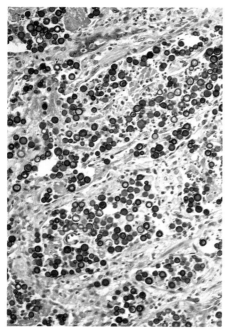

FIGURE 18.

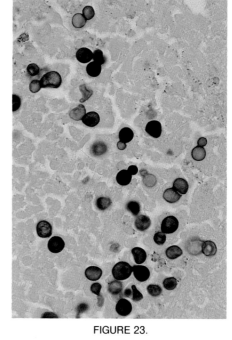

FIGURE 23.

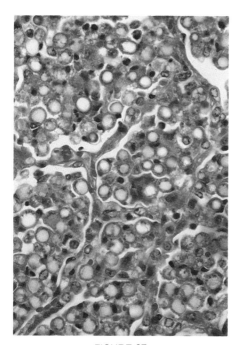

FIGURE 27.

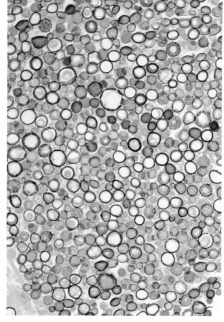

FIGURE 29.

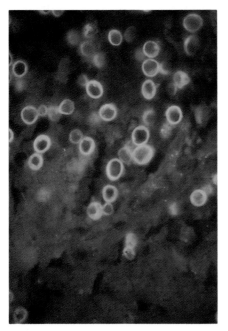

FIGURE 30.

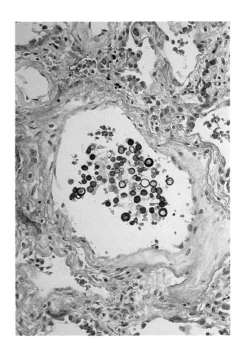

FIGURE 33.

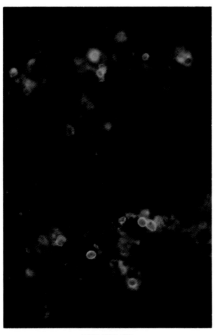

FIGURE 34.

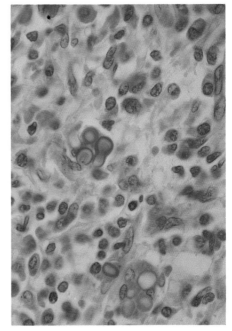

FIGURE 35.

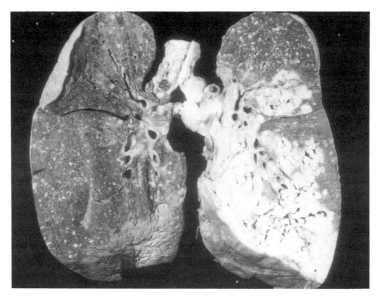

FIGURE 3. Pulmonary lesions of systemic blastomycosis. Sectioned surfaces of lungs reveal miliary nodules. Multiple confluent abscesses and granulomas involve the left lower and middle lobes. (Courtesy of Dr. Norman L. Goodman.)

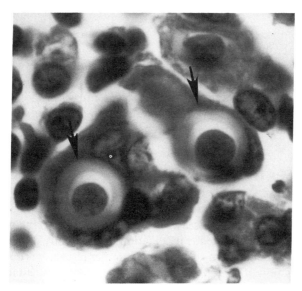

FIGURE 5. *Blastomyces dermatitidis* cells (arrows) within epithelioid histiocytes of pulmonary granuloma. The yeast cells are spherical, hyaline, 8 to 15 μm in diameter, and have thick, "doubly contoured" walls and retracted cytoplasmic contents. (Hematoxylin and eosin, ×250.)

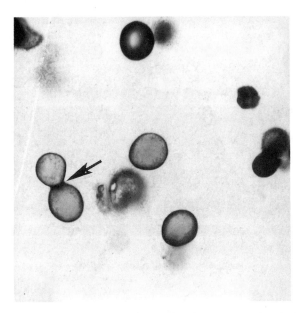

FIGURE 6. Acute blastomycotic pneumonia. An alveolar space contains single and budding yeast cells of *Blastomyces dermatitidis*. The thick walls of the blastomyces cells may not be readily apparent when special stains for fungi are used. Broad-based budding (arrow) is diagnostic of this fungus in tissue sections. (Gomori methenamine silver, ×160.)

disseminate more often and is more rapidly progressive in patients who are immunocompromised. Widespread dissemination of primary cutaneous blastomycosis, which in the immunocompetent individual is a localized and self-limited infection, also has been reported in an immunocompromised patient.[53] Unlike cryptococcosis and histoplasmosis, blastomycosis is seldom encountered as an opportunistic infection in patients with AIDS or other profound T-cell immunodeficiencies.

2. GROSS PATHOLOGY

The gross pathologic findings in blastomycosis vary according to the clinical presentation of the disease. Lesions of primary cutaneous blastomycosis acquired by percutaneous inoculation are distinctly different from the secondary cutaneous lesions that result from hematogenous dissemination. After introduction of *B. dermatitidis* into the skin and subcutaneous tissue, an erythematous papule develops within 1–2 weeks. The papule gradually

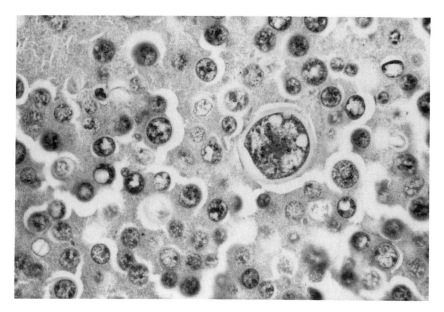

FIGURE 7. Pulmonary blastomycosis in an immunocompromised patient. Myriad intracellular and extracellular *Blastomyces dermatitidis* cells are spherical, multinucleated, and have vacuolated cytoplasm and thick "doubly contoured" walls. Generally, the larger the number of fungal cells, the greater is the variation in size and shape. (Hematoxylin and eosin, ×160.)

enlarges over several months, and it may eventually ulcerate and resemble a chancre. Regional lymphangitis and lymphadenopathy are common, resulting in a linear chain of nodules along the course of lymphatics that drain the primary skin lesion. Epidermal hyperplasia is not a prominent feature of these lesions, which usually contain numerous organisms.

In patients who have chronic blastomycosis with minimal or no apparent pulmonary involvement, the secondary lesions of the skin (Figs. 1 and 2) and squamous mucosal surfaces that result from hematogenous dissemination are often multiple. When biopsy specimens are sectioned, the epithelial thickening caused by florid pseudoepitheliomatous hyperplasia resembles squamous cell carcinoma; the presence of small abscesses, best seen at the periphery of the lesions, may be the only clue to an infectious etiology. Lymphangitis and lymphadenitis are infrequent, and, unlike the rare primary skin lesions, organisms are usually sparse. At autopsy, the primary pulmonary blastomycotic lesion is often undetectable or appears only as a focus of pulmonary scarring or pleural fibrosis. Calcified fibrocaseous nodules, as seen in histoplasmosis and coccidioidomycosis, are almost never

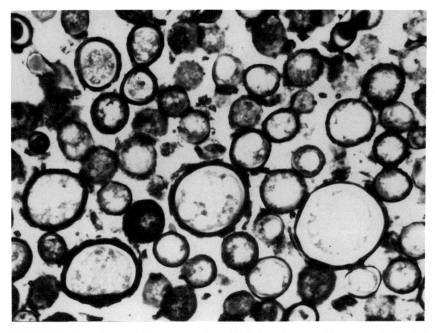

FIGURE 12. Giant forms of *Blastomyces dermatitidis* in pulmonary blastomycosis. Typical fungal cells, 8 to 15 μm in diameter, are mixed with unusually large yeast forms, 20 to 40 μm in diameter. Both the conventionally sized and enlarged blastomyces cells have thick walls and bud by a broad base. (Gomori methenamine silver, ×250.)

found. In blastomycosis, a primary pulmonary–lymph node complex is rarely encountered at autopsy.[15,29,43] When present, the lymph node component is generally less severe than that in tuberculosis and histoplasmosis.

The lesions of progressive systemic blastomycosis are suppurative or mixed suppurative and granulomatous, and fungal cells are usually numerous. In the lungs, blastomycotic lesions can appear as focal or diffuse areas of pneumonic consolidation; small, discrete, yellow to grayish-white miliary nodules; large abscesses; necrotic nodules; and focal or confluent granulomas (Figs. 3 and 4). Cavitation and caseation are sometimes seen but are much less frequent than in tuberculosis and histoplasmosis. In one series of 152 patients with blastomycosis, about 20% had one or more pulmonary cavities.[15] Although cavities are usually small, some measure up to 7 cm in diameter. When the lungs are sectioned, the firm, confluent granulomatous nodules and infiltrative pattern of blastomycotic lesions can resemble bronchogenic carcinoma.[54] The distinction between the two can be difficult until histopathologic studies are completed. Pleuritis and pleural fibrosis are fre-

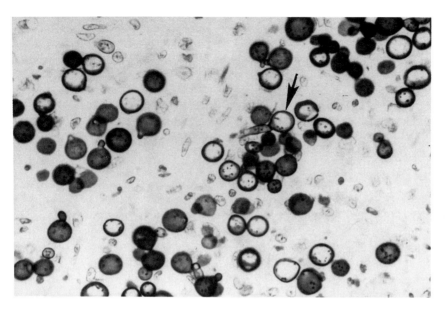

FIGURE 13. Pulmonary blastomycosis. Single cells, budding cells, and a germinating yeastlike cell (arrow) of *Blastomyces dermatitidis* are located within the suppurative center of a granuloma. (Gomori methenamine silver with hematoxylin and eosin counterstain, ×160.)

quent when pulmonary lesions are severe, and infection may extend directly from the pleural cavity to adjacent vertebrae and ribs, and through the chest wall to the subcutaneous tissue and skin. Pericarditis, myocarditis, and endocarditis have been reported rarely and are presumed to result from either direct extension of pulmonary lesions or hematogenous dissemination.[29] Draining sinus tracts that connect subcutaneous and osseous lesions have also been described. These tracts drain pinkish or greenish-yellow pus that usually contains numerous organisms.

After the skin, bone is the second most frequent site of extrapulmonary blastomycosis; osseous lesions are reported to occur in about one-third of cases.[55,56] Radiographs usually reveal sharply outlined lesions and prominent osteolysis, and several bones can be involved simultaneously. Sites most frequently involved include the vertebral bodies (especially thoracic, lumbar, and sacral) followed by the long bones of the lower extremities, ribs, pelvis, skull, and short bones. Examination of the bone marrow often reveals abscesses, granulomas, or dispersed inflammatory infiltrates that contain large numbers of organisms. The epiphysis is the favored site of infection in long bones, and direct extension of infection to the contiguous joint space

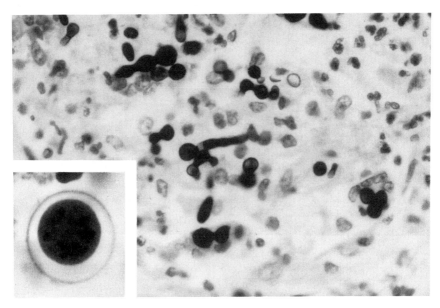

FIGURE 14. Cutaneous blastomycosis in an Israeli farmer. Germinating cells, cells with multiple buds, and pseudohyphae of *Blastomyces dermatitidis* are mixed with typical yeast forms. Inset: Thin-walled yeast form of *B. dermatitidis* that might represent a cell-wall-deficient spheroplast in dermal granuloma. (Gomori methenamine silver with hematoxylin and eosin counterstain, ×160; inset, hematoxylin and eosin, ×250.)

sometimes occurs. The posterior elements of the vertebrae are especially susceptible to *B. dermatitidis* infection. Psoas abscesses result from direct extension of vertebral or pelvic lesions.

Blastomycotic lesions of the prostate gland, epididymis, and testes range from small, firm, sharply circumscribed, yellowish-white nodules to almost complete involvement of the entire parenchyma accompanied by marked enlargement.[29,57,58] Often, the sectioned surfaces of these organs reveal multiple abscesses that are confluent and of varying sizes. Lesions of the seminal vesicles occur either by direct extension from the prostate or by hematogenous dissemination from a primary pulmonary focus of infection. In renal blastomycosis, both kidneys are usually affected, and typical suppurative and granulomatous lesions are most frequently seen in the cortices. Blastomycotic emboli have been described in the glomerular tufts, and numerous compact yeast forms of *B. dermatitidis* occasionally fill the lumens of renal tubules.

Involvement of the CNS has been reported to occur in 6 to 33% of cases

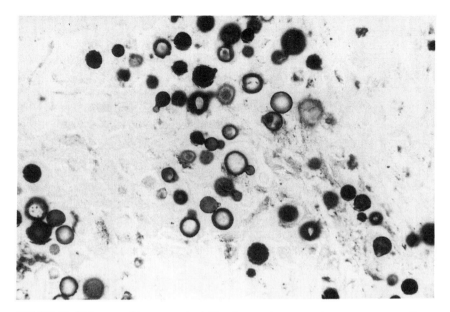

FIGURE 15. Pulmonary blastomycosis. A fibrotic granuloma contains numerous yeast forms that are distorted, fragmented, and unevenly contoured. Note the persistent broad-based budding. (Gomori methenamine silver, ×160.)

of systemic blastomycosis.[46,59–63] The most common neuropathologic finding is chronic, focal or diffuse leptomeningitis. Solitary or multiple abscesses and large granulomas that often present as mass lesions ("blastomycomas") have been described in the cerebrum, cerebellum, basal ganglia, and spinal cord.

Although the skin, bone, male genitourinary tract, and CNS, in descending order of frequency, are the most frequent sites of extrapulmonary involvement in systemic blastomycosis, virtually any organ can be affected. Additional sites of involvement include the larynx, trachea, lymph nodes, heart and pericardium, eye, adrenal glands, female reproductive tract, thyroid, spleen, liver, and gastrointestinal tract.[64–80]

3. MORPHOLOGIC AND TINCTORIAL FEATURES OF *B. DERMATITIDIS* IN TISSUE SECTIONS

Because *B. dermatitidis* is dimorphic, it grows as nonencapsulated yeast cells both in host tissues and *in vitro* at 37°C and as a white-to-tan, downy-to-

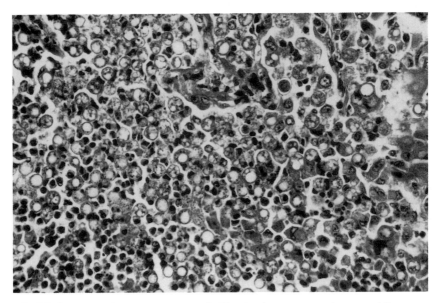

FIGURE 16. Acute pulmonary blastomycosis. The alveolar spaces contain neutrophils, macrophages, and many intra- and extracellular blastomyces cells that have vacuolated cytoplasm and thick walls. (Hematoxylin and eosin, ×100.)

fluffy mold at room temperature. In tissue sections stained with hematoxylin and eosin (H&E), typical yeastlike cells are morphologically distinctive.[81–83] They are spherical, 8 to 15 μm in diameter, multinucleated, and have vacuolated cytoplasm and thick "doubly contoured" walls with sharply defined inner and outer tables (Figs. 5–8). Because of fixation, the cytoplasm is sometimes retracted from the rigid cell wall, leaving a clear space that surrounds all or part of the internal contents (Fig. 5). The yeastlike cells reproduce by budding in which the buds (blastoconidia) are attached to their parent cells by a broad base (Fig. 6). Generally, only one bud is produced, and the broad-based buds are often connected to parent cells by large (4- to 5-μm diameter) bud pores (Fig. 8). Very small (2 to 4 μm) but morphologically typical microforms of B. dermatitidis are occasionally found in blastomycotic lesions.[82–85] In our experience, these microforms are usually numerous and may represent the majority of the fungal cell population (Figs. 9 and 10). However, they are always present as part of a continuous series of sizes ranging from the unusually small to the larger yeast forms typical of this fungus (Fig. 11). Rarely, giant forms of B. dermatitidis are also encountered in the lesions of blastomycosis.[86] These abnormally large yeast forms measure 20 to 30 μm in

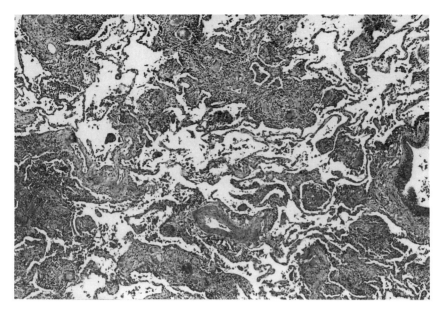

FIGURE 19. Miliary pulmonary blastomycosis. The interstitial pattern of granulomatous inflammation and fibrosis resembles hypersensitivity pneumonitis. Sparse and poorly stained fungal cells are not visible at this magnification. (Hematoxylin and eosin, ×25.)

diameter and occasionally reach 40 μm (Fig. 12). Their morphology is otherwise similar to that of adjacent, typical blastomyces cells. The giant forms, which usually lack blastoconidia, form a minor part of a continuous series of sizes ranging from the usual to the gigantic. Germ tubes, chainlike budding, cells with multiple buds, hyphae, and thin-walled yeast forms of *B. dermatitidis* that might represent cell-wall-deficient spheroplasts are produced rarely in tissue (Figs. 13 and 14).[15,82,83,87,88] When these aberrant forms are encountered, typical budding blastomyces cells are also usually present. In several African cases of culture-proven blastomycosis, we have observed cells whose buds were so unusually broad-based that they were initially mistaken for septate cells rather than budding cells. In each of these cases, *B. dermatitidis* cells with conventional buds were also observed.

   Blastomyces dermatitidis can be readily identified in H&E-stained sections of blastomycotic lesions when numerous organisms are present. H&E is the stain of choice to demonstrate the thick, hyaline cell wall and multiple hematoxylinophilic nuclei within the centrally retracted, amphophilic and vacuolated cytoplasm of individual organisms (Figs. 5 and 7). H&E is also the stain of choice to demonstrate the intensely eosinophilic, clublike Splen-

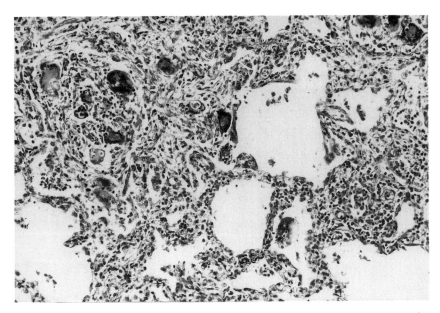

FIGURE 20. Miliary pulmonary blastomycosis. A mixed suppurative and granulomatous in-flammatory response is accompanied by mild interstitial fibrosis. The blastomyces cells appear as spherical vacuoles within the multinucleated giant cells. (Hematoxylin and eosin, ×50.)

dore–Hoeppli material that occasionally ensheathes individual *B. dermatiti-dis* cells in chronic lesions.[89] Special stains for fungi such as the Gomori methenamine silver (GMS), periodic acid–Schiff reaction (PAS), and Grid-ley fungus (GF) procedures are helpful to locate organisms and delineate their morphology, especially when fungal cells are sparse. The staining reac-tions of these procedures are based on the principle that adjacent hydroxyl groups of the complex polysaccharides in fungal cell walls are oxidized, by chromic or periodic acid, to aldehydes. In the GMS procedure, the aldehydes reduce the methenamine silver nitrate complex, and fungal cell walls are colored brownish-black because reduced silver is deposited wherever alde-hydes are located. In our experience, the GMS stain is best for screening because it provides higher contrast and stains degenerated and fragmented organisms better than the other special stains for fungi (Fig. 15). Because *B. dermatitidis* cells often stain intensely and uniformly with GMS, it may be difficult to discern their thick cell walls and characteristic internal morphol-ogy with this stain. Except for the PAS reaction, special stains for fungi do not adequately demonstrate the host reaction to fungal invasion. To circum-vent this, a GMS-stained section can be counterstained with H&E for simul-

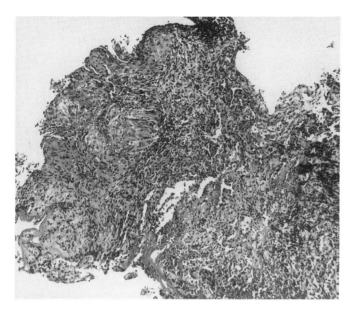

FIGURE 21. Chronic pulmonary blastomycosis. A transbronchial biopsy specimen reveals tuberculoid granulomas composed of compact epithelioid histiocytes, fibroblasts, and lymphocytes. Intracellular fungal elements are not clearly seen at this magnification. (Hematoxylin and eosin, ×25.)

taneous demonstration of a mycotic agent and the tissue response. Fungal cell walls stain brownish-black, while background tissue components stain as expected for H&E. *B. dermatitidis* is not reliably demonstrated with the modified Gram stains.

Foci within the cytoplasm of certain fungi in tissue sections, especially the yeast cells of *B. dermatitidis* and *Histoplasma capsulatum* var. *capsulatum,* are variably acid-fast.[90] However, this staining property is inconsistent and should not be used for diagnosis. The cell walls of the pathogenic fungi are not acid-fast.

When viewed under ultraviolet light, *B. dermatitidis* and certain other pathogenic fungi in H&E- and PAS-stained tissue sections are autofluorescent.[91] This property may help delineate sparse or poorly stained fungal elements but, in our experience, fungal autofluorescence is inconsistent and should not be used in the place of special stains and immunohistologic procedures. Many fungi in frozen or formalin-fixed paraffin-embedded tissue sections also stain nonspecifically with whitening agents such as Calcofluor white and Hiltamine white that fluoresce under ultraviolet light.[92,93] Tissue sections are usually stained for one minute with one of these fluorescent

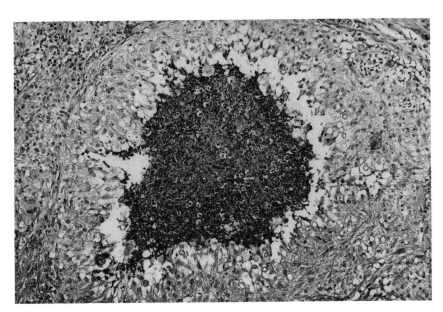

FIGURE 22. Blastomycotic lymphadenitis. A mediastinal lymph node contains a large caseated granuloma. Poorly stained blastomyces cells are located in the wall and central caseous material of the granuloma. (Hematoxylin and eosin, ×50.)

brighteners and then counterstained with Evan's blue. This very rapid and simple fluorescence procedure is useful in the intraoperative examination of fresh-frozen tissues for fungi, but it should not be used for definitive diagnosis.

4. MICROSCOPIC PATHOLOGY

Microscopically, the predominant inflammatory reaction in the lesions of acute blastomycosis is suppurative, with infiltration of neutrophils and abscess formation (Figs. 16 and 17); occasionally, eosinophils are present also. Large numbers of fungal cells are scattered throughout the lesion or localized to well-defined abscesses (Fig. 18). In chronic lesions, a mixed suppurative and granulomatous inflammatory reaction is seen; either component may predominate, depending on the age of the lesion and the immunologic status of the host (Figs. 19–22). Fungal cells in these lesions are usually sparse and sometimes distorted (Fig. 23); examination of several GMS-stained serial sections may be necessary to detect typical organisms

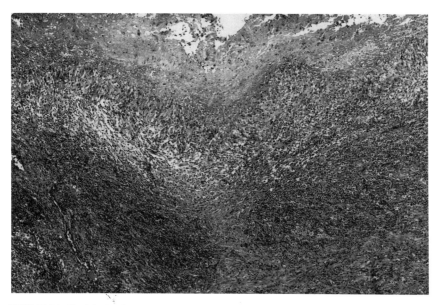

FIGURE 24. Residual pulmonary blastomycosis. This section of a surgically excised pulmonary nodule reveals central caseous material (top) enclosed by a zone of active fibrogranulomatous inflammation (bottom). (Hematoxylin and eosin, ×25.)

with diagnostic broad-based buds. In the lungs, classical tuberculoid granulomas composed of compact epithelioid histiocytes, lymphocytes, and fibroblasts can be seen in interstitial or intraalveolar locations (Figs. 19–21), but caseation is uncommon (Figs. 24 and 25). Focal or confluent granulomas with suppurative and necrotic centers also can be found in the lungs as well as in other organs. Epithelioid histiocytes and varying numbers of multinucleated giant cells of both the Langhans and foreign body types are concentrated about the periphery of suppurative and necrotic foci. When fungal cells are present, they can be found lying free in abscesses and the suppurative or necrotic centers of granulomas, and within the cytoplasm of epithelioid histiocytes and multinucleated giant cells (Figs. 23 and 25). Because the fungal cell walls are hyaline in H&E-stained sections, empty or poorly stained organisms appear as large, spherical vacuoles within the giant cells. In other instances, amorphous, GMS-positive granular material that represents the residuum of fungal cell wall degradation can be seen within the cytoplasm of phagocytes. Some authors have speculated that the large size of typical *B. dermatitidis* cells stimulates the formation of multinucleated giant cells, but in our experience, microforms of the fungus evoke a similar re-

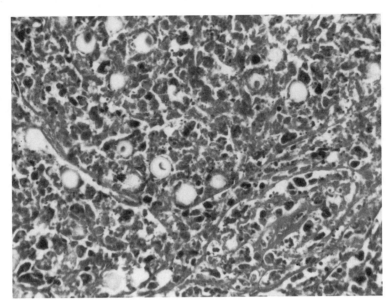

FIGURE 25. Residual pulmonary blastomycosis. Empty, distorted, and poorly stained yeast forms of *Blastomyces dermatitidis* are seen within the necrotic center of an excised pulmonary nodule. (Hematoxylin and eosin, ×160.)

sponse. Fibrosis and hyalinization of granulomatous foci occur frequently in long-standing infections, and, in the lungs, may be accompanied by cavitation.

In acute, rapidly expanding lesions or in the profoundly immunodeficient host, *B. dermatitidis* cells sometimes proliferate in great numbers, and solid sheets or compact clusters of fungal cells with minimal inflammatory reaction (so-called "yeast lakes") may be found in many organs; epithelioid cell granulomas are rarely formed (Figs. 26–29). In the lungs, alveolar spaces are sometimes filled with and distended by myriad, rapidly proliferating yeast forms that elicit little or no inflammatory response, resembling the paucireactive pattern often seen in cryptococcosis. The *B. dermatitidis* cells in these lesions are generally uniform in size. However, the larger the number of fungal cells, the greater is the variation in size and shape. Occasionally, fungal cells can be demonstrated within the lumens of arteries and veins, providing evidence of fungemia (Fig. 30). In the prostate, ducts and glands are sometimes distended by numerous fungal elements and few inflammatory cells.

In cutaneous blastomycosis, most investigators believe that the fungus

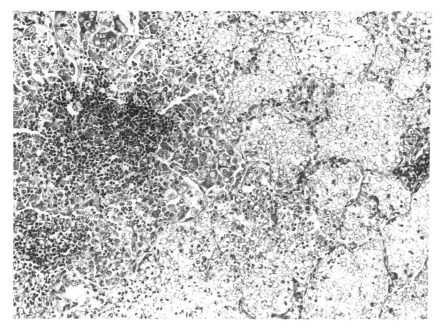

FIGURE 26. Acute blastomycotic pneumonia. The alveolar spaces are filled with and distended by neutrophils, multinucleated giant cells, and myriad intra- and extracellular yeast forms. (Hematoxylin and eosin, ×50.)

is carried in the bloodstream to the papillary dermis by macrophages. Through unknown mechanisms, the *B. dermatitidis* cells then incite florid pseudoepitheliomatous hyperplasia that is usually more extensive than that seen in chromoblastomycosis, sporotrichosis, and coccidioidomycosis (Fig. 31). Intraepidermal microabscesses result from extensive downgrowth of rete pegs and incorporation of dermal microabscesses or their draining sinuses. Fungal cells can be found in microabscesses in the dermis and epidermis, within giant and epithelioid cells at the periphery of microabscesses (Fig. 32), and in the hyperkeratotic layer of the epidermis. Similar lesions can occur in the larynx or on other mucous membranes lined by stratified squamous epithelium. Although not pathognomonic, the histologic pattern should alert the pathologist to the possibility of blastomycosis.

Whenever possible, microbiologic culture should always complement histopathologic studies. The mycelial form of *B. dermatitidis* can be isolated from various types of specimens (see Chapter 6), including material massaged from an infected prostate gland. Diagnosis by direct examination of

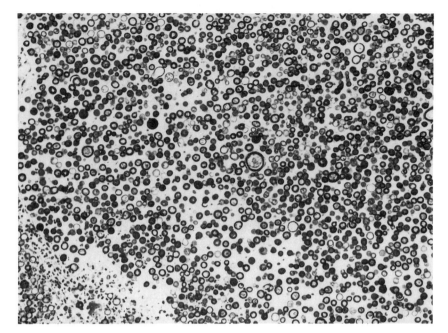

FIGURE 28. Acute pulmonary blastomycosis in an immunocompromised patient. Myriad, proliferating blastomyces cells efface the normal pulmonary architecture and elicit little or no inflammatory response. (Gomori methenamine silver, ×100.)

Papanicolaou-stained smears of respiratory secretions has been reported.[94-97] When atypical fungal cells are observed, direct immunofluorescence using a specific conjugate directed against the cell wall polysaccharide antigens of *B. dermatitidis* is useful for the rapid definitive identification of the fungus in smears and tissue sections.[98-100]

5. IMMUNOHISTOLOGIC DIAGNOSIS: APPLICATIONS AND CURRENT STATUS

The Division of Mycotic Diseases, Centers for Disease Control, Atlanta, and certain other specialized laboratories have developed a battery of sensitive and relatively specific immunofluorescence (IF) reagents for the detection and identification of the common pathogenic fungi, including *B. dermatitidis*.[98-100] Because of the added dimension of immunologic specificity,

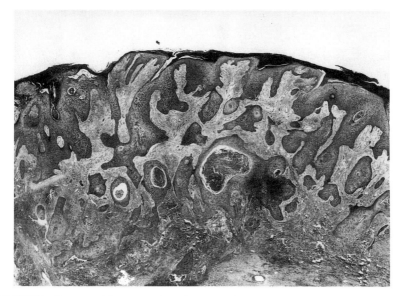

FIGURE 31. Cutaneous blastomycosis. This section of a surgically excised nodular skin lesion reveals florid pseudoepitheliomatous hyperplasia of the epidermis and a mixed suppurative and granulomatous inflammatory reaction in the dermis. (Hematoxylin and eosin, ×5.)

IF can greatly increase the accuracy of direct microscopic examination. It can be used to detect and identify fungi in smears of clinical materials and in deparaffinized sections of formalin-fixed tissue (Figs. 33 and 34). IF is especially helpful to confirm a presumptive histopathologic diagnosis, especially when only atypical forms of a fungus are present or when fungal elements are sparse (Fig. 34). It is also useful to identify a suspected fungal pathogen in contaminated specimens.

Before IF staining, localization and morphologic characterization of fungal elements by light microscopy using conventional and special histologic stains are recommended; this enables the pathologist to establish a preliminary differential diagnosis and then to select the most appropriate IF reagents needed for rapid confirmation. The method for direct IF staining is rapid, reliable, and straightforward. Replicate paraffin sections are mounted on glass microscope slides coated with 3'-aminopropyltriethoxysilane (Sigma Chemical Co., St. Louis, Mo.), deparaffinized by passage through two changes of xylol, and hydrated through graded concentrations of alcohol to phosphate-buffered saline (PBS), pH 7.2. Direct IF of deparaffinized tissue sections works best when the sections are uniformly thin (3 to 5 μm), when

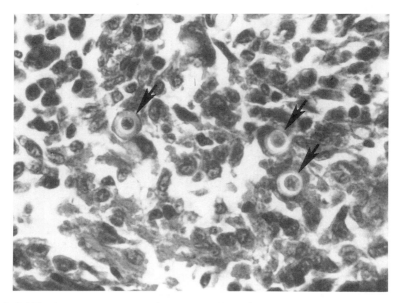

FIGURE 32. Cutaneous blastomycosis. Three spherical, thick-walled blastomyces cells (arrows) are seen within a dermal granuloma. Note retraction of the fungal cell cytoplasm from the rigid cell wall. (Hematoxylin and eosin, ×160.)

fungal elements are intact and easily located in replicate sections stained with GMS, and when the tissue is not calcified or necrotic. When these desirable conditions are not present, enhanced fungal fluorescence and reduced background staining can be achieved by digesting the deparaffinized, decalcified sections in a 1% trypsin solution at pH 8.0 for 1 h at 37°C prior to application of the immune conjugates. Following application of the appropriate conjugates, the sections are incubated at room temperature for 30 to 60 min and are then washed in two changes of PBS. Coverslips are mounted with a drop of buffered glycerol–saline, pH 7.8, and the sections are examined with an ultraviolet (UV) microscope. Positive and negative control sections are processed with each batch of slides.

Because the cell wall antigens of *B. dermatitidis* and most other pathogenic fungi survive formalin fixation and processing into paraffin quite well, IF can be performed retrospectively on archival material. Unstained sections, paraffin blocks, or formalin-fixed "wet" tissue can be shipped to specialized reference centers for IF if the appropriate conjugates are not available locally. If the number of sections available is limited, those already stained with H&E, Giemsa, or tissue Gram stains can be decolorized in

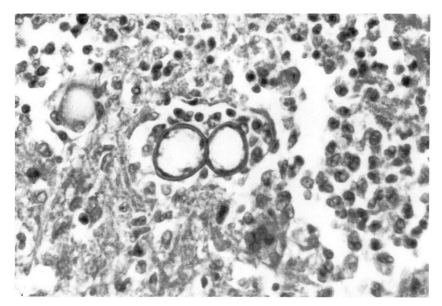

FIGURE 36. Acute coccidioidal pneumonia. Immature, empty spherules of *Coccidioides immitis* can be mistaken for large forms of *Blastomyces dermatitidis.* When appressed, as illustrated here, the spherules give the false impression of a budding yeast form. (Hematoxylin and eosin, ×160.)

acid–alcohol and restained with specific immune conjugates as outlined above. Sections stained with GMS, PAS, or GF procedures are not suitable for this purpose, because oxidation of the cell wall polysaccharides irreparably alters the antigenicity of the fungal cells.

Immunoperoxidase techniques that do not require a fluorescence microscope can also be used to identify certain fungi in cytologic preparations and formalin-fixed paraffin-embedded tissues.[101–103] However, to date, these techniques have been applied to only a few pathogens and have had limited diagnostic use. With time and resources, highly specific immunohistochemical reagents should become commercially available for use in most laboratories.

6. DIFFERENTIAL DIAGNOSIS

When typical multinucleated yeast forms with single, broad-based buds are found in tissue sections, *B. dermatitidis* can be identified with confidence

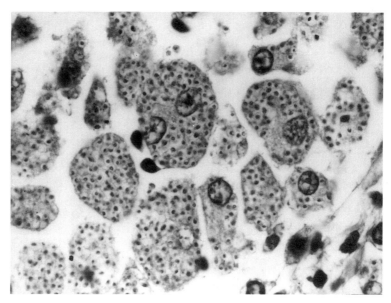

FIGURE 37. Acute pulmonary histoplasmosis capsulati. Intracellular yeast forms of *Histoplasma capsulatum* var. *capsulatum* are 2 to 4 μm in diameter and resemble the microforms of *Blastomyces dermatitidis*. However, the histoplasma cells are uninucleate, have thin walls, and bud by a narrower base. (Hematoxylin and eosin, ×250.)

and a definitive histopathologic diagnosis made. If such forms are not seen, this fungus can be confused with others. For example, nonbudding capsule-deficient cells of *Cryptococcus neoformans* can be mistaken for *B. dermatitidis*. In such instances, mucin stains such as mucicarmine, Alcian blue, and colloidal iron should be used to demonstrate the mucopolysaccharide capsular material of the former pathogen. However, the cell walls of *B. dermatitidis* sometimes react positively with mucin stains (Fig. 35); nevertheless, in our experience, the intensity of staining is usually weak and not as great as that of typical *C. neoformans* cells, especially when a mucicarmine stain is used. Because *B. dermatitidis* cells lack a true capsule, the staining reaction is confined to the thick cell wall rather than to pericellular capsular material, which among human yeast pathogens is only produced by the *Cryptococcus* spp. Blastoconidia of *C. neoformans* can be differentiated from those of *B. dermatitidis* because the former are attached to the parent cells by a narrow base. Giant forms of *B. dermatitidis* that are devoid of blastoconidia and lack internal contents can be easily mistaken for immature or empty spherules of *Coccidioides immitis* (Figs. 12 and 36). When these giant blastomyces cells,

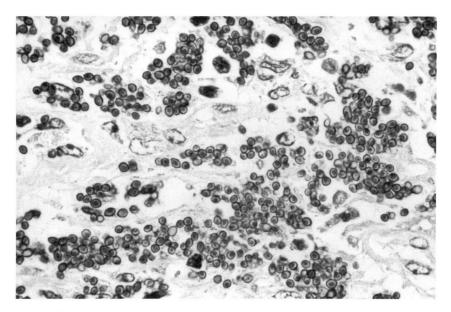

FIGURE 38. Disseminated histoplasmosis capsulati in an AIDS patient. This section of prostate gland contains extracellular aggregates or "yeast lakes" of histoplasma cells that resemble microforms of *Blastomyces dermatitidis* with centrally retracted cytoplasm. (Gomori methenamine silver with hematoxylin and eosin counterstain, ×250.)

which can attain diameters of 30 to 40 μm, do contain multiple prominent nuclei, as best seen with the H&E stain, they resemble small endosporulating spherules of *C. immitis.* In such instances, replicate tissue sections stained with GMS must be carefully screened for intact or broken spherules of *C. immitis* that either contain or are in the process of releasing endospores. Coccidioidal endospores are GMS-positive, whereas nuclei are GMS-negative. Microforms of *B. dermatitidis* can be confused with *H. capsulatum* var. *capsulatum,* especially when they are intracellular (Figs. 9, 37, and 38). However, in the microforms, several nuclei may be seen in H&E-stained sections, the budding is by a much broader base, and other yeast forms that vary in size ranging up to that of typical *B. dermatitidis* cells usually are present. The mixture of unusually small and large, conventional forms of *B. dermatitidis* should not be mistaken for coexisting mycoses (Figs. 10 and 11).[104]

The greatest challenge in the histopathologic differential diagnosis of blastomycosis is histoplasmosis duboisii, a progressive mycosis that has a pulmonary inception with a marked tendency to disseminate to bones and skin.[105–108] It is caused by the large-celled or *duboisii* variety of *H. capsula-*

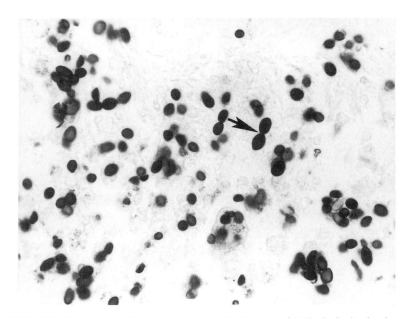

FIGURE 39. Disseminated histoplasmosis duboisii. Because of their similarity in size and shape, the yeast forms of *Histoplasma capsulatum* var. *duboisii* and *Blastomyces dermatitidis* can be mistaken for each other in tissue sections. However, the former bud by a narrow base, producing characteristic "double-cell" forms (arrow). (Gomori methenamine silver, ×160.)

tum. With the exception of two reported cases—one from Japan and the other from Madagascar (Malagasy)—natural infection by this fungus is known to occur only in humans and nonhuman primates from Africa. However, the disease is occasionally seen in the United States in persons who previously lived or traveled in Africa. In cultures grown at 25°C, the mycelial forms of the two varieties of *H. capsulatum* cannot be distinguished from each other either macroscopically or microscopically. The *in vitro* yeast forms of the two varieties grown at 37°C are also morphologically identical. Cultures of the two varieties can be distinguished with certainty only by infecting laboratory animals and observing the difference in size of the respective yeast forms produced in tissue. In tissue sections, the cells of *H. capsulatum* var. *duboisii* are spherical to oval, uninucleate, 8 to 15 μm in diameter, have relatively thick walls and vacuolated cytoplasm, and bud by a narrow base (Figs. 39 and 40). The budding daughter cells commonly enlarge until they are approximately equal in size to the parent cells to which they remain attached, thus creating classical "hourglass," "double-cell," or "figure-eight" forms (Fig. 39).

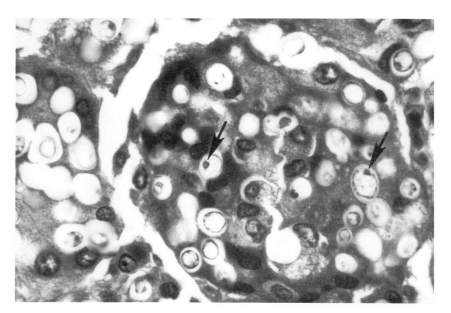

FIGURE 40. Disseminated histoplasmosis duboisii. The spherical to oval yeastlike cells of *Histoplasma capsulatum* var. *duboisii* contain a single, eccentric nucleus (arrows), whereas the yeastlike cells of *Blastomyces dermatitidis* are multinucleate. (Hematoxylin and eosin, ×250.)

Because of their similarity in size and shape and their thick cell walls, the yeast forms of *H. capsulatum* var. *duboisii* and *B. dermatitidis* can be mistaken easily for each other in tissue sections. However, the former usually bud by a narrower base with typical "hourglass" forms, whereas the diagnostic budding form of *B. dermatitidis* is broad-based (Figs. 6 and 39). When stained with H&E, the cells of *H. capsulatum* var. *duboisii* are uninucleate (Fig. 40), whereas *B. dermatitidis* cells each contain multiple nuclei (Fig. 7). The only other yeastlike pathogens that have multiple nuclei are *Paracoccidioides brasiliensis* and *Loboa loboi,* both of which are indigenous to South America and are almost never encountered in the United States. When these differentiating features are equivocal, a presumptive morphologic diagnosis can be confirmed by immunofluorescence or microbiologic culture.

REFERENCES

1. McDonough ES: Blastomycosis: Epidemiology and biology of its ecologic agent, *Ajellomyces dermatitidis. Mycopathologia* 41:195–201, 1970

2. Tenenbaum MJ, Greenspan J, Kerkering TM: Blastomycosis. *CRC Crit Rev Microbiol* 9:139–163, 1982

3. Emmons CW, Binford CH, Utz JP, et al: *Medical Mycology,* ed 3. Philadelphia, Lea & Febiger, 1977, p 342

4. Rippon JW: *Medical Mycology: The Pathogenic Fungi and the Pathogenic Actinomycetes,* ed 3. Philadelphia, WB Saunders, 1988, p 474

5. Schwarz J: Epidemiology and epidemics of blastomycosis. *Mykosen* 16:7–14, 1983

6. Sekhon AS, Jackson FL, Jacobs HJ: Blastomycosis: Report of the first case from Alberta, Canada. *Mycopathologia* 79:65–69, 1982

7. Kane J, Righter J, Krajden S, et al: Blastomycosis: A new endemic focus in Canada. *Can Med Assoc J* 129:728–731, 1983

8. Emmons CW, Murray IG, Lurie HL, et al: North American blastomycosis: Two autochthonous cases from Africa. *Sabouraudia* 3:306–311, 1964

9. Bhagwandeen SB: North American blastomycosis in Zambia. *Am J Trop Med Hyg* 23:231–234, 1974

10. Fragoyannis S, Van Wyk G, DeBeer M: North American blastomycosis in South Africa. *S Afr Med J* 51:169–171, 1977

11. Emerson PA, Higgins E, Branfoot A: North American blastomycosis in Africans. *Br J Dis Chest* 78:286–291, 1984

12. Kuttin ES, Beemer AM, Levu T, et al: Occurrence of *Blastomyces dermatitidis* in Israel: First autochthonous Middle Eastern case. *Am J Trop Med Hyg* 27:1203–1205, 1978

13. Randhawa HS, Khan Z, Gaur S: *Blastomyces dermatitidis* in India: First report of its isolation from clinical material. *Sabouraudia* 21:215–221, 1983

14. Denton JF, McDonough ES, Ajello L, et al: Isolation of *Blastomyces dermatitidis* from soil. *Science* 133:1126–1127, 1961

15. Schwarz J, Salfelder K: Blastomycosis: A review of 152 cases. *Curr Top Pathol* 65:165–200, 1977

16. Landay ME, Schwarz J: Primary cutaneous blastomycosis. *Arch Dermatol* 104:408–411, 1971

17. Wilson JW, Cawley EP, Weidman FD, et al: Primary cutaneous North American blastomycosis. *Arch Dermatol Syphilol (Chicago)* 71:39–45, 1955

18. Larsh HW, Schwarz J: Accidental inoculation blastomycosis. *Cutis* 19:334–337, 1977

19. Graham WR, Callaway JL: Primary inoculation blastomycosis in a veterinarian. *J Am Acad Dermatol* 7:785–786, 1982

20. Larson DM, Eckman MR, Alber RL, et al: Primary cutaneous (inoculation) blastomycosis: An occupational hazard to pathologists. *Am J Clin Pathol* 79:253–255, 1983

21. Gnann JW, Bressler GS, Bodet CA, et al: Human blastomycosis after a dog bite. *Ann Intern Med* 98:48–49, 1983

22. Baum GL, Lerner PI: Primary pulmonary blastomycosis: A laboratory acquired infection. *Ann Intern Med* 73:263–265, 1970

23. Schwarz J, Baum GL: Blastomycosis. *Am J Clin Pathol* 21:999–1029, 1951

24. Kunkel WM Jr, Weed LA, McDonald JR, et al: Collective review: North American blastomycosis—Gilchrist's disease. Clinicopathologic study of ninety cases. *Int Abstr Surg* 99:1–26, 1954

25. Cherniss EI, Weisbren BA: North American blastomycosis. A clinical study of 40 cases. *Ann Intern Med* 44:105–123, 1956

26. Busey JF, Baker RD, Birch L, et al: Blastomycosis: 1. A review of 198 collected cases in Veterans Administration hospitals. *Am Rev Respir Dis* 89:659–672, 1964

27. Witorsch P, Utz JP: North American blastomycosis: A study of 40 patients. *Medicine (Baltimore)* 47:169–200, 1968
28. Vanek J, Schwarz J, Haken S: North American blastomycosis. *Am J Clin Pathol* 54:384–400, 1970
29. Chick EW: North American blastomycosis, in Baker RD (ed): *Human Infection with Fungi, Actinomycetes and Algae.* Berlin, Springer-Verlag, 1971, p 465
30. Sarosi GA, Davies SF: Blastomycosis. *Am Rev Respir Dis* 120:911–938, 1979
31. Steel RW, Abernathy RS: Systemic blastomycosis in children. *Pediatr Infect Dis* 2:304–307, 1983
32. Abernathy RS: Clinical manifestations of pulmonary blastomycosis. *Ann Intern Med* 51:707–727, 1959
33. Sarosi GA, Hammerman KJ, Tosh FE, et al: Clinical features of acute pulmonary blastomycosis. *N Engl J Med* 290:540–543, 1974
34. Recht LD, Philips JR, Eckman MR, et al: Self limited blastomycosis. A report of thirteen cases. *Am Rev Respir Dis* 120:1109–1112, 1979
35. Schwarz J, Baum GL: Fungus diseases of the lungs. North American blastomycosis. *Semin Roentgenol* 5:40–48, 1970
36. Cush R, Light RW, George RB: Clinical and roentgenographic manifestations of acute and chronic blastomycosis. *Chest* 69:345–349, 1976
37. Laskey W, Sarosi GA: The radiologic appearance of pulmonary blastomycosis. *Radiology* 126:351–357, 1978
38. Halvorsen RA, Duncan JD, Merten DJ, et al: Pulmonary blastomycosis: Radiologic manifestations. *Radiology* 150:1–5, 1984
39. Stelling CB, Woodring JH, Rehm SR, et al: Miliary pulmonary blastomycosis. *Radiology* 150:7–13, 1984
40. Sheflin JR, Campbell JA, Thompson GP: Pulmonary blastomycosis: Findings on chest radiographs in 63 patients. *AJR* 154:1177–1180, 1990
41. Griffith JE, Campbell GD: Acute miliary blastomycosis presenting as fulminating respiratory failure. *Chest* 75:630–632, 1979
42. Sarosi GA, Davies SF: *Blastomyces dermatitidis* pneumonia, in Pennington JE (ed): *Respiratory Infections: Diagnosis and Management.* New York, Raven Press, 1983, p 381
43. Chandler FW, Watts JC: Fungal infections, in Dail DH, Hammar SP (eds): *Pulmonary Pathology.* Berlin, Springer-Verlag, 1987, p 201
44. Landis FB, Varkey B: Late relapse of pulmonary blastomycosis after adequate therapy with amphotericin B. *Am Rev Respir Dis* 113:77–81, 1976
45. Green NB, Baughman RP, Kim CK, et al: Failure of ketoconazole in an immunosuppressed patient with pulmonary blastomycosis. *Chest* 88:640–641, 1985
46. Pitrak DL, Andersen BR: Cerebral blastomycoma after ketoconazole therapy for respiratory tract blastomycosis. *Am J Med* 86:713–714, 1989
47. Kinasewitz GT, Penn RL, George RB: The spectrum and significance of pleural disease in blastomycosis. *Chest* 86:580–584, 1984
48. Laskey WL, Sarosi GA: Endogenous reactivation in blastomycosis. *Ann Intern Med* 88:50–52, 1978
49. Murray JJ, Clark CA, Lands RH, et al: Reactivation blastomycosis presenting as a tuboovarian abscess. *Obstet Gynecol* 64:828–830, 1984
50. Ehni W: Endogenous reactivation in blastomycosis. *Am J Med* 86:831–832, 1989
51. Onal E, Lopata M, Lourence RV: Disseminated pulmonary blastomycosis in an immunosuppressed patient: Diagnosis by fiberoptic bronchoscopy. *Am Rev Respir Dis* 113:83–86, 1976

52. Recht LD, Davies SF, Eckman MR, et al: Blastomycosis in immunosuppressed patients. *Am Rev Respir Dis* 125:359–362, 1982
53. Butka BJ, Bennett SR, Johnson AC: Disseminated inoculation blastomycosis in a renal transplant recipient. *Am Rev Respir Dis* 130:1180–1183, 1984
54. Poe RH, Vassalo CL, Plessingar VA: Pulmonary blastomycosis versus carcinoma: A challenging differential. *Am J Med Sci* 263:145–155, 1972
55. Carnesdale PL, Stegman KF: Blastomycosis of bone. Report of four cases. *Ann Surg* 144:252–257, 1956
56. Rhangos WC, Chick EW: Mycotic infections of bone. *South Med J* 57:664–674, 1964
57. Burr AH, Huffiness R: Blastomycosis of the prostate with miliary dissemination treated by stilbamidine. *J Urol* 71:464–468, 1954
58. Inoshita T, Youngberg GA, Boelen LJ, et al: Blastomycosis presenting with prostatic involvement: Report of 2 cases and review of the literature. *J Urol* 130:160–162, 1983
59. Fetter BF, Klintworth GK, Hendry WS: *Mycoses of the Central Nervous System.* Baltimore, Williams & Wilkins, 1967
60. Buechner HA, Clawson CM: Blastomycosis of the central nervous system. II. A report of nine cases from the Veterans Administration cooperative study. *Am Rev Respir Dis* 95:820–826, 1967
61. Rippon JW, Zvetina JR, Reyes C: Case report: Miliary blastomycosis with cerebral involvement. *Mycopathologia* 60:121–125, 1977
62. Gonyea EF: The spectrum of primary blastomycotic meningitis: A review of central nervous system blastomycosis. *Ann Neurol* 3:26–39, 1978
63. Bell RM, Starshak RJ, Sty JR, et al: Solitary intracranial blastomycotic abscess. *Wis Med J* 82:23–25, 1983
64. Hamblen EC, Baker RD, Martin DS: Blastomycosis of the female reproductive tract with report of a case. *Am J Obstet Gynecol* 30:345–356, 1935
65. Cassady JV: Uveal blastomycosis. *Arch Ophthalmol* 35:84–97, 1946
66. Ranier A: Primary laryngeal blastomycosis. A review of the literature and report of a case. *Am J Clin Pathol* 21:444–450, 1951
67. Pond NE, Humphreys RJ: Blastomycosis with cardiac involvement and peripheral embolization. *Am Heart J* 43:615–620, 1952
68. Sinskey RM, Anderson WB: Miliary blastomycosis with metastatic spread to posterior uvea of both eyes. *Arch Ophthalmol* 54:602–604, 1955
69. Lester GF, Conrad FG, Atwell RJ: Primary laryngeal blastomycosis. Review of the literature and presentation of a case. *Am J Med* 24:305–309, 1958
70. Abernathy RS, Melby JC: Addison's disease in North American blastomycosis. *N Engl J Med* 266:552–554, 1962
71. Kent DC, Collier TM: Addison's disease associated with North American blastomycosis. A case report. *J Clin Endocrinol* 25:164–169, 1965
72. Font RL, Spaulding AG, Green WR: Endogenous mycotic panophthalmitis caused by *Blastomyces dermatitidis. Arch Ophthalmol* 77:217–222, 1967
73. Chandler PT: Addison's disease secondary to North American blastomycosis. *South Med J* 70:863–864, 1977
74. Dumich PS, Neel HB: Blastomycosis of the larynx. *Laryngoscope* 93:1266–1270, 1983
75. Payne J, Koopmann CF Jr: Laryngeal carcinoma—or is it laryngeal blastomycosis? *Laryngoscope* 94:608–611, 1984
76. McKenzie R, Khakow R: Blastomycosis of the esophagus presenting with gastrointestinal bleeding. *Gastroenterology* 88:1271–1273, 1984
77. Kaufman J: Tracheal blastomycosis. *Chest* 93:424–425, 1988

78. Lewis H, Aaberg TM, Fary DR, et al: Latent disseminated blastomycosis with choroidal involvement. *Arch Ophthalmol* 106:527–530, 1988
79. Christie AJ, Binns PM, Kredo KR: Long-standing indolent blastomycosis at internal opening of tracheostomy. *Chest* 95:932–933, 1989
80. Ryan ME, Kirchner JP, Sell T, et al: Cholangitis due to *Blastomyces dermatitidis. Gastroenterology* 96:1346–1349, 1989
81. Benham RW: Fungi of blastomycosis and coccidioidal granuloma. *Arch Dermatol* 30:385–400, 1934
82. Chandler FW, Kaplan W, Ajello L: *Color Atlas and Text of the Histopathology of Mycotic Diseases.* Chicago, Year Book Medical Publishers, 1980, pp 39, 158
83. Chandler FW, Watts JC: *Pathologic Diagnosis of Fungal Infections.* Chicago, ASCP Press, 1987, p 149
84. Moore M: Morphologic variation in tissue of the organisms of the blastomycoses and of histoplasmosis. *Am J Pathol* 31:1049–1063, 1955
85. Tuttle JG, Lichtwardt HE, Altshuler CH: Systemic North American blastomycosis. Report of a case with small forms of blastomycetes. *Am J Clin Pathol* 23:890–897, 1953
86. Watts JC, Chandler FW, Mihalov ML, et al: Giant forms of *Blastomyces dermatitidis* in the pulmonary lesions of blastomycosis. Potential confusion with *Coccidioides immitis. Am J Clin Pathol* 93:119–122, 1990
87. Hardin HF, Scott DJ: Blastomycosis: Occurrence of filamentous forms in vivo. *Am J Clin Pathol* 62:104–106, 1974
88. Atkinson JB, McCurley TL: Pulmonary blastomycosis: Filamentous forms in an immunocompromised patient with fulminating respiratory failure. *Hum Pathol* 14:186–188, 1983
89. Liber AF, Choi HS: Splendore–Hoeppli phenomenon about silk sutures in tissue. *Arch Pathol Lab Med* 95:217–220, 1973
90. Wages DS, Wear DJ: Acid-fastness of fungi in blastomycosis and histoplasmosis. *Arch Pathol Lab Med* 106:440–441, 1982
91. Graham AR: Fungal autofluorescence with ultraviolet illumination. *Am J Clin Pathol* 79:231–234, 1983
92. Monheit JG, Cowan DF, Moore DG: Rapid detection of fungi in tissues using Calcofluor White and fluorescence microscopy. *Arch Pathol Lab Med* 108:616–618, 1984
93. Monheit JG, Brown G, Kott MM, et al: Calcofluor White detection of fungi in cytopathology. *Am J Clin Pathol* 85:222–225, 1986
94. Johnson WW, Mantulli J: The role of cytology in the primary diagnosis of North American blastomycosis. *Acta Cytol* 17:200–204, 1970
95. Sanders JS, Sarosi GA, Nollet DJ, et al: Exfoliative cytology in the rapid diagnosis of pulmonary blastomycosis. *Chest* 72:193–196, 1977
96. Trumbull ML, Chesney TM: The cytological diagnosis of pulmonary blastomycosis. *JAMA* 245:836–838, 1981
97. Dyer ML, Young TL, Kattine AA, et al: Blastomycosis in a Papanicolaou smear. Report of a case with possible venereal transmission. *Acta Cytol* 27:285–287, 1983
98. Kaplan W, Kaufman L: Specific fluorescent antiglobulins for the detection and identification of *Blastomyces dermatitidis* yeast phase cells. *Mycopathologia* 19:173–180, 1963
99. Kaplan W, Kraft DE: Demonstration of pathogenic fungi in formalin fixed tissues by immunofluorescence. *Am J Clin Pathol* 52:420–432, 1969
100. Kaplan W: Practical application of fluorescent antibody procedures in medical mycology, in: *Mycoses.* PAHO Sci Publ No 304, Washington, DC, 1975, pp 178–185
101. Russell B, Beckett JH, Jacobs PH: Immunoperoxidase localization of *Sporothrix schenckii*

and *Cryptococcus neoformans:* Staining of tissue sections fixed in 4% formaldehyde solution and embedded in paraffin. *Arch Dermatol* 115:433–435, 1979

102. El Nageeb S, Hay RJ: Immunoperoxidase staining in the recognition of *Aspergillus* infections. *Histopathology* 5:437–444, 1981
103. Moskowitz LB, Ganjei P, Ziegels-Weissman J, et al: Immunohistologic identification of fungi in systemic and cutaneous mycoses. *Arch Pathol Lab Med* 110:433–436, 1986
104. Brandsberg JW, Tosh FE, Furcolow ML: Concurrent infection with *Histoplasma capsulatum* and *Blastomyces dermatitidis. N Engl J Med* 270:874–877, 1964
105. Cockshott WP, Lucas AO: Histoplasmosis duboisii. *Q J Med* 33:223–238, 1964
106. Clark BM, Greenwood BM: Pulmonary lesions in African histoplasmosis. *J Trop Med Hyg* 71:4–10, 1968
107. Lucas AD: Cutaneous manifestations of African histoplasmosis. *Br J Dermatol* 82:435–447, 1970
108. Nethercott JR, Schachter RK, Givan KF, et al: Histoplasmosis due to *Histoplasma capsulatum* var *duboisii* in a Canadian immigrant. *Arch Dermatol* 114:595–598, 1978

11

Experimental Blastomycosis

George C. Cozad

1. INTRODUCTION

Pathogenicity of mycotic agents of disease is a summation of many different interrelated factors. Some are directly dependent upon the parasite and its ability to survive in living tissue. Others have to do with the nature of the host and its various immune responses. The parasite, through its life processes or antigen properties, may influence in some fashion host immune responses, which play a vital role in the tenuous balance between survival of the parasite and the well-being of the host.

Experimental blastomycosis in animals has given and will continue to provide information essential to understanding the multipotential mycotic pathogen, *Blastomyces dermatitidis.*

2. EXPERIMENTAL INFECTION AND PATHOGENICITY

In exudate from lesions, sputum, and tissue sections from animals infected with blastomycosis, large, round, thick-walled yeast cells are seen, 5–15 μm in diameter, with reproduction by formation of a single bud. The

Blastomycosis, edited by Yousef Al-Doory and Arthur F. DiSalvo, Plenum Medical Book Company, New York, 1992.

mycelial form has branching, septate hyphae with lateral, spherical to pyriform conidia, 5–8 μm in diameter.

Under natural conditions in soil the fungus exists in the mycelial form, with these microconidia the proper size for entering the alveolar spaces of the lungs upon inhalation. The organisms may infect and cause lesions in practically any organ of the body, including the skin.[1]

Spontaneous blastomycosis has been reported in dogs,[2–4] horses,[5] and a sea lion[6] and other animals. Animals experimentally infected have been guinea pigs,[7,8] hamsters,[9,10] rats,[10] and mice.[11,12] Based upon studies by Spencer[13] and others, mice appear to be the experimental animal of choice.

Spring[14] compared seven isolates of B. dermatitidis with respect to their resistance to dyes, ability to ferment carbohydrates, and virulence for laboratory animals.

Baker[15] found the mycelial fragments of B. dermatitidis to be as effective as yeast in causing death of mice when equal doses were injected intraperitoneally (i.p.). Hitch[16] attempted to induce primary cutaneous blastomycosis in mice, without success. A heavy suspension of yeast cells of the organism was painted on their shaved abdomens and multiple dermal punctures were applied.

Heilman[17] and later Schwarz and Baum[18] reported the organism to cause embolic pneumonia in mice. Heilman showed that intravenous (i.v.) injection of 1.8×10^5 yeast cells killed mice in an average of 7 days. With i.p. injection it took 44 days to produce death.

Smith et al.[10] injected conidia and mycelial fragments i.p. into rabbits, guinea pigs, rats, hamsters, and mice. Hamsters were most susceptible, followed by mice. Rabbits were more resistant. The authors determined the infective dose 50% (ID_{50}) for mice to be 1×10^5 conidia and mycelial fragments.

The recovery of B. dermatitidis from mice inoculated i.v. and i.p. with yeast cells was studied by Spencer.[13] Mice injected with 1290 cells by the i.v. route contained approximately one million organisms in their lungs 2 weeks after infection. The number of organisms in the liver and spleen of these mice ranged from 100 to 10,000 at this time. Intraperitoneally inoculated mice receiving 1290 yeast cells did not contain organism in the lungs at any autopsy period. Organisms were not recovered from the lungs of mice receiving this i.p. dosage until the second week and only 544 cells were found 3 weeks after injection. The number of organisms in livers and spleens of these mice ranged from about 300 at 2 days to 10,000 organisms 3 weeks after injection.

The 21-day i.v. LD_{50} was 1.23×10^3 yeast cells, and the i.p. LD_{50} for the same time period was 1.28×10^6 yeast cells. By the i.p. route it took 1000 times more organisms to kill an equal number of mice in the same length of time.

These studies found that progressive multiplication of *B. dermatitidis* occurs more readily in the lungs of i.v. infected mice than in the liver or spleen. The predilection of fungal pathogens for growth in a particular organ was suggested by Larsh and Cozad in 1965.[19] These investigators, studying *Histoplasma capsulatum* infection in mice by the aerosolized intranasal (i.n.) route, found the highest number of organisms in the liver.

With i.p. inoculation of blastomyces yeast cells, the organisms do not readily invade the lung in the early phase of the infection. Additionally, the finding that it took 1000 times more yeast cells to kill an equivalent number of animals by the i.p. route compared to the i.v. route, suggests extensive infection of the lungs to be a primary cause of death in mice. This predilection for lungs may help to partially explain a puzzling phenomenon in rabbits. It has been found that rabbits experimentally infected by i.v. injection of *B. dermatitidis* yeast cells often show no visible effects but then die rapidly, often within hours after appearing perfectly normal (unpublished data).

3. IMPORTANCE OF CELLULAR IMMUNITY IN BLASTOMYCOSIS

Blastomyces dermatitidis is a systemic pathogen, with ability to infect a wide variety of animal tissues. The pulmonary infection may disseminate to other internal organs, as well as bones and skin. Mild clinical forms of the disease may occur, as is the case with other systemic mycoses. An understanding of the major host defense mechanisms is of prime importance to predicting the outcome and severity of the disease.

Smith[20] early recognized that blastomycosis patients with delayed hypersensitivity (DH) to blastomycin had a better prognosis. Many investigators have reported that mice develop DH to proteins[21] and fungal antigens.[22–24] Resistance to systemic fungal diseases may be determined in mice by noting increased survival after lethal challenge, suppression of fungal dissemination, or modification in the course of reinfection.

Many experimental animals have been infected with *B. dermatitidis*,[25,26] but mice have been found particularly useful for these studies.[27,28] Salvin[24] and Box and Briggs[22] sensitized mice with live or dead cells of *H. capsulatum*. Kong *et al.*[23] detected DH to *Coccidioides immitis* by footpad inoculation of spherulin or mycelial extracts. In a series of studies, Spencer and Cozad[29] reported that C57BL/6J mice sensitized to *B. dermatitidis* were protected from the lethal effects of blastomyces infection. Solid protection was seen following a lethal i.p. challenge with viable yeast cells 15 days after subcutaneous (s.c.) inoculation with 3.9×10^4 viable cells. Tissue hypersensitivity was induced by two injections of merthiolate-killed yeast cells in incomplete Freund adjuvant or by a single injection of 3.9×10^4 viable cells. Development of hypersensitivity, which peaked at 15 days, was determined by footpad injection of killed yeast cells. The results from this study indicate that cellular immunity plays a significant role in host defense against blastomycosis, and firmly established the mouse as a useful experimental model for study of host–parasite relationships in this fungal disease.

These early studies provided a protocol vital to further investigation, by demonstration that:

1. C57BL/6J mice were the preferred strain.
2. These animals could be sensitized by a single s.c. injection of a small number (3.9×10^4) of live *B. dermatitidis* yeast cells, or by two s.c. injections of a yeast cell–incomplete Freund adjuvant emulsion containing 2 mg of merthiolate-killed yeast cells.
3. Footpad testing could be used to assay for tissue sensitivity and the optimal inoculum was 45 μg of killed yeast cells contained in 0.03 ml.
4. Results of footpad sensitivity tests were best read after 48 h.
5. The earliest detection of DH was found at 12 days after s.c. inoculation with either viable cells or killed cells in adjuvant. The peak reaction was after 15 days for viable cells, 20 days for killed cells in adjuvant. Subcutaneous inoculation was superior to i.p. inoculation for both preparations.

A continuation of studies on the importance of cellular immunity in blastomycosis was reported by Scillian, Cozad, and Spencer.[30] These investigators used two inbred mouse strains to demonstrate passive transfer of DH by transfer of spleen cells from sensitized donors to normal recipients. They also sought to demonstrate another important correlate of cellular immunity, the *in vitro* migration inhibition of peritoneal exudate cells (macrophages) in the presence of specific antigen.

To sensitize animals, groups of C57BL/6J and BALB/cJ mice were injected s.c. with 3.9×10^4 viable *B. dermatitidis* yeast cells. This equaled 0.1 of a 21-day i.p. mean lethal dose.[29] Fifteen days later, spleen cells and blood sera were obtained for transfer to recipient mice, and peritoneal exudate (PE) cells collected for migration inhibition testing. Methods of Yamamato and Anacker[31] were used for migration inhibition (MI) tests, and the procedure described by Spencer and Cozad[29] was used for footpad testing. After 24 h, mice that had received spleen cells or serum from sensitized animals were tested by the footpad using killed *B. dermatitidis* yeast cell antigen.

Mice that had received i.v. injection of spleen cells from sensitized animals had a significant increase in footpad thickness 24–48 h after testing. Those receiving only serum were negative. The presence of blastomycin antigen was shown to inhibit migration of PE cells from blastomyces-sensitized donor mice.

Neither passively sensitized mice nor PE cells from blastomyces-sensitized animals reacted with mycobacterial antigen (PPD). Passive transfer of DH to *B. dermatitidis* was thus accomplished in C57BL/6J and BALB/cJ mice using 10^8 spleen cells from sensitized donor mice of the same strain.

The observed migration inhibition of PE cells from sensitized animals in the presence of blastomycin was evidence that positive footpad reaction was cell-mediated. These investigators also were successful in sensitizing mice with killed yeast-form *B. dermatitidis* without adjuvant, which lasted at least 42 days after footpad injection.

Results from these animal studies correlate well with resistance factors in human disease in that prognosis in blastomycosis seems to be dependent upon the cell-mediated resistance state of the patient. Smith[32] reported that positive skin test reactions indicate good prognosis and recovery. Proven blastomycosis cases with high complement fixation titers and negative skin test reaction have a poor prognosis. A similar pattern has been reported in a coccidioidomycosis study in rats.[33]

4. CELL-MEDIATED IMMUNOPROTECTION IN BLASTOMYCOSIS (WHOLE ANIMAL STUDY)

Cellular immunity, the host resistance obtained through interactions of thymus derived lymphocytes and mononuclear phagocytes through cytokine mediation, involves particularly facultative intracellular parasites.[34]

Viable cells of *B. dermatitidis,* as well as *C. immitis, Cryptococcus neoformans,* and *H. capsulatum* have been reported to induce resistance as measured by increase in 50% lethal dose (LD_{50}) in experimental animals.[27,29,35–37] Immunization for blastomycosis using killed cells seemed to have equivocal results, as evidenced by early work by Landay *et al.*[38] These researchers reported that mice injected i.p. with killed *B. dermatitidis* cells were protected when challenged with mycelial-form cells but not from yeast-form effects.

As has been previously demonstrated,[29] cellular immunity can be accomplished by single injection of viable cells or by two s.c. injections of killed yeast cells of *B. dermatitidis* in incomplete Freund adjuvant, and mice at the time of greatest sensitivity are protected from lethal challenge. The assumption was that this resistance is due to inhibition or killing of parasites.

Additional studies substantiating this finding were reported by Cozad and Chang.[39]

Mice were sensitized by s.c. inoculation of killed *B. dermatitidis* yeast antigen emulsified in incomplete Freund adjuvant on days 0 and 7. Mice were footpad tested at various time intervals by injection of 45 μg of killed yeast into the right hind footpads. Footpads were measured at zero time and 48 h after testing. The mean differences in thicknesses between right and left hind footpads served as the measure of tissue sensitivity. Mice were negative to day 3, sharply increased in hypersensitivity to day 18, and then sensitivity waned, although lasting to at least day 56.

A sensitive measure of immunity is obtained by determining the extent of suppression of parasite multiplication in host tissue. With this in mind, the "index of resistance" (IR) as described by Blanden *et al.* was used.[40] In brief, a group of mice were inoculated with antigen emulsion on days 0 and 7. At various intervals, mice were inoculated i.v. with 1.5×10^5 viable *B. dermatitidis* yeast cells. At 1 or 48 h after this challenge, mice were killed, lungs, livers, and spleens homogenized separately, diluted, cultured, and the number of fungal cells in each organ determined. The IR represents the log value of the ratio of *B. dermatitidis* increasing rate and unit time between control group and antigen emulsion-inoculated group. In other words, this measures the growth inhibition of *B. dermatitidis* cells in sensitized animals versus nonsensitized animals during this early stage of infection.

There was no protection in sensitized mice at day 3 of the experiment. The IR for the spleens, livers, and lungs increased progressively thereafter, and peaked between day 18 and 21. The IR then fell rapidly, although a low level of resistance persisted until day 49. Thus, all three organs contained cells capable of handling the parasite, although with different efficiency. The largest numbers of fungal cells were found in the lungs. An important observation was that the IR followed almost exactly the tissue sensitivity pattern, with both reaching maximum intensity at 18 to 21 days.

This study also showed effectiveness of s.c. sensitization of mice using killed cell antigen emulsion in protecting mice from lethal challenge, i.v. and i.p. After 3 days (when animals were not sensitive) there was no protective effect. At 18 days, there was significant protective effect to challenge with 0.5 LD_{50} given both i.v. and i.p. Protective effects were still noted at 35 days.

These studies strongly suggested that blastomyces antigen suitably administered results in a population of sensitized T lymphocytes with the capacity to interact with deposited antigen. This would result in a typical tissue hypersensitivity, and stimulate the sequence of events that leads to destruction of parasites, presumably through interaction with macrophages.

It was hoped that the findings from this mouse model would provide some insight into the human disease. That this may be so is suggested from the findings of Sarosi *et al.*,[41] who described the clinical spectrum of the acute self-limited infection observed during an epidemic of blastomycosis.

5. IMMUNE MONITORING IN BLASTOMYCOSIS

Because mice were shown to be most resistant to blastomycosis when cellular immunity was highest, studies were done to monitor lymphocyte numbers and functional activity of T and B lymphocytes during this period.[42–44]

The objectives of these studies were to develop procedures and reagents to allow enumeration of mouse T and B lymphocytes. These procedures were used to determine relative numbers of lymphocytes in blood and inguinal lymph nodes of mice at various times after receiving sensitizing doses of *B. dermatitidis* antigen. Functional activity of sensitized lymphocytes was also monitored by lymphocyte transformation studies with various specific and nonspecific mitogens at various stages of tissue sensitivity.

Mice were sensitized to *B. dermatitidis* and their footpad swelling was tested over a 35-day period, using the method of Cozad and Chang.[39] Mouse lymphocytes were quantitated by immunofluorescent techniques: T lymphocytes by indirect immunofluorescence and B lymphocytes by direct immunofluorescence. In these experiments, peak tissue sensitization occurred at day 15; the numbers of T lymphocytes in both peripheral blood and inguinal lymph nodes peaked at 15–18 days. A corresponding decrease in numbers of B lymphocytes was found in peripheral blood and lymph nodes, reaching the lowest percentages between days 15 and 18. Thus, there was a direct correlation between T- and B-lymphocyte percentages and the extent of tissue sensitivity.

In transformation studies, cells were removed from inguinal lymph nodes of the animals and cultured with blastomycin or phytohemagglutinin (PHA) and blast transformation measured by uptake of tritiated thymidine. PHA stimulated transformation of lymphocytes from sensitized or unsensitized mice. Sensitized lymphocytes cultured with blastomycin showed a peak isotope incorporation index of 3.5 on day 18 of the experiment. Thus, the peak proliferation paralleled the time of maximum resistance and the peak of tissue sensitivity.

Immune monitoring in blastomycosis could be helpful in predicting outcome of the disease. Figures 1–4 show how well two *in vitro* methods and the one *in vivo* method for determining cell-mediated immunity can predict capability of the host to respond to *B. dermatitidis* infection.

In short, increased numbers of T lymphocytes, increased functional

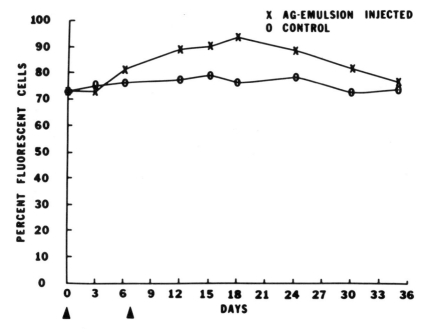

FIGURE 1. Quantitation of T lymphocytes in peripheral blood of mice inoculated with Blasto yeast antigen-emulsion (incomplete Freund adjuvant).

activity of those T lymphocytes, as well as ability to respond by tissue reactivity with specific antigen indicates killing of parasites.

6. THYMOSIN, LYMPHOTOXIN, AND IMMUNE REACTION

Studies of thymosin restoration of cellular immunity to *B. dermatitidis* in T-cell-depleted mice have been reported by Longley and Cozad.[45] Collins and Morrison demonstrated that thymosin could restore tissue hypersensitivity responses of thymectomized, lethally irradiated, and bone marrow-reconstituted mice (ThyXBM) to a sensitizing dose of sheep erythrocytes.[46] Goldstein *et al.* partially purified a water-soluble polypeptide, thymosin, derived from bovine thymus.[47] This material has proven effective in bringing about maturation of immunocompetent T lymphocytes in thymectomized, lethally irradiated animals, and human lymphocyte cultures.[48–50] Thymosin had not previously been reported to restore tissue sensitivity of ThyXBM mice.

Longley and Cozad's study[45] was prompted by the correlation between

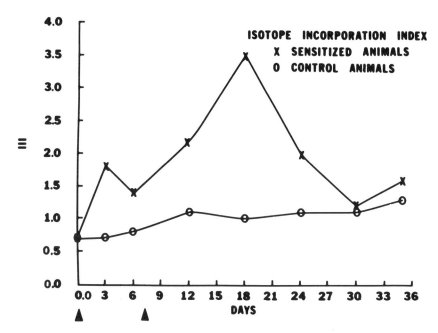

FIGURE 2. Isotope incorporation index of lymph node lymphocytes cultured with blastomycin.

high levels of tissue sensitivity to *B. dermatitidis* antigen and enhanced resistance to this fungus. Further studies[42–44,51] indicated that increasing tissue sensitivity closely followed increases in T-lymphocyte numbers in peripheral blood; increases in number of sensitized T lymphocytes as measured by blast transformation; increases in lymphotoxin activity. Since these activities are T-cell dependent, as expected, ThyXBM mice were unable to respond to *B. dermatitidis* yeast antigen in footpad swelling tests. Normal mice had tissue hypersensitivity to killed yeast cells of *B. dermatitidis* when footpad tested at day 12, following sensitization at days 0 and 7. The footpad response of normal mice treated with thymosin 2 weeks before and 12 days after initial sensitization was similar to that of normal, non-thymosin-treated mice. ThyXBM mice failed to show a significant footpad response when similarly sensitized and tested. ThyXBM mice that received the 2-week and 12-day treatments with thymosin responded to footpad testing on day 12 at a level that was 62% greater than the response seen in non-thymosin-treated ThyXBM mice. Results indicated that thymosin could restore immunocompetence to a T-cell-depleted host by inducing maturation of functional T lymphocytes from lymphoid precursor pools in the transplanted bone marrow. Recovery from blastomycosis is dependent upon a competent cel-

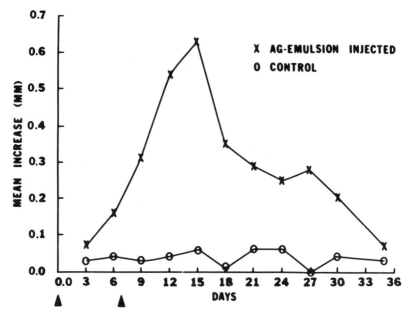

FIGURE 3. Tissue sensitivity induced by subcutaneous inoculation of killed *B. dermatitidis* yeast emulsified in incomplete Freund adjuvant.

lular immune apparatus and it appears that thymosin may be useful in potentiating a cellular immune response to aid in the recovery of these individuals.

Quantitation of lymphotoxin activity in murine blastomycosis was reported by Gorcyca and Cozad.[52] Numerous studies have shown that supernatants from lymphocyte cultures stimulated with either a nonspecific mitogen or a specific antigen contain a toxic substance, lymphotoxin (LT).

The objectives of this work were to show the susceptibility of yeast cells of *B. dermatitidis* to LT and to quantitate LT activity during the induction of tissue type hypersensitivity to blastomyces antigens. The quantitation of LT activity was performed on monolayers of L-929 cells in microwells at various day intervals during tissue sensitivity. The cytotoxicity against *B. dermatitidis* yeast was demonstrated by comparing the number of viable cells recovered from supernatants of stimulated lymphocyte cultures to that recovered from nonstimulated lymphocyte cultures. Supernatants from cultures of lymphocytes stimulated with either PHA or blastomycin were toxic for *B. dermatitidis* yeasts. The quantity of LT activity paralleled the *in vivo* pattern of tissue sensitivity as shown by footpad swelling tests in the murine blastomycosis model.

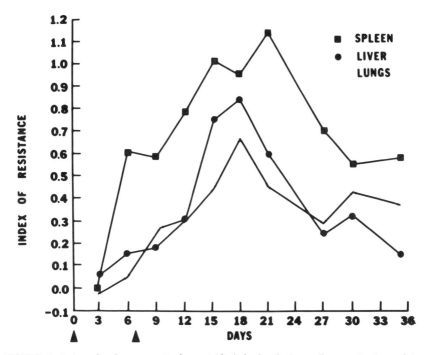

FIGURE 4. Index of resistance to *B. dermatitidis* infection in lungs, liver, and spleen of Ag-emulsion-injected mice. Arrowheads indicate days on which the subcutaneous inoculations were made. The index expresses the efficiency of host tissue in suppression of parasites when organs are cultured at 1 and at 48 h after a challenge with live *B. dermatitidis* yeast cells.

7. *B. DERMATITIDIS* AS A BIOLOGIC RESPONSE MODULATOR

As previously indicated, cell-mediated immunity plays the dominant role in the immune response of mice to *B. dermatitidis* infections. The macrophage is the key cell, being the processor of antigen and the destroyer of fungal cells through phagocytosis. In early studies,[53] peritoneal macrophages from mice sensitized to *B. dermatitidis* by the method of Cozad and Chang[39] were examined for morphological or quantitative functional differences. Observations were made using scanning electron microscopy (SEM). Phagocytic activity of sensitized macrophages was followed, using latex particles and *B. dermatitidis* yeast cells.

Peak phagocytic activity was found 15 days after the sensitizing dose, paralleling the extent of cellular immunity. *In vivo* challenge provided a more accurate presentation of phagocytosis than *in vitro* methods. Observations by SEM revealed that latex particles or yeast cells were actually engulfed rather than merely attached to macrophages. These SEM studies demonstrated the multipotential of blastomyces-activated macrophages with regard to morphology and functional activity.

Interactions between blastomyces-sensitized murine peritoneal macrophages and yeast-form cells of *B. dermatitidis* were investigated by McDaniel and Cozad.[54] SEM observations showed that sensitized macrophages readily phagocytized *B. dermatitidis* yeast cells in *in vitro* studies. The increased chemiluminescence activity during phagocytosis indicated activation of metabolic pathways within the sensitized macrophages. There was a rapid increase in emitted light from blastomyces-sensitized macrophages during interaction with *B. dermatitidis* yeast cells.

Sensitized macrophages were found to be significantly more efficient in controlling intracellular proliferation of the yeast cells, as determined by description of macrophages and plating for viable yeasts. SEM studies offered more substantiation of these results. Studies using *Candida albicans* as the challenge organism indicated that *B. dermatitidis* nonspecifically activated macrophages. Thirty percent fewer *C. albicans* yeast cells were found to produce germ tubes when phagocytized by blastomyces-sensitized macrophages. Immunomodulation by killed cells of *B. dermatitidis* yeast in incomplete Freund adjuvant was thus firmly established.

8. IMMUNOADJUVANT EFFECTS OF *B. DERMATITIDIS* AGAINST EL4 LYMPHOMA

Immunomodulation was first established as a potential means of treating tumors in studies utilizing bacillus Calmette-Guerin (BCG).[55] Success in these early experiments prompted the search for immunomodulators that did not pose the risk associated with living bacteria. Killed *Corynebacterium parvum* and methanol extraction residue (MER) of tubercle bacilli have been investigated most extensively in recent years.[56,57] Studies with *B. dermatitidis* indicated that this organism greatly stimulates the cell-mediated immune system, and suggested its use as an immunomodulator for suppression of tumor cell growth.

As reported in studies by McDaniel and Cozad,[58] *B. dermatitidis* yeast cells are remarkably effective in promoting control of EL4 lymphoma. Mice were injected i.p. with 10^2 to 10^6 EL4 cells or 10^2 to 10^6 EL4 cells mixed with thimerosal-killed *B. dermatitidis* yeast cells. None of the animals receiving tumor cells alone survived. Mice receiving *B. dermatitidis* were protected from as many as 10^4 tumor cells. Complete suppression of tumor growth was found in treated animals that received 10^2 or 10^3 tumor cells. Ten days after treatment, peritoneal macrophages from mice that showed complete suppression of tumors were tested for the ability to prevent *in vitro* cell proliferation. These macrophages gave 90% inhibition of [^{3}H]thymidine incorporation by EL4 tumor cells. Macrophages from *B. dermatitidis* yeast-treated animals gave a twofold increase in specific lysis of EL4 at 10 and 15 days. Spleen and lymph node cells from protected animals gave no cytotoxic activity against EL4 in a ^{51}Cr release assay.

When mice were preimmunized with *B. dermatitidis* in incomplete Freund adjuvant, animals challenged with EL4 cells after 3 days showed a significant increase in survival time. This protective effect was found at 3 to 6 days after s.c. or i.p. injection of *B. dermatitidis.*

Killed *B. dermatitidis* yeast antigen appears to be more effective than *C. parvum* at preventing growth of EL4 tumor *in vivo,* and would appear to merit further investigation as an immunostimulant for therapy of other forms of tumors.

REFERENCES

1. Salvin SB: *Progress in Allergy: Immunologic Aspects of the Mycoses,* vol 7. Basel, Karger, 1963
2. Menges RW, Furcolow ML, Selby LA, et al: Clinical and epidemiological studies on seventy nine canine blastomycosis cases in Arkansas. *Am J Epidemiol* 81:164–179, 1964
3. Menges RW, Selby LA, Habermann RT: Survey for blastomycosis and histoplasmosis among stray dogs in Arkansas. *Am J Vet Res* 28:345–349, 1967
4. Menges RW: Blastomycosis in animals. *Vet Med* Dec 1967:45–54
5. Benbrook EA, Bryant JB, Saunders LZ: A case of blastomycosis in the horse. *J Am Vet Med Assoc* 124:475–478, 1948
6. Williamson WM, Lombard LA, Gethy RE: North American blastomycosis in a northern sea lion. *J Am Vet Med Assoc* 135:513–515, 1959
7. Howell A: Isolation of pathogenic fungi from experimentally inoculated guinea pigs. *Am Rev Tuberc* May 1948:602–617
8. Maldonado WE, Felton FG: Experimental North American blastomycosis. *Am J Med* July 1963:89–94
9. Salfelder K, Schwarz J, Johnson CE: Experimental South American blastomycosis in hamsters. *Arch Dermatol* 97:69–77, 1968
10. Smith CD, Brandesberg JW, Selby LA, et al: A comparison of the relative susceptibilities of laboratory animals to infection with the mycelial phase of *B. dermatitidis. Sabouraudia* 5:126–131, 1966
11. Sethi K, Salfelder K, Schwarz J: Cross reactions to *B. dermatitidis* in mice. *Mycopathol Mycol Appl* 24:70–72, 1964
12. Williams TW, Emmons CW: Hamycin treatment of experimental blastomycosis in mice. *Proc Soc Exp Biol Med* 120:481–484, 1965
13. Spencer HD: Recovery of *Blastomyces dermatitidis* from intravenously and intraperitoneally inoculated mice. MS thesis, University of Oklahoma, Norman, 1968
14. Spring D: Comparison of seven strains of organism causing blastomycosis in man. *J Infect Dis* 44:169–185, 1929

15. Baker RD: Comparison of mice by mycelial and yeast forms of *B. dermatitidis. J Infect Dis* 63:324, 1938
16. Hitch JM: Experimental blastomycosis in mice. *J Invest Dermatol* 5:41–45, 1941
17. Heilman FR: Experimental production of rapidly fatal blastomycosis in mice for testing chemotherapeutic agents. *J Invest Dermatol* 5:87–90, 1947
18. Schwarz J, Baum GL: Blastomycosis. *Am J Clin Pathol* 21:999–1029, 1951
19. Larsh HW, Cozad GC: Respiratory infection of mice with *H. capsulatum. Mycopathol Mycol Appl* 27:305–310, 1965
20. Smith DT: Immunologic types of blastomycosis: A report on 40 cases. *Ann Intern Med* 31:463–469, 1949
21. Crowle AJ, Hu CC: Duration of some cutaneous hypersensitivities in mice. *J Immunol* 93:132–134, 1964
22. Box E, Briggs NT: Endotoxin susceptibility and delayed hypersensitivity in experimental histoplasmosis. *J Immunol* 87:485–491, 1961
23. Kong YM, Savage DC, Kong LNL: Delayed dermal hypersensitivity in mice to spherule and mycelial extracts of *Coccidioides immitis. J Bacteriol* 91:876–883, 1966
24. Salvin SB: Hypersensitivity in mice with experimental histoplasmosis. *J Immunol* 75:1–6, 1955
25. Conti-Dias IA, Smith CD, Furcolow ML: Comparison of infection of laboratory animals with *Blastomyces dermatitidis* using different routes of inoculation. *Sabouraudia* 7:279–283, 1970
26. Smith CD, Brandesberg JW, Selby LA, et al: A comparison of the relative susceptibilities of laboratory animals to infection with the mycelial phase of *Blastomyces dermatitidis. Sabouraudia* 5:126–131, 1966
27. Kong Yi-Chi M, Levine HB: Experimentally induced immunity in the mycoses. *Bacteriol Rev* 31:35–53, 1967
28. Martin DS: Serologic studies on North American blastomycosis. *J Immunol* 71:192–201, 1955
29. Spencer HD, Cozad GC: Role of delayed hypersensitivity in blastomycosis of mice. *Infect Immun* 7:329–334, 1973
30. Scillian JJ, Cozad GC, Spencer HD: Passive transfer of delayed hypersensitivity to *Blastomyces dermatitidis* between mice. *Infect Immun* 10:705–711, 1974
31. Yamamoto K, Anacker RL: Macrophage migration inhibition studies with cells from mice vaccinated with cell walls of *Mycobacterium bovis* (BCG): Characterization of the experimental system. *Infect Immun* 1:587–594, 1970
32. Smith DT: Immunologic types of blastomycosis: A report on 40 cases. *Ann Intern Med* 31:463–469, 1949
33. Sharbough RJ, Grogan JB: Suppression of reticuloendothelial function in the rat with cyclophosphamide. *J Bacteriol* 100:117–122, 1969
34. Mackaness GB: The relationship of delayed hypersensitivity to acquired cellular resistance. *Br Med Bull* 23:52–54, 1967
35. Louria DB: Specific and non-specific immunity in experimental cryptococcosis in mice. *J Exp Med* 111:643–665, 1960
36. Pappagianis D, Levine HB, Smith CE, et al: Immunization of mice with viable *Coccidioides immitis. J Immunol* 86:28–34, 1961
37. Salvin SB: Resistance to reinfection in experimental histoplasmosis. *J Immunol* 74:214–221, 1955
38. Landay ME, Hotchi M, Soares N: Effect of prior vaccination on experimental blastomycosis. *Mycopathol Mycol Appl* 46:61–64, 1972

39. Cozad GC, Chang CT: Cell-mediated immunoprotection in blastomycosis. *Infect Immun* 28:398–403, 1980
40. Blanden RV, Lefford MJ, Mackaness GB: The host response to Calmette-Guerine bacillus infection in mice. *J Exp Med* 129:1079–1101, 1969
41. Sarosi GA, Hammerman KJ, Tosh FE, et al: Clinical features of acute pulmonary blastomycosis. *N Engl J Med* 290:540–543, 1974
42. Cozad GC, Andrew SA, Thompson EM: Immune monitoring in blastomycosis. *Abstr Annu Meet Am Soc Microbiol* F28, 1977, p 123
43. Thompson EM: The role of cell mediated immunity in blastomycosis: Quantitation of B and T-lymphocytes. MS thesis, University of Oklahoma, Norman, 1976
44. Andrew SA: Lymphocyte transformation in murine blastomycosis. MS thesis, University of Oklahoma, Norman, 1976
45. Longley RE, Cozad GC: Thymosin restoration of cellular immunity to *Blastomyces dermatitidis* in T-cell depleted mice. *Infect Immun* 26:187–192, 1979
46. Collins FM, Morrison NE: Restoration of delayed hypersensitivity to sheep erythrocytes by thymosin treatment of T-cell depleted mice. *Infect Immun* 13:564–568, 1975
47. Goldstein AL, Slater FD, White A: Preparation assay and partial purification of a thymic lymphopoietic factor (thymosin). *Proc Natl Acad Sci USA* 56:1010–1017, 1966
48. Hooper JA, McDaniel MC, Thurman GB, et al: Purification and properties of bovine thymosin. *Ann NY Acad Sci* 249:125–144, 1975
49. Touraine JL, Touraine F, Incefy GS, et al: Effect of thymic factors on the differentiation of human marrow cells into T-lymphocytes in-vitro in normals and patients with immunodeficiencies. *Ann NY Acad Sci* 249:335–342, 1975
50. Wybran J, Levine AS, Fudenberg HH, et al: Thymosin: Effects on normal human blood T-cells. *Ann NY Acad Sci* 249:300–307, 1975
51. Gorcyca DE: Quantitation of lymphotoxin activity in murine blastomycosis. MS thesis, University of Oklahoma, Norman, 1977
52. Gorcyca DE, Cozad GC: Quantitation of lymphotoxin activity in murine blastomycosis. *Abstr Annu Meet Am Soc Microbiol* F30, 1977, p 123
53. Cozad GC, Kronholm LM: Scanning electron microscope studies of macrophages activated by *Blastomyces dermatitidis. Abstr Annu Meet Am Soc Microbiol* F51, 1979, p 371
54. McDaniel LS, Cozad GC: Immunomodulation by *Blastomyces dermatitidis:* Functional activity of murine peritoneal macrophages. *Infect Immun* 40:733–740, 1983
55. Zbar B: Specific and nonspecific immunotherapy: Use of BCG, in *Recent Results in Cancer Research* 47, *Investigation and Stimulation of Immunity in Cancer Patients.* Berlin, Springer, 1974, p 350
56. Currie GA, Bagshawe KD: Active immunotherapy with *Corynebacterium parvum* and chemotherapy in murine fibrosarcomas. *Br Med J* 1:541, 1970
57. Starzl TE, Halgrimson GC: Immunosuppression and malignant neoplasms. *N Engl J Med* 283:934, 1970
58. McDaniel LS, Cozad GC: Immunoadjuvant effects of *Blastomyces dermatitidis* against EL4 lymphoma in C57BL/6J mice. *J Natl Cancer Inst* 68:1337–1342, 1982

12

Prognosis and Therapy of Blastomycosis

Robert W. Bradsher

1. INTRODUCTION

It has become clear that blastomycosis is very similar to histoplasmosis and coccidioidomycosis with respect to the epidemiology and immunology of the infection. As late as 1945, histoplasmosis was considered to be a uniformly fatal infection with less than 75 disseminated cases reported.[1] With the advent of histoplasmin skin testing, it became clear that many persons without a clinical history had, indeed, been infected with the fungus.[2] Similar findings are being discovered with blastomycosis. Patients with acute infection who recovered despite no therapy with an antifungal agent have been reported. The majority of those cases have been associated with point-source epidemics such as those at Big Fork, Minnesota, and Eagle River, Wisconsin.[3,4] In that latter epidemic of blastomycosis, only 9 patients with culture-proven infection were treated with an antifungal agent.[4] The other 35 patients with immunologic evidence of infection were not treated; none have had relapse of infection. Edson and Keys reported a number of patients

Blastomycosis, edited by Yousef Al-Doory and Arthur F. DiSalvo, Plenum Medical Book Company, New York, 1992.

who had no deleterious effects with only observation following surgical resection of a solitary pulmonary nodule as long as no other disease was present.[5]

The incidence of disease currently depends on reporting of clinical cases of infection. However, there have been limited but clear reports of subclinical infection with *Blastomyces dermatitidis*. In the Eagle River epidemic, only a few of those with immune markers of infection had signs and symptoms characteristic of blastomycosis.[4] During immune studies using cells from treated blastomycosis patients,[6,7] two control persons with no history of blastomycosis had evidence of immunity. Cells from these controls showed lymphocyte responses to a blastomyces antigen and macrophage phagocytosis and inhibition of intracellular growth similar to those with culture-proven infections and dissimilar to other controls with no history of exposure. This prompted studies of other persons who had analogous environmental exposures to patients with clinical blastomycosis. In a group of seven forestry workers with daily exposure to woods within the endemic area, all had evidence of previous blastomycosis with none having had a history of clinical disease.[8] Avid hunters from the same endemic area had a 60% prevalence of immune markers indicating previous infection with this fungus.[8] Since these studies were performed with persons from overlapping endemic areas of exposure with blastomycosis and histoplasmosis, studies using lymphocytes from forestry workers by Vaaler *et al.*[9] were performed in areas endemic for only blastomycosis (northern Minnesota and Wisconsin). Thirty percent of the workers had *in vitro* markers of immunity as evidence of subclinical infection with no question of cross-reactions due to *Histoplasma capsulatum*.[9] Blastomycosis appears to have comparable patterns of subclinical infection as occurs with histoplasmosis and coccidioidomycosis.

2. INITIATION OF THERAPY

The first consideration for the patient with blastomycosis is whether or not to treat with an antifungal agent. The clinical presentation of the patient and the toxicity of the antifungal agent are the major determinants of whether or not to observe the infection or use the antifungal agent. Relapse of the initial infection either with or without treatment has been reported so that careful following of the patient for a prolonged period is required if therapy is not given.[10,11]

Because such resolution of the infection without therapy[12] may occur in patients involved with either an epidemic focus of infection or in an endemic area, observation of the pneumonia for 1 to 2 weeks may be considered (Table 1). If the patient has deterioration or progression, antifungal therapy should begin. Occasionally the diagnosis of blastomycosis had not been con-

TABLE 1
Treatment of Blastomycosis

No antifungal therapy, observation
Mild acute pulmonary infection
Point-source epidemic of infection
Ketoconazole
Progressive untreated acute pulmonary infection
Extrapulmonary infection (i.e., skin, bone, prostate)
Disseminated infection but not life-threatening
Itraconazole (pending FDA approval)
Ketoconazole failure or relapse
First-line therapy in place of ketoconazole
Amphotericin B
Noncompliant patient
Life-threatening infection (i.e., ARDS)
Central nervous system involvement
Progression of infection while on oral therapy

sidered in a patient with pneumonia until the culture of respiratory secretions (sputum, bronchoscopy washings or brushings) grows the organism. Observation alone may also be indicated in such a patient who has already improved while the culture was incubating. As noted above, surgical resection of a solitary pulmonary nodule may cure the infection without further therapy.[5] It must be emphasized that the presence of pleural disease or any extrapulmonary infection during the course of illness requires antifungal treatment. All other forms of blastomycosis should also be treated with systemic therapy.

3. AMPHOTERICIN B

The mortality rate of untreated blastomycosis depends on the disease manifestations. Before antifungal therapy was available, a case-fatality ratio of 78% was documented.[13] In more recent reports, 21 and 28% of untreated patients died from the fungal infections.[14,15] Since amphotericin B was introduced in 1956, this polyene antifungal drug has been shown to be effective in the treatment of blastomycosis. In five large series of patients with this fungal infection, intravenous amphotericin B in a dosage of at least 1.0 g resulted in cure without relapse in 16 of 19, 21 of 27, 32 of 35, 13 of 15, and 37 of 41 patients.[16–20] A dosage of 2 g has been associated with cure rates of up to 97%. A brief summary of clinical aspects of amphotericin B treatment for blastomycosis is listed in Table 2. The mechanism of action of amphotericin B is interaction of the agent with components of the surface of the cell which then

TABLE 2
Amphotericin B Therapy for Blastomycosis

Begin with 1 mg test dose, rapid escalation of dose to 35–50 mg per day

Maintain adequate hydration since dehydration and amphotericin B
are synergistically nephrotoxic

Acetaminophen and antihistamines for premedication; heparin, steroids,
or meperidine used if needed

A total dose of 2 g is the goal

Laboratory assessment of electrolytes, blood counts, and renal function
performed twice a week

Temporary cessation for creatinine values above 3 mg%, hematocrit
below 24%, or uncorrectable hypokalemia

alters the integrity of the fungal cell membrane.[21] Amphotericin B has also been associated with antitumor activity as well as immune stimulation activity.[21]

The antifungal activity is responsible for the high cure rates in blastomycosis with amphotericin B. However, this high degree of antimycotic activity is associated with significant toxicity. In a group of patients with blastomycosis reported by Abernathy, almost three-fourths (71%) experienced a decline in renal function[22]; a number of other toxicities were also reported including anemia (53%), anorexia and nausea (53%), fever (49%), hypokalemia (37%), and thrombophlebitis (19%). Interruption of therapy during some point in the course was required in 41% of patients and termination of therapy with amphotericin B before reaching the desired total dose was mandatory because of toxicity in 14% of the patients.[22] Similarly, all 21 courses of amphotericin B treatment in patients with blastomycosis reported by Witorsch and Utz[16] were complicated by both azotemia and anemia. Therefore, other agents have been sought.

Relapse of blastomycosis following amphotericin B therapy occurs only rarely and appears to be dose-dependent when it does occur.[11,23] In one large retrospective series, relapse occurred in only 2 of 30 patients who received more than 1.5 g of the drug, whereas 5 of 19 patients who received a smaller dose had relapse.[18] Most of the cases of relapse described by Witorsch and Utz occurred shortly after completion of amphotericin B therapy.[16] However, patients have had relapse of disease as long as 9 years following treatment. As discussed above, patients have also been described with relapse of infection many years after spontaneous resolution.[24] The main reason for withholding or postponing treatment of pulmonary blastomycosis has been the toxicity of amphotericin B, the mainstay of therapy until recent years.

Other agents have been tried in an attempt to lessen toxicity. Although 2-hydroxystilbamidine given orally was reported to be marginally effective, it is now of historic interest only. Miconazole is an intravenously administered imidazole that has activity against *B. dermatitidis.* However, adequate trials in this infection have not been performed primarily because of the adverse effects of miconazole.

4. KETOCONAZOLE

Ketoconazole is an imidazole antifungal agent with *in vitro* activity against *B. dermatitidis* similar to that of amphotericin B.[25] The drug works by disrupting the cell membranes following interactions with cytochrome P-450 enzymes which ultimately reduces the concentration of ergosterol, the major sterol of the membrane of the fungus.[21,25] Ketoconazole is well absorbed from the gastrointestinal tract and has been generally well tolerated in clinical studies of patients with other fungal infections. The drug has been used to treat blastomycosis in canines,[26,27] and moderate effectiveness has been shown in a murine model of *B. dermatitidis* infection.[28] The major advantage of the drug is that it is absorbed from the gastrointestinal tract and is generally well tolerated.

Adverse effects include those that are severe and those that are less of a problem. One severe toxicity is hepatocellular damage which appears to be a very rare occurrence[29]; liver transaminase enzymes should be monitored during ketoconazole therapy. Hormonal abnormalities have been described at higher dosages of the drug, such as gynecomastia, dysfunctional uterine bleeding, and oligospermia.[25,30,31] More common but less severe adverse effects include nausea and vomiting when the drug is taken without a meal, as well as dizziness, pruritus, and headache.[31] The absorption of ketoconazole requires an acidic gastric content so that antacids or H_2 blocking agents such as cimetidine or ranitidine are contraindicated while the patient is taking ketoconazole. Other agents such as rifampin, oral contraceptives, cyclosporine, phenobarbital, and dilantin may interfere with ketoconazole therapy.[21]

With its lower potential of toxicity than amphotericin B, ketoconazole has been viewed with considerable enthusiasm for treatment of blastomycosis. However, the initial trial from the National Institutes of Health (NIH) Mycoses Study Group was not optimistic. Of 16 patients with blastomycosis, 7 were cured, 4 were considered to have treatment failures, and 5 had relapse of infection.[32] The adequacy of the dose and the duration of ketoconazole therapy were questioned. Ten of the twenty-five patients with relapses of infection with the various fungi treated received 200 mg of ketoconazole per day as the maximal dose. Some received the drug for only a month before failure was declared. Following that report, there have been scattered case reports of ketoconazole therapy,[33-38] two prospective trials with the agent,[31,39] and one retrospective review of ketoconazole treatment of blasto-

TABLE 3
Ketoconazole Therapy for Blastomycosis

Begin with 400 mg per day as single dose with a meal

Avoid antacids, histamine-2 blockers

If no response in 2–4 weeks, increase dose to 600 mg/day

If no response in 2–4 weeks at the higher dose, increase dose to 800 mg/day in split doses

With progressive disease or no response to 800 mg/day, switch to i.v. amphotericin B or consider itraconazole

Continue ketoconazole for at least 6 months and consider a 12-month course if resolution was slow

Monitor liver function tests, blood counts, and electrolytes on a monthly basis

mycosis.[10] These reports with ketoconazole at a dosage of 400 to 800 mg per day for at least 6 months were more promising than the initial reports. A summary of the use of ketoconazole for blastomycosis is listed in Table 3.

The NIH Mycoses Study Group summarized the results of the 80 blastomycosis patients enrolled into its second trial of ketoconazole as successful with 89% of the patients cured, provided that treatment with 400 or 800 mg per day was used for at least 6 months.[39] Relapse occurred 2, 7, 18, and 24 months following therapy. Cure without relapse was obtained in 35 of 44 patients over a 2-year period in Arkansas, a state with a high rate of endemic cases of blastomycosis. They were treated at a dose of 400 mg given as a single daily dose with breakfast.[31] Six patients had relapses after therapy but three were protocol inadherent. As an example, one patient had both pulmonary blastomycosis and alcoholic hepatitis and was protocol inadherent. She responded to the initial 14 days of in-hospital therapy with a loss of fever, but she discontinued therapy after discharge and did not keep follow-up appointments. She was hospitalized 3 weeks later with progression of infiltrates to five lobes and a high yeast count on sputum smears. Despite mechanical ventilation and intensive treatment with amphotericin B, she began to have delirium tremens, became hypotensive, and died. An additional two patients had lesions that did not totally resolve so that both were considered treatment failures. One patient died from gastric surgery complications after 1 month of therapy but his pulmonary blastomycosis had already been cured. Since that report, only one further case of relapse of infection has occurred with an additional $5\frac{1}{2}$ years of follow-up for a total of up to 87 months.

Because ketoconazole is the only available oral agent at the present time, further details of this trial are given.[31] All patients showed initial improvement after starting ketoconazole therapy. Of those with chronic pneumonia, 13 of 16 were cured. More than 6 months of ketoconazole treatment was given because of relapse after previous therapy with amphotericin B in one patient and because of massive pleural effusion in two of the patients. Six of the eight patients with acute blastomycosis pneumonia were cured with 6 months of ketoconazole therapy in this trial.[31] Ketoconazole therapy cured 14 of 18 patients with extrapulmonary blastomycosis. Two of those not cured had relapse while the other two had primary treatment failure. One of those is detailed as an example. She had extensive pulmonary infection and associated bone infection in her calcaneus. Her fever, pulmonary infiltrate, and hypoxia responded to ketoconazole therapy over a 2-month period, but she developed new cutaneous lesions with histopathologic evidence of *B. dermatitidis* during therapy despite adequate serum levels of ketoconazole. Treatment with amphotericin B resolved the lesions.[31] Other patients with primary drug failure despite compliance have been reported.[40]

The reason for failure of some patients to respond to ketoconazole despite adequate serum concentrations of the agent and susceptible organisms remains obscure. The clinical value of measuring inhibitory levels for *B. dermatitidis* or measuring serum concentrations of either amphotericin B or ketoconazole remains unclear.[21] Until further large clinical studies are performed comparing the assays with clinical outcomes, routine testing for these laboratory measurements is not recommended.

Noncompliance may be a major reason for failure. One of the patients with chronic pneumonia who was noncompliant had recurrence of the infection in the central nervous system.[31] Pitrak and Andersen reported a similar patient with a cerebral blastomycoma following an inadequate course of ketoconazole.[41] Ketoconazole does not cross the blood–brain barrier so that neurological manifestations of blastomycosis should not be treated with the agent.

McManus and Jones[10] reported success in treating blastomycosis with ketoconazole and commented on the potential cost savings with this form of therapy compared to amphotericin B given in the hospital. The length of stay according to diagnosis-related group (DRG) for blastomycosis in 1985 was 8.8 days.[10] Expenses would likely exceed payments to hospitals for a 6- to 8-week course of amphotericin B if outpatient therapy could not be arranged.

5. ITRACONAZOLE

Itraconazole is a triazole that is also given orally with relatively good absorption.[25,42,43] The mechanism of action and the pharmacokinetics are similar to those of ketoconazole. The major theoretical advantage with itraconazole has been a lower rate of toxicity in the investigational trials, particularly with regards to the endocrinopathies associated with ketoconazole.[25] The drug was used at a dose of 200 to 400 mg per day in the Mycoses Study Group of the NIH beginning in 1985. Of the 40 patients with blastomycosis treated with the agent, only 2 patients were not considered to be cured.[43] The drug was used at a dose of 200 mg per day to treat an additional 41 patients with blastomycosis with a good response.[44] This includes 12 patients who had either progression of disease while on ketoconazole or relapse following cure of the blastomycosis with ketoconazole. All of the patients had a rapid initial response with itraconazole. Five patients out of the thirty-four who have concluded therapy have had a less than satisfactory response while seven remain on therapy. One man with preexisting pancreatitis and malabsorption had rapid clearing of the pulmonary infiltrate but had relapse of blastomycosis documented 9 months later. This relapse responded to a second course of itraconazole. Another patient (who had quiescent myeloma) treated on the NIH protocol had relapse of infection after itraconazole but was cured with retreatment with the same agent. One patient was found to have intracerebral lesions by computed tomographic scans after being on itraconazole for only 4 days; amphotericin B was used since itraconazole has no better penetration into spinal fluid than ketoconazole.[25] Two patients of the twelve who had a relapse of blastomycosis after ketoconazole therapy had relapses following itraconazole. One was receiving immunosuppressive therapy for a renal transplant but the other patient had no obvious reason for the relapse after itraconazole. Both were cured with amphotericin B.

6. OTHER MODES OF THERAPY

Newer imidazole and triazole antifungal agents are being developed. There has been very limited experience in *B. dermatitidis* infections with fluconazole. With a low dose of 50 mg per day in an NIH Mycoses Study Group trial, the agent in a small number of patients was not associated with the same cure rates for blastomycosis as with ketoconazole or itraconazole. This failure is considered to be more an inadequacy of the dose that was given than a deficiency of the agent itself. Trials are currently underway with 200 to 400 mg per day of fluconazole. Other agents also are in early investigations. Comparative trials of various antifungal agents, such as itraconazole or fluconazole versus ketoconazole, will be required for full assessment.[45]

Generally, 6 months of therapy with the various azole antifungal agents has been recommended but there are no trials with a shorter span of therapy. Comparative lengths of therapy should also be studied to determine the optimal duration of therapy. Difficulty in designing suitable trials between amphotericin B and imidazoles has centered on the intravenous administration and relative toxicity of amphotericin B versus the oral medicines. Comparisons may be possible in the future with severely ill patients with blastomycosis if itraconazole or other agents continue to have the same efficacy rates. Because relatively few cases of this infection occur from a single location, multicenter trials similar to those performed by the NIH Mycoses Study Group will likely be required.

7. SUMMARY

The results of oral therapy of blastomycosis are encouraging. In the very ill patient, amphotericin B remains the treatment of choice, but after improvement with 500 mg or so of amphotericin B, a switch to an oral agent like ketoconazole for the remainder of the treatment may be appropriate. One major disadvantage of oral therapy is the potential of noncompliance.[31,39] The majority of patients who have had ketoconazole treatment failures had not taken the drug as they were instructed, a problem that is usually not encountered with intravenous therapy with amphotericin B. In addition, central nervous system infection with blastomycosis may occur while on ketoconazole[31,41] since penetration into the brain is thought to be minimal. Cases have been reported with clearing of the cutaneous or pulmonary infection with ketoconazole but subsequent diagnosis of central nervous system infection.

On the basis of available information, ketoconazole, at a dose of 400 mg per day for 6 months, should replace amphotericin B as therapy in compliant patients with less-than-overwhelming, life-threatening blastomycosis (Table 1). Itraconazole may well replace ketoconazole for first-line therapy when the drug is released based on the successful treatment of ketoconazole failures. However, for the patient with life-threatening manifestation of infection, such as the appearance of adult respiratory distress syndrome (ARDS), or the person with central nervous system involvement with blastomycosis, amphotericin B remains the treatment of choice.

REFERENCES

1. Parsons RJ, Zaronfontis CJD: Histoplasmosis in man: Report of 7 cases and review of 71 cases. *Arch Intern Med* 75:1–23, 1945
2. Christie A, Peterson JC: Pulmonary calcifications in negative reactors to tuberculin. *Am J Public Health* 35:1131–1147, 1945
3. Tosh FE, Hammerman KJ, Weeks RJ, et al: A common source epidemic of North American blastomycosis. *Am Rev Respir Dis* 109:525–529, 1974

4. Klein BS, Vergeront JM, Weeks RJ, et al: Isolation of *Blastomyces dermatitidis* in soil associated with a large outbreak of blastomycosis in Wisconsin. *N Engl J Med* 314:529–534, 1986

5. Edson RS, Keys TF: Treatment of primary pulmonary blastomycosis. *Mayo Clin Proc* 56:683–685, 1981

6. Bradsher RW, Ulmer WC, Marmer DJ, et al: Intracellular growth and phagocytosis of *Blastomyces dermatitidis* by monocyte-derived macrophages from previously infected and normal subjects. *J Infect Dis* 151:57–64, 1985

7. Bradsher RW, Balk RA, Jacobs RF: Growth inhibition of *Blastomyces dermatitidis* in alveolar and peripheral macrophages from patients with blastomycosis. *Am Rev Respir Dis* 135:412–417, 1987

8. Taft EF, Bradsher RW: Subclinical blastomycosis detected by lymphocyte transformation to *Blastomyces* antigen. *Am Rev Respir Dis* 136:A267, 1987

9. Vaaler AK, Bradsher RW, Davies SF: Evidence of subclinical blastomycosis in forestry workers in northern Minnesota and northern Wisconsin. *Am J Med* 89:470–475, 1990

10. McManus EJ, Jones JM: The use of ketoconazole in the treatment of blastomycosis. *Am Rev Respir Dis* 133:141–143, 1986

11. Landis FB, Varkey B: Late relapse of pulmonary blastomycosis after adequate treatment with amphotericin B. *Am Rev Respir Dis* 113:77–81, 1976

12. Recht LD, Philips JR, Eckman MR, et al: Self-limited blastomycosis: A report of 13 cases. *Am Rev Respir Dis* 120:1109–1112, 1979

13. Martin DS, Smith DT: Blastomycosis: I. A review of the literature. *Am Rev Tuberc* 39:275–304, 1939

14. Abernathy RS: Clinical features of pulmonary blastomycosis. *Ann Intern Med* 51:707–727, 1959

15. Furcolow ML, Watson KA, Tisdall OF, et al: Some factors affecting survival in systemic blastomycosis. *Dis Chest* 54(suppl):285–296, 1968

16. Witorsch P, Utz JP: North American blastomycosis: A study of 40 patients. *Medicine* 47:169–200, 1968

17. Lockwood WR, Allison F Jr, Batson BE, et al: The treatment of North American blastomycosis: Ten years' experience. *Am Rev Respir Dis* 100:314–320, 1969

18. Parker JD, Doto IL, Tosh FE: A decade of experience with blastomycosis and its treatment with amphotericin B. *Am Rev Respir Dis* 99:895–902, 1969

19. Seaburg JH, Dascomb HE: Results of the treatment of systemic mycosis. *JAMA* 188:509–513, 1964

20. Busey JF: Blastomycosis. III. A comparative study of 2-hydroxystilbamidine and amphotericin B therapy. *Am Rev Respir Dis* 105:812–818, 1972

21. Bennett JE: Antifungal agents, in Mandell GL, Douglas RG Jr, Bennett JE (eds): *Principles and Practice of Infectious Diseases,* ed 3. Edinburgh, Churchill Livingstone, 1990, pp 361–370

22. Abernathy RS: Amphotericin therapy of North American blastomycosis. *Antimicrob Agents Chemother* 3:208–211, 1967

23. Sarosi GA, Davies SF: Blastomycosis. State of the art. *Am Rev Respir Dis* 120:911–938, 1979

24. Laskey WL, Sarosi GA: Endogenous activation in blastomycosis. *Ann Intern Med* 88:50–52, 1978

25. Saag MS, Dismukes WE: Azole antifungal agents: Emphasis on new triazoles. *Antimicrob Agents Chemother* 32:1–8, 1988

26. Dunbar M Jr, Pyle RL, Boring JG, et al: Treatment of canine blastomycosis with ketoconazole. *J Am Vet Med Assoc* 182:156–157, 1983

27. Legendre AM, Selcer BA, Edwards DF, et al: Treatment of canine blastomycosis with amphotericin B and ketoconazole. *J Am Vet Med Assoc* 184:1249–1254, 1984
28. Harvey RP, Isenberg RA, Stevens DA: Molecular modifications of imidazole compounds: Studies of activity and synergy in vitro and of pharmacology and therapy of blastomycosis in a mouse model. *Rev Infect Dis* 2:559–569, 1980
29. Lewis JH, Zimmerman HJ, Benson GD, et al: Hepatic injury associated with ketoconazole therapy. *Gastroenterology* 86:503–513, 1984
30. Pont A, Graybill JR, Craven PC, et al: High-dose ketoconazole therapy and adrenal and testicular function in humans. *Arch Intern Med* 144:2150–2153, 1984
31. Bradsher RW, Rice DC, Abernathy RS: Ketoconazole therapy of endemic blastomycosis. *Ann Intern Med* 103:872–879, 1985
32. Dismukes WE, Stamm AM, Graybill JR, et al: Treatment of systemic mycoses with ketoconazole: Emphasis on toxicity and clinical response in 52 patients. *Ann Intern Med* 98:13–20, 1983
33. Symoens J, Moens M, Dom J, et al: An evaluation of two years of clinical experience with ketoconazole. *Rev Infect Dis* 2:674–687, 1980
34. Scheld WM: Grand Rounds: North American blastomycosis. *Va Med Mon* 110:240–248, 1983
35. Gnann JW Jr, Bressler GS, Bodet CA, et al: Human blastomycosis after a dog bite. *Ann Intern Med* 98:48–49, 1983
36. Hii JH, Legault L, DeVeber G, et al: Successful treatment of systemic blastomycosis with high-dose ketoconazole in a renal transplant recipient. *Am J Kidney Dis* 15:595–597, 1990
37. Tuthill S: Disseminated blastomycosis treated with ketoconazole. *South Med J* 79:1188–1189, 1986
38. Moore RM, Green NE: Blastomycosis of bone: A report of six cases. *J Bone Jt Surg* 64A:1097–1101, 1983
39. National Institute of Allergy and Infectious Diseases Mycosis Study Group: Treatment of blastomycosis and histoplasmosis with ketoconazole: Results of a prospective, randomized clinical trial. *Ann Intern Med* 103:861–872, 1985
40. Hevert CA, King J, George RB: Late dissemination of pulmonary blastomycosis during ketoconazole therapy. *Chest* 95:240–242, 1989
41. Pitrak DL, Andersen BR: Cerebral blastomycoma after ketoconazole therapy for respiratory tract blastomycosis. *Am J Med* 86:713–714, 1989
42. Van Cauteren HJ, Heykants J, De Coster R, et al: Itraconazole: Pharmacologic studies in animals and humans. *Rev Infect Dis* 9:S43–46, 1987
43. Dismukes W, Bradsher R, Girard W, et al: Itraconazole therapy for blastomycosis and histoplasmosis [abstract 798]. NIAID Mycosis Study Group. 26th Interscience Conference on Antimicrobial Agents and Chemotherapy, 1986
44. Bradsher RW: Itraconazole therapy of blastomycosis: Cure following progression or relapse after ketoconazole [abstract 1351]. New York, 27th Interscience Conference on Antimicrobial Agents and Chemotherapy, 1987
45. Dismukes W, Bennett JE, Drutz DJ, et al: Criteria for evaluation of therapeutic response to antifungal drugs. *Rev Infect Dis* 2:535–545, 1980

13

Blastomycosis in Animals

Alfred M. Legendre

1. INTRODUCTION

Infection with *Blastomyces dermatitidis* can be induced in a variety of laboratory animal species. Mice have been used extensively to study experimental
infection. A number of different mouse models have been utilized.[1-4] These
models have demonstrated differences in virulence among strains of *B. dermatitidis.*[5-7] Murine blastomycosis has also been useful in studying the immune response of the host to the organism.[8,9] Thymectomized mice[10] and
athymic nude mice[11] have been used to evaluate the role of cell-mediated
immunity in blastomycosis. Hamsters,[12-14] guinea pigs,[15] and dogs[16,17] have
also been used to study blastomycosis.

Blastomycosis occurs in a variety of wild species. A wild wolf in Minnesota died of blastomycosis.[18] The incidence of blastomycosis is very difficult
to ascertain in animals in the wild, but blastomycosis is not uncommon in
captive wild animals. Captive marine mammals appear to be at significant
risk when in endemic areas. Blastomycosis occurs in dolphins (*Tursiops
truncatus*),[19,20] sea lions (*Eumetopias jubata*),[19,21] and has recently been diagnosed in a captive polar bear (*Ursus maritimus*).[22] Other captive wild ani-

Blastomycosis, edited by Yousef Al-Doory and Arthur F. DiSalvo, Plenum Medical Book Company, New York, 1992.

mals that have developed blastomycosis include an African lion[23] and a ferret (*Mustela putorjus furo*).[24]

This chapter will focus on naturally occurring disease in animals. Of the domestic animals, dogs have the highest incidence of blastomycosis. Participating colleges of veterinary medicine in the Veterinary Medical Data Program reported 324 canine cases of blastomycosis in the 5-year period of 1977 through 1981.[25] Three cats with blastomycosis were identified during the same period of time. The disease is rare in the horse and there are no reports of cows or other domestic animals with blastomycosis.[26]

2. EPIDEMIOLOGY OF BLASTOMYCOSIS IN ANIMALS

Dogs are the only species of animals where adequate numbers of cases are available for epidemiologic conclusions. The geographic distribution in dogs parallels that previously described for people.[27,28] In endemic areas, the canine infection rate is estimated at about ten times the human rate or 6.5 per 100,000 per year.[27] The difference in incidence between man and dog may be even greater as some owners of sick dogs do not pursue diagnosis and treatment. Most reports of blastomycosis in cats are from endemic areas, but blastomycosis has been seen in cats from nonendemic areas such as Florida[29] and New York.[30]

Sandy, acid soil appears to favor the growth of *B. dermatitidis* in the environment.[31] The enzootic areas identified in Wisconsin[31] have similar soil characteristics to the areas of southwest Arkansas[32] where canine blastomycosis is common. Exposure to wet environments is associated with canine blastomycosis. In one study, 69% of Wisconsin dogs with blastomycosis lived within 500 yards of water.[31] Many of the other infected dogs that did not live close to water were used for hunting in the wetlands.[31] This association with water in canine blastomycosis is not surprising. Sites of *B. dermatitidis* growth near water have been identified in human exposure.[33,34] A common-source infection in wetlands, of dogs and their owners during raccoon and duck hunting, was suspected in two studies.[35,36] Most of these dogs developed signs of blastomycosis prior to or at the same time their owners developed disease. Owners of dogs with blastomycosis should be alerted by their veterinarians to the possibility of common-source exposure.

Blastomyces dermatitidis does not appear to be uniformly distributed within an endemic area. There appear to be foci of the fungus within endemic areas. Menges *et al.*[32] identified multiple dogs with blastomycosis on certain farms. The animals developed the disease over a period of 2 years.

These findings are consistent with the author's clinical observation of high incidence of canine blastomycosis in certain neighborhoods.

Seasonal differences in the incidence of canine blastomycosis have been identified. A national survey of canine blastomycosis seen at veterinary colleges between 1964 and 1976 showed the lowest frequency of newly diagnosed cases in June and July and the highest frequency in September.[37] An Arkansas study showed the highest frequency in summer and fall, but there were no significant seasonal differences.[32] Archer et al.[31] in Wisconsin showed most cases occurred in late spring through early fall, but a second incidence peak was seen in late fall and early winter. The second peak was attributed to exposure during the fall hunting season. Foster and Dunn[38] evaluating 26 cases in Wisconsin found the lowest incidence in spring and the highest incidence in late summer, fall, and early winter. No significant seasonal variation was found by the author in Tennessee in dogs seen between 1977 and 1982. There are considerable variations in the reported seasonal occurrence of canine blastomycosis, which may be attributable to the region, use of the dogs (hunting or pet), and weather conditions during a certain year.

Male dogs are more frequently infected with B. dermatitidis than female dogs with reported rates that range from 54%,[31] 63%,[37] 67%,[28] 67%,[39] to 72%.[25] One study of five infected dogs showed higher sex-specific attack rates in females.[40]

Blastomycosis is more common among dogs under 4 years of age and is rare in dogs over 10 years.[25,28,31,39] Infection has occurred in dogs as young as $2\frac{1}{2}$ months of age[39] with the peak between 2 and 3 years. A review of feline blastomycosis cases showed no sex predilection and an age range of 2 to 7 years.[41]

Large purebred dogs are most frequently infected with blastomycosis.[25,31,39] Size appears to be a significant factor with no dog under 9 kg (20 pounds) in one study of 47 infected dogs.[42] This is in contrast with an early study where beagles were the most frequently infected breed.[39] In a Wisconsin study, 44% of infected dogs were Labrador and golden retrievers, probably reflecting the popularity of these dogs for hunting rather than a breed susceptibility.[31] Saint Bernards, Labradors, and beagles were found to be at increased risk in one study.[37] Another study found the Doberman pinscher (a nonsporting breed) and the Labrador retriever to be overrepresented compared to the general clinic population of dogs.[25] These studies suggest that use of the dogs and the tendency of large dogs to roam may be more important factors than breed.

Infection in animals occurs by the inhalation of the conidia from the environmental mycelial form of the fungus. The infection is established in the lungs and disseminates throughout the body. Infection by inoculation from a puncture wound has been suspected by the author in some dogs but appears to be a rare situation. Self-limited blastomycosis as seen in man[43] probably occurs in the dog, but it is rarely recognized. Experimental exposure of dogs to soil inoculated with *B. dermatitidis* resulted in the death of 18% of the dogs. Seventy-seven percent of the dogs developed eye and skin lesions, but recovered spontaneously from the blastomycosis by the 68th week after exposure. No organisms were recovered at 120 weeks after exposure in spite of prednisone and azathioprine immunosuppression.[17] This study supports the hypothesis that self-limiting blastomycosis occurs in the dog.

Subclinical disease appears to be uncommon in blastomycosis compared to other fungal infections such as histoplasmosis. In surveys of stray dogs in areas of Kentucky and Arkansas where both organisms are endemic, *B. dermatitidis* was identified at necropsy in the tissues of 1–2% of the dogs.[44–46] This compares to the presence of *Histoplasma capsulatum* in 34–40% of the dogs necropsied.

Naturally infected dogs that show signs of blastomycosis rarely recover without treatment. Mild infections are probably not recognized by the owners or the veterinarian as blastomycosis. Menges *et al.*[32] followed the course of 12 untreated dogs with blastomycosis. Ten died and two were euthanatized from 7 days to 9 months (mean 59 days, median 35 days) after diagnosis. All symptomatic dogs should be treated aggressively for blastomycosis.

The incubation period for naturally occurring canine blastomycosis is not known. Experimental aerosol infection resulted in clinical signs of disease in 2–4 weeks in one study[16] and 7 weeks in another.[47] Three dogs developed signs of blastomycosis 3 weeks after a suspected exposure while hunting. The exposure resulted in infection of the dogs and the owners.[35] The disease may also be quite indolent with clinical signs in untreated cases persisting up to a year.[39] Menges *et al.*[32] found that 10 of 70 untreated dogs had been sick 5 months or longer.

3. CLINICAL ASPECTS OF ANIMAL BLASTOMYCOSIS

Canine blastomycosis was first recognized at necropsy by Meyer[48] in 1912. The organism was first isolated from a dog by Martin and Smith[49] in 1936. The clinical signs in 55 cases of canine blastomycosis were described by Ausherman *et al.*[50] in 1957. There were numerous reports of canine blastomycosis which were reviewed with an additional ten new cases added by Menges[39] in 1960. He presented an overview of the breed, sex, age, geographic distribution, and clinical presentation of canine blastomycosis. The Menges review is consistent with subsequent descriptions of the clinical signs of canine blastomycosis.[31,32,42] A current review of clinical blastomycosis of the dog and cat supports the previous findings.[51]

Fever, anorexia, weight loss, respiratory disease, cutaneous and subcutaneous abscesses, generalized lymphadenopathy, lameness, and ocular disease are the most commonly observed signs in the dog. Testicular enlargement, prostatitis, mammary gland abscess, seizures, regurgitation, nasal discharge, and gingivitis are less commonly seen. There is radiographic evidence of involvement of the lungs in 85% of the dogs.[42] This is consistent with a respiratory portal of entry of the organism. Lymphadenopathy either generalized or in regional lymph nodes, draining areas of skin and subcutaneous infection occurs in approximately 60% of infected dogs.

A nodular interstitial lung pattern is most commonly seen on thoracic radiographs with bronchointerstitial and mixed alveolar interstitial patterns also seen.[52,53] Thoracic lymphadenopathy occurs in approximately 20% of dogs with blastomycosis and is less common than in histoplasmosis and coccidioidomycosis.[53] Pneumomediastinum,[52] pleural effusion,[52] and chylothorax[54] occur occasionally. Cavitary lesions and solid pulmonary masses have also been seen. The lung lesions in canine blastomycosis are difficult to differentiate radiographically from other mycotic diseases and from some metastatic neoplastic lesions.

Ocular disease is common in canine blastomycosis with approximately 40% of dogs having eye disease.[42] There have been numerous case reports of canine ocular blastomycosis.[55-60] The eye changes in 21 dogs with ocular blastomycosis were described by Buyukmihci.[61] Uveitis was most common with retinal separation, panophthalmitis, and glaucoma commonly seen. Histologically, choroiditis and separation of the sensory retina were prominent lesions. Inflammation of the anterior ocular tissues was intense but rarely associated with organisms.[62] Early treatment of ocular blastomycosis is essential to maintaining vision.

Fungal osteomyelitis is common in blastomycosis with approximately 30% of dogs having lameness and bony lesions.[63] In half of the dogs with bone involvement, lameness was the only sign of disease. The bone lesions were mainly osteolytic changes in the tubular bones of the distal portion of the limbs. About half of the lesions had periosteal and soft tissue reactions. Two-thirds of the dogs had solitary bone lesions. Blastomycosis of the bone can easily be mistaken for a malignancy.

Brain infection with blastomycosis appears to be uncommon.[42] Among

47 dogs with blastomycosis, it was suspected in only one dog with seizures. Blastomyces meningoencephalitis has been found in association with widely disseminated disease.[64] Although clinical neurologic disease is usually associated with lung and other sites of infection, brain involvement as a solitary site of disease has been identified by the author.

There are various other case reports describing the spectrum of signs in blastomycosis.[65-71] Shull et al.[72] found prostatic blastomycosis by biopsy and identification of the organisms in the urine. A variety of atypical sites have been identified at necropsy which include: renal cortex, spleen, thyroid, parathyroid, heart, liver, and ovary.[64,73]

Canine blastomycosis has also been associated with systemic amyloidosis[74] and arterial thromboembolic disease from erosion of the left atrium by a granulomatous mass originating in the hilar lymph nodes.[75]

The hematology and clinical chemistry findings are generally not helpful in the diagnosis of blastomycosis. Hematologic findings in canine blastomycosis are suggestive of inflammation and are similar to any chronic infection. Mild to moderate neutrophilia with a left shift is expected. Approximately 35% of dogs had mild anemia attributed to chronic inflammation. Lymphopenia and monocytosis were seen in 35 and 47% of dogs, respectively.[42] Hypercalcemia associated with granulomatous disease has been seen in canine blastomycosis.[76]

Immunologic changes in canine blastomycosis include polyclonal gammopathy with increases in IgG and decreases in IgM. One study showed a significant depression of mitogen-induced lymphocyte blastogenesis when lymphocytes from dogs with blastomycosis are stimulated in autologous sera.[77] Another study did not identify a suppression of lymphocyte mitogenesis by autologous sera.[40]

Feline blastomycosis produces mainly respiratory, neurologic, ocular, lymph node, and skin disease.[30,78-85] Brain and spinal cord involvement appear to be much more common in the cat than in the dog. Pleural effusion with granulomatous pleuritis was found in two cats.[81,85] There are sites of blastomycosis in cats that have not been reported in the dog. One cat had a granulomatous mass of the larynx.[85] Involvement of the gastrointestinal tract and spleen, which is rare in the dog, occurred in two cats.[29,85] Fungal osteomyelitis has not been reported in the cat. The widely disseminated clinical disease differs markedly from the localized pulmonary disease noted in cats experimentally exposed to infected soil.[86]

The radiographic lung changes in the cat are similar to those of the dog. Inadequate numbers of laboratory studies of cats have been done to generalize about the changes.

There are an inadequate number of reports in other species to provide an overview of blastomycosis except for sea lions. Six captive sea lions have been diagnosed with blastomycosis at a facility on the coast of Mississippi.[87] The most common sites of lesions were the skin and the respiratory tract. Some animals died acutely without significant signs of illness while others developed ulcerative skin lesions and some respiratory signs. One animal from this facility responded well to 90 days of itraconazole but died a year later.[88]

4. DIAGNOSTIC PROCEDURES

Because therapy is costly and has the potential for significant toxicity, a definitive diagnosis should be made when possible. Identification of *B. dermatitidis* in the tissues histologically or cytologically is preferred. A fine-needle aspirate is the easiest and least invasive approach to diagnosis. This diagnostic technique has also been recommended for diagnosis of blastomycosis in people.[89] There is usually an abundance of organisms in the disseminated form of the disease. Impression smears of discharges from fistulous tracts and ulcerative skin lesions as well as aspiration biopsies of peripheral lymph nodes and subcutaneous lesions identified organisms in 52% of the infected dogs.[42] Aspirates of the posterior segment of blind eyes or histologic examination of enucleated eyes will also identify *B. dermatitidis* as the cause of the ocular disease. Tracheal wash will only identify organisms in about half of the dogs with respiratory blastomycosis, because organisms are not consistently found in the bronchi. Aspiration of the lung parenchyma, though somewhat more invasive, will often yield a cytologic diagnosis in dogs with disease restricted to the lungs. The organism can usually be identified on a urinalysis in dogs with prostatic disease. Dogs uncommonly develop fibrotic lung masses in response to blastomycosis. These masses contain few organisms; open biopsy and diligent searching for the organism within the mass is required for diagnosis. In one series of cases, 82% of dogs with blastomycosis were diagnosed by histology and cytology, and only 18% of dogs were diagnosed by characteristic radiographic lung lesions and positive serology.[42]

The tissue form of the organism is usually a thick-walled, round to oval budding yeast cell, but filamentous forms of *B. dermatitidis* have been seen in the tissues of the dog.[90] Giant forms of the *B. dermatitidis* yeast have been seen in pulmonary lesions in man.[91] In-office culturing for *B. dermatitidis* is not recommended for the veterinary practitioner because of the potential hazard to laboratory personnel.[92,93]

Skin testing for the diagnosis of canine blastomycosis is unreliable.[32,47,65,94] Serologic evaluation should be done to support a diagnosis of blastomycosis if the organism cannot be identified by direct examination.

Serologic diagnosis of blastomycosis was initially done with the precipitin and complement fixation tests. These tests were not very effective in identifying infected dogs.[46] Cross-reactions in dogs with other fungal infections were a problem.[46,95] Canine serum often has anticomplementary activity, which precludes doing the complement fixation test.

The specific immunodiffusion test was shown in people to be more sensitive and specific than the complement fixation test[96] and is currently most frequently used in diagnosis of canine blastomycosis. In the dog, the agar gel immunodiffusion (AGID) test has a sensitivity and specificity of over 90%.[97,98] The test is probably less sensitive early in the disease process. Many dogs with blastomycosis, that were positive on AGID in our facility, had a history of a prior negative AGID in other labs. The specificity and sensitivity of the counterimmunoelectrophoresis test are similar to the AGID test, but the results are obtained more quickly.[99] The immunodiagnostics in fungal diseases of animals have been reviewed.[100] A preliminary study of an enzyme-linked immunosorbent assay (ELISA) in the diagnosis of human and canine blastomycosis suggests improved sensitivity and specificity.[101] More extensive studies will be needed to evaluate the ELISA method of identifying dogs with clinical blastomycosis.

The AGID method is useful in the diagnosis of disease but cannot be used to evaluate response to therapy. Antibodies persisted for up to 33 months after successful treatment of canine blastomycosis.[98]

There are two few reports of the use of the AGID in other species to generalize about the test. Antibodies against *B. dermatitidis* were found on the microimmunodiffusion test on a dolphin with blastomycosis.[20] A polar bear with blastomycosis was initially negative and become strongly positive by AGID during the course of the disease.[22] A ferret with blastomycosis was also positive by AGID.[24] Only one cat with blastomycosis was evaluated serologically by AGID, and it was positive.[85] Further studies will be needed to determine the reliability of the AGID in cats and exotic species.

5. THERAPY

Early reports about canine blastomycosis discouraged treatment because of concerns that people treating infected dogs could become infected with blastomycosis.[50,102] After the epidemiology of blastomycosis became better understood, therapy of dogs was attempted.

The studies of Butler and Hill showed that alternate day therapy using

0.25 to 0.5 mg/kg of amphotericin B could be safely given to dogs.[103] Renal toxicosis was the most significant adverse effect of amphotericin B. The dose relationship to renal toxicosis and the nature of amphotericin B-induced renal damage were evaluated in the dog.[104-107] Careful monitoring of renal function during therapy is required to prevent severe renal damage. McMurry successfully treated a pointer with blastomycosis using amphotericin B.[108] Ausherman[109] made recommendations on an effective treatment protocol using approximately 0.5 mg/kg doses three times a week to a cumulative dose of 7 mg/kg of amphotericin B. Therapy was discontinued when blood urea nitrogen (BUN) values exceeded 1.5 times normal. Foster and Dunn[38] using a similar protocol but giving cumulative doses of 8 to 20 mg/kg of amphotericin B, reported cures in 23 of 26 dogs treated. Two dogs had recurrence of disease requiring retreatment.[38] In a review of the treatment of 62 dogs with blastomycosis, approximately 75% responded well to amphotericin B given three times a week at 1 mg/kg to a cumulative dose of 8 to 9 mg/kg. Approximately 20% of the dogs had relapses and required retreatment.[110] Ketoconazole at 10 mg/kg per day for 60 days produced responses in 65% of the dogs, but half of the responding dogs subsequently relapsed.[110] Ketoconazole used at 30 mg/kg per day in divided doses for 2 months was effective in treating 4 of 5 dogs with blastomycosis.[111,112] Two of the dogs were euthanatized 1 month after terminating the therapy, and no organisms were found at necropsy.

Ketoconazole is not without toxicity in animals. Anorexia and liver toxicosis can occur in the dog and cat. Cats appear especially susceptible to anorexia and depression.[113] Ketoconazole also inhibits production of testosterone and cortisol in the dog.[114,115] These endocrinological effects can significantly interfere with fertility in breeding dogs. Cats do not have significant changes in hormone concentrations.[116]

A combination of amphotericin B and ketoconazole appears as effective as amphotericin B alone in the treatment of blastomycosis.[110] This reduces the amount of amphotericin B needed thereby reducing the potential for renal toxicosis and reducing the logistic problems with an intravenously administered drug. The author's current recommendation for the treatment of blastomycosis is initiation of therapy using amphotericin B at 0.5 mg/kg in 60 to 120 ml of 5% dextrose given over 5 to 10 min intravenously. The amphotericin B is given every other day. A cumulative dose of 4 to 6 mg/kg is given depending on severity of the disease. The BUN is monitored before each dose, and the therapy is temporarily discontinued when the BUN exceeds 50 mg/dl. The amphotericin B should produce a fairly rapid improvement in the dog's condition. The amphotericin B therapy should be followed by ketoconazole at 10 mg/kg BID for 60 days. In severe disease, an additional 2 to 3 mg/kg of amphotericin B can be given at 0.5 mg/kg per dose after the course of ketoconazole to reduce the likelihood of recurrence. This treatment protocol takes advantage of the more rapid onset of response produced by the amphotericin B while limiting the dose and potential renal toxicosis of this drug.

There is no information about the successful therapy of cats with blastomycosis. Ketoconazole at 10 mg/kg BID for 60 days would be recommended. Therapy should be temporarily discontinued if anorexia and hepatic toxicosis occur. After improvement in the appetite in cats that cannot tolerate a full dose, therapy should be continued at 10 mg/kg per day until the disease is cured.

Itraconazole, a triazole, will become, when approved for use in the United States, the treatment of choice for canine and feline blastomycosis. Given at 5 mg/kg per day orally in food for 60 days, it appears to produce responses equal to treatment with amphotericin B or amphotericin B and ketoconazole. The ease of administration, the minimal adverse reactions, and the efficacy of the drug in dogs and cats make it a very promising treatment. A polar bear has been cured with a 90-day course of itraconazole therapy.[22]

6. PROGNOSTIC FACTORS

Severity of the lung disease at initial diagnosis is the most significant prognostic factor for death and recurrence of disease in canine blastomycosis.[110] Dogs with severe lung disease must be treated longer to obtain a cure. Leukocytosis with a left shift is also an adverse prognostic factor. Brain involvement carries a guarded prognosis, but dogs with brain involvement can be effectively treated with amphotericin B and ketoconazole or itraconazole. The dose of ketoconazole should be increased to 30 to 40 mg/kg per day if the dog will tolerate the dose.

Female dogs are more likely to survive than male dogs with a similar severity of lung involvement. The reason for the better response in female dogs is not known. Most dogs that die of blastomycosis die of respiratory failure during the first week of treatment.[110]

7. PUBLIC HEALTH ASPECTS OF ANIMAL BLASTOMYCOSIS

Animals with blastomycosis are usually not considered a source of infection for people by the usual respiratory route of infection. At least three human infections have occurred from inoculation of *B. dermatitidis* by bites of infected dogs.[117-119] Veterinarians have also become infected from cuts that occurred during necropsy of infected dogs.[120,121] Aerosol transmission or transmission by contact with discharges has not been reported.

REFERENCES

1. Conti-Diaz IA, Smith CD, Furcolow ML: Comparison of infection of laboratory animals with *Blastomyces dermatitidis* using different routes of inoculation. *Sabouraudia* 7:279–283, 1970
2. Harvey RP, Schmid ES, Carrington CC, et al: Mouse model of pulmonary blastomycosis: Utility, simplicity, and quantitative parameters. *Am Rev Respir Dis* 117:695–702, 1978
3. Williams JE, Moser SA: Chronic murine pulmonary blastomycosis induced by intratracheally inoculated *Blastomyces dermatitidis* conidia. *Am Rev Respir Dis* 135:17–25, 1987
4. Sugar AM, Picard M: Experimental blastomycosis pneumonia in mice by infection with conidia. *J Med Vet Mycol* 26:321–326, 1988
5. Cox RA, Mills LR, Best GK, et al: Histologic reactions to cell walls of an avirulent and a virulent strain of *Blastomyces dermatitidis*. *J Infect Dis* 129:179–186, 1974
6. Brass C, Volkmann CM, Klein HP, et al: Pathogen factors and host factors in murine pulmonary blastomycosis. *Mycopathologia* 78:129–140, 1982
7. Moser SA, Koker PJ, Williams JE: Fungal-strain-dependent alterations in the time course and mortality of chronic murine pulmonary blastomycosis. *Infect Immun* 56:34–39, 1988
8. Spencer HD, Cozad GC: Role of delayed hypersensitivity in blastomycosis of mice. *Infect Immun* 7:329–334, 1973
9. Scillian JJ, Cozad GC, Spencer HD: Passive transfer of delayed hypersensitivity to *Blastomyces dermatitidis* between mice. *Infect Immun* 10:705–711, 1974
10. Longley RE, Cozad GC: Thymosin restoration of cellular immunity to *Blastomyces dermatitidis* in T-cell-depleted mice. *Infect Immun* 26:187–192, 1979
11. Frey CL, DeMarsh PL, Drutz DJ: Divergent patterns of pulmonary blastomycosis induced by conidia and yeasts in athymic and euthymic mice. *Am Rev Respir Dis* 140:118–124, 1989
12. Salfelder K: Experimental cutaneous North American blastomycosis of hamsters. *J Invest Dermatol* 45:409–418, 1965
13. Landay ME, Lowe EP, Mitten J, et al: Disseminated blastomycosis in hamsters after intramuscular, subcutaneous and intraperitoneal injection. *Sabouraudia* 6:318–323, 1968
14. Korkij W, Soltanj K, Chyu JY, et al: Immunohistopathological studies of blastomycosis: The use of labeled specific antigens in a hamster model of disease. *Mycopathologia* 85:17–20, 1984
15. Deighton F, Cox RA, Hall NK, et al: In vivo and in vitro cell-mediated immune responses to a cell wall antigen of *Blastomyces dermatitidis*. *Infect Immun* 15:429–435, 1977
16. Ebert JW, Jones V, Jones RD, et al: Experimental canine histoplasmosis and blastomycosis. *Mycopathol Mycol Appl* 45:285–300, 1971
17. Smith CD, Furcolow ML, Hulker P: Effect of immunosuppressants on dogs exposed two and one-half years previously to *Blastomyces dermatitidis*. *Am J Epidemiol* 104:299–305, 1976

18. Thiel RP, Mech LD, Ruth GR, et al: Blastomycosis in wild wolves. *J Wildl Dis* 23:321–323, 1987

19. Sweeney JC, Migaki G, Vainik PM, et al: Systemic mycoses in marine mammals. *J Am Vet Med Assoc* 169:946–948, 1976

20. Cates MB, Kaufman L, Grabau JH, et al: Blastomycosis in an Atlantic bottlenose dolphin. *J Am Vet Med Assoc* 189:1148–1150, 1986

21. Williamson WM, Lombard LS, Getty RE: North American blastomycosis in a northern sea lion. *J Am Vet Med Assoc* 135:513–515, 1959

22. Morris PJ, Legendre AM, Bowersock TL, et al: Diagnosis and treatment of systemic blastomycosis in a polar bear (*Ursus maritimus*). *J Zoo Wildl Med* 20:336–345, 1989

23. Stroud RK, Coles BM: Blastomycosis in an African lion. *J Am Vet Med Assoc* 177:842–844, 1980

24. Lenhard L: Blastomycosis in a ferret. *J Am Vet Med Assoc* 186:70–72, 1985

25. Legendre AM: System mycotic infections of dogs and cats, in Scott FW (ed): *Infectious Diseases. Contemporary Issues in Small Animal Practice,* vol 3. Edinburgh, Churchill Livingstone, 1986, pp 29–53

26. Benbrook EA, Bryant JB, Saunders LZ: A case of blastomycosis in the horse. *J Am Vet Med Assoc* 112:475–477, 1948

27. Furcolow ML, Busey JF, Menges RW, et al: Prevalence and incidence studies of human and canine blastomycosis. *Am J Epidemiol* 92:121–131, 1970

28. Furcolow ML, Chick EW, Busey JF, et al: Prevalence and incidence studies of human and canine blastomycosis. *Am Rev Respir Dis* 102:60–67, 1970

29. Jasmin AM, Carroll JM, Baucom JN, et al: Systemic blastomycosis in Siamese cats. *Vet Med Small Anim Clin* 64:33–37, 1969

30. Meschter C, Heiber K: Blastomycosis in a cat in lower New York State. *Cornell Vet* 79:259–262, 1989

31. Archer JR, Trainer DO, Schell RF: Epidemiologic study of canine blastomycosis in Wisconsin. *J Am Vet Med Assoc* 190:1292–1295, 1987

32. Menges RW, Furcolow ML, Selby LA, et al: Clinical and epidemiologic studies on seventy-nine canine blastomycosis cases in Arkansas. *Am J Epidemiol* 81:164–179, 1965

33. Klein BS, Vergeront JM, Weeks RJ, et al: Isolation of *Blastomyces dermatitidis* in soil associated with a large outbreak of blastomycosis in Wisconsin. *N Engl J Med* 314:529–534, 1986

34. Klein BS, Vergeront JM, DiSalvo AF, et al: Two outbreaks of blastomycosis along rivers in Wisconsin. Isolation of *Blastomyces dermatitidis* from riverbank soil and evidence of its transmission along waterways. *Am Rev Respir Dis* 136:1333–1338, 1987

35. Sarosi GA, Eckman MR, Davies SF, et al: Canine blastomycosis as a harbinger of human disease. *Ann Intern Med* 91:733–735, 1979

36. Armstrong CW, Jenkins SR, Kaufman L, et al: Common-source outbreak of blastomycosis in hunters and their dogs. *J Infect Dis* 155:568–570, 1987

37. Selby LA, Becker SV, Hayes HW: Epidemiologic risk factors associated with canine systemic mycoses. *Am J Epidemiol* 113:133–139, 1981

38. Foster RC, Dunn TJ: Blastomycosis: A practical therapeutic approach. *Vet Med Small Anim Clin* 76:200–204, 1981

39. Menges RW: Blastomycosis in animals: A review of an analysis of 116 canine cases. *Vet Med Small Anim Clin* 55:45–54, 1960

40. Czuprynski CJ, Thomas CB, Yang WC, et al: Epidemiologic and immunologic evaluation of an outbreak of canine blastomycosis. *J Med Vet Mycol* 26:243–252, 1988

41. Legendre AM: Systemic mycotic infections, in Sherding RG (ed): *The Cat: Diseases and Clinical Management,* vol 1. Edinburgh, Churchill Livingstone, 1989, pp 427–437

42. Legendre AM, Walker M, Buyukmihci N, et al: Canine blastomycosis: A review of 47 clinical cases. *J Am Vet Med Assoc* 178:1163–1168, 1981

43. Recht LD, Philips JR, Eckman MR, et al: Self-limited blastomycosis: A report of thirteen cases. *Am Rev Respir Dis* 120:1109–1112, 1979

44. Selby LA, Menges RW, Habermann RT: Survey for blastomycosis and histoplasmosis among stray dogs in Arkansas. *Am J Vet Res* 28:345–349, 1967

45. Turner C, Smith CD, Furcolow ML: Frequency of isolation of *Histoplasma capsulatum* and *Blastomyces dermatitidis* from dogs in Kentucky. *Am J Vet Res* 33:137–141, 1972

46. Turner C, Smith CD, Furcolow ML: The efficiency of serologic and cultural methods in the detection of infection with *Histoplasma* and *Blastomyces* in mongrel dogs. *Sabouraudia* 10:1–5, 1972

47. Smith CD, Furcolow ML, Hulker PW: Distribution of *Blastomyces dermatitidis* in dogs with skin test and serologic results following airborne infection. *Sabouraudia* 13:192–199, 1975

48. Meyer KF: Blastomycosis in dogs. *Proc Pathol Soc Philadelphia* 15:10, 1912

49. Martin DS, Smith DT: The laboratory diagnosis of blastomycosis. *J Lab Clin Med* 21:1289, 1936

50. Ausherman RJ, Sutton HH, Oakes JT: Clinical signs of blastomycosis in dogs. *J Am Vet Med Assoc* 130:541–542, 1957

51. Legendre AM: Blastomycosis, in Greene CE (ed): *Infectious Diseases of the Dog and Cat.* Philadelphia, WB Saunders Co, 1990

52. Walker MA: Thoracic blastomycosis: A review of its radiographic manifestations in 40 dogs. *Vet Radiol* 22:22–26, 1981

53. Ackerman N, Spencer CP: Radiologic aspects of mycotic diseases. *Vet Clin NA Small Anim Pract* 12:175–191, 1982

54. Willard MD, Conroy JD: Chylothorax associated with blastomycosis in a dog. *J Am Vet Med Assoc* 186:72–73, 1985

55. Trevino GS: Canine blastomycosis with ocular involvement. *Pathol Vet* 3:652–658, 1966

56. Simon J, Helper LC: Ocular disease associated with blastomycosis in dogs. *J Am Vet Med Assoc* 157:922–925, 1970

57. Wilson RW, van Dreumel AA, Henry JNR: Urogenital and ocular lesions in canine blastomycosis. *Vet Pathol* 10:1–11, 1973

58. Carlton WW, Austin WL: Ocular blastomycosis in a dog with lymph node and testicular lesions. *J Am Anim Hosp Assoc* 12:502–506, 1976

59. Peiffer RL, Gelatt KN, Mehlhoff T: Ocular blastomycosis in a dog. *Canine Pract* 5:26–30, 1978

60. Albert RA, Whitley RD, Crawley RR: Ocular blastomycosis in the dog. *Comp Cont Educ* 3:303–311, 1981

61. Buyukmihci N: Ocular lesions of blastomycosis in the dog. *J Am Vet Med Assoc* 180:426–431, 1982

62. Buyukmihci NC, Moore PF: Microscopic lesions of spontaneous ocular blastomycosis in dogs. *Comp Pathol* 97:321–328, 1987

63. Roberts RE: Osteomyelitis associated with disseminated blastomycosis in nine dogs. *Vet Radiol* 20:124–134, 1979

64. Kurtz HJ, Sharpnack S: *Blastomyces dermatitidis* meningoencephalitis in a dog. *Pathol Vet* 6:375–377, 1969

65. Selby LA, Habermann RT, Breshears DE: Canine blastomycosis. *Vet Med Small Anim Clin* 59:1221–1227, 1964
66. Hoff B: North American blastomycosis in two dogs in Saskatchewan. *Can Vet J* 14:122–123, 1973
67. Herman PH, Stedham MA: Blastomycosis in a dog in Maryland. *J Am Vet Med Assoc* 164:488–489, 1974
68. Shatto NL: Canine pulmonary blastomycosis (a case report). *Vet Med Small Anim Clin* 71:47–51, 1976
69. Dunn TJ: Blastomycosis in a dog. *Vet Med Small Anim Clin* 72:1443–1445, 1977
70. Pyle RL, Dunbar M, Nelson PD, et al: Canine blastomycosis. *Comp Cont Educ* 11:963–974, 1981
71. Nagaraj MP: Cutaneous blastomycosis in a dog. *Canine Pract* 8:65–66, 1981
72. Shull RM, Hayden DW, Johnston GR: Urogenital blastomycosis in a dog. *J Am Vet Med Assoc* 171:730–735, 1977
73. Robbins ES: North American blastomycosis in the dog. *J Am Vet Med Assoc* 125:391–397, 1954
74. Sherwood BF, LeMay JC, Castellanos RA: Blastomycosis with secondary amyloidosis in the dog. *J Am Vet Med Assoc* 150:1377–1381, 1967
75. Ware WA, Fenner WR: Arterial thromboembolic disease in a dog with blastomycosis localized in a hilar lymph node. *J Am Vet Med Assoc* 193:847–849, 1988
76. Dow SW, Legendre AM, Stiff M, et al: Hypercalcemia associated with blastomycosis in dogs. *J Am Vet Med Assoc* 188:706–709, 1986
77. Legendre AM, Becker PU: Immunologic changes in acute canine blastomycosis. *Am J Vet Res* 43:2050–2053, 1982
78. Easton KL: Cutaneous North American blastomycosis in a Siamese cat. *Can Vet J* 2:350–351, 1961
79. Sheldon WG: Pulmonary blastomycosis in a cat. *Lab Anim Care* 16:280–285, 1966
80. Alden CL, Mohan R: Ocular blastomycosis in a cat. *J Am Vet Med Assoc* 164:527–528, 1974
81. Hatkin JM, Phillips WE, Utroska WR: Two cases of feline blastomycosis. *J Am Anim Hosp Assoc* 15:217–220, 1979
82. Campbell KL, Humphrey JA, Ramsey GH: Cutaneous blastomycosis. *Feline Pract* 10:28–32, 1980
83. Neunzig RJ: Epidemiology, diagnosis, and treatment of canine and feline blastomycosis. *Vet Med Small Anim Clin* 78:1081–1088, 1983
84. Nasisse MP, van Ee RT, Wright B: Ocular changes in a cat with disseminated blastomycosis. *J Am Vet Med Assoc* 187:629–631, 1985
85. Breider MA, Walker TL, Legendre AM: Blastomycosis in cats: Five cases (1979–1986). *J Am Vet Med Assoc* 193:570–572, 1988
86. Denton JF, DiSalvo AF: Respiratory infection of laboratory animals with conidia of *Blastomyces dermatitidis*. *Mycopathol Mycol Appl* 36:129–136, 1968
87. Dr. Joe W Alexander, Personal communication, Stillwater, Oklahoma, 1989
88. Sweeney JC, Samansky TS, Solange MA: Course of therapy utilized in a California sea lion with blastomycosis. *Proc Int Assoc Aquatic Anim Med* 1987
89. Mamikunian C, Gatti WM, Reyes CV: Subcutaneous blastomycosis: Diagnosis by fine-needle aspiration cytology. *Otolaryngol Head Neck Surg* 101:607–610, 1989
90. Kaufmann AF, Kaplan W, Kraft DE: Filamentous forms of *Ajellomyces* (*Blastomyces*) *dermatitidis* in a dog. *Vet Pathol* 16:271–273, 1979
91. Watts JC, Chandler FW, Mihalov ML, et al: Giant forms of *B. dermatitidis* in the pulmo-

nary lesions of blastomycosis. Potential confusion with *Coccidioides immitis. Am J Clin Pathol* 93:575–578, 1990

92. Baum GL, Lerner PI: Primary pulmonary blastomycosis: A laboratory-acquired infection. *Ann Intern Med* 73:263–265, 1970

93. Larsh HW, Schwarz J: Accidental inoculation blastomycosis. *Cutis* 19:334–345, 337, 1977

94. Kaplan W: Epidemiology of the principal systemic mycoses of man and lower animals and the ecology of their etiologic agents. *J Am Vet Med Assoc* 163:1043–1047, 1973

95. Balows A, Ausherman RJ, Hopper JM: Practical diagnosis and therapy of canine histoplasmosis and blastomycosis. *J Am Vet Med Assoc* 148:678–684, 1966

96. Kaufman L, McLaughlin DW, Clark MJ: Specific immunodiffusion test for blastomycosis. *Appl Microbiol* 26:244–247, 1973

97. Phillips WE, Kaufman L: Cultural and histopathologic confirmation of canine blastomycosis diagnosed by an agar-gel immunodiffusion test. *Am J Vet Res* 41:1263–1265, 1980

98. Legendre AM, Becker PU: Evaluation of the agar-gel immunodiffusion test in the diagnosis of canine blastomycosis. *Am J Vet Res* 41:2109–2111, 1980

99. Barta O, Hubbert NL, Pier AC: Counterimmunoelectrophoresis (immunoelectroosmosis) and serum electrophoretic pattern in serologic diagnosis of canine blastomycosis. *Am J Vet Res* 44:218–222, 1983

100. Jackson JA: Immunodiagnosis of systemic mycoses in animals: A review. *J Am Vet Med Assoc* 188:702–705, 1986

101. Turner S, Kaufman L, Jalbert M: Diagnostic assessment of an enzyme-linked immunosorbent assay for human and canine blastomycosis. *J Clin Microbiol* 23:294–297, 1986

102. Newberne JW, Neal JE, Heath MK: Some clinical and microbiological observations on four cases of canine blastomycosis. *J Am Vet Med Assoc* 127:220–223, 1955

103. Butler WT, Hill GJ: Intravenous administration of amphotericin B in the dog. *J Am Vet Med Assoc* 144:399–402, 1964

104. Butler WT: Changes in renal function. *Ann Intern Med* 61:344–348, 1964

105. Butler WT, Bennett JE, Hill GJ: Electrocardiographic and electrolyte abnormalities caused by amphotericin B in dog and man. *Proc Soc Exp Biol Med* 116:857–863, 1964

106. Butler WT, Hill GJ, Szwed CF, et al: Amphotericin B renal toxicity in the dog. *J Pharmacol Exp Ther* 143:47–56, 1964

107. Hill GJ, Butler WT, Szwed CF, et al: Lethal toxicity and dose-related azotemia due to amphotericin B in dogs. *Proc Soc Exp Biol Med* 114:76–79, 1963

108. McMurry TS: Successful clinical treatment of localized blastomycosis in a dog. *Vet Med Small Anim Clin* 62:341–344, 1967

109. Ausherman RJ: Treatment of blastomycosis and histoplasmosis in the dog. *J Am Vet Med Assoc* 163:1048–1049, 1973

110. Legendre AM, Selcer BA, Edwards DF, et al: Treatment of canine blastomycosis with amphotericin B and ketoconazole. *J Am Vet Med Assoc* 184:1249–1254, 1984

111. Dunbar M, Pyle RL: Ketoconazole treatment of osseous blastomycosis in a dog. *Vet Med Small Anim Clin* 76:1593–1595, 1981

112. Dunbar M, Pyle RL, Boring JG, et al: Treatment of canine blastomycosis with ketoconazole. *J Am Vet Med Assoc* 182:156–157, 1983

113. Moriello KA: Ketoconazole: Clinical pharmacology and therapeutic recommendations. *J Am Vet Med Assoc* 188:303–306, 1986

114. DeCoster R, Beerens D, Dom J, et al: Endocrinological effects of single daily ketoconazole administration in male beagle dogs. *Acta Endocrinol (Copenhagen)* 107:275–281, 1984

115. Willard MD, Nachreiner R, McDonald R, et al: Ketoconazole-induced changes in selected canine hormone concentrations. *Am J Vet Res* 47:2504–2509, 1986
116. Willard MD, Nachreiner RF, Howard VC, et al: Effect of long-term administration of ketoconazole in cats. *Am J Vet Res* 47:2510–2513, 1986
117. Scott MJ: Cutaneous blastomycosis. *Northwest Med* 54:255–257, 1955
118. Jaspers RH: Transmission of blastomyces from animals to man. Letter to the Editor. *J Am Vet Med Assoc* 164:8, 1974
119. Gnann JW, Bressler GS, Bodet CA, et al: Human blastomycosis after a dog bite. *Ann Intern Med* 98:48–49, 1983
120. Ramsey FK, Carter GR: Canine blastomycosis in the United States. *J Am Vet Med Assoc* 120:93–98, 1952
121. Graham WR, Callaway JL: Primary inoculation blastomycosis in a veterinarian. *J Am Acad Dermatol* 7:785–786, 1982

Index